T0200382

Talley & O'Connor's Clinical OSCEs

Guide to passing the OSCEs

Talley & O'Connor's Clinical OSCEs

Guide to passing the OSCEs

Nicholas J Talley

MBBS (Hons) (NSW), MD (NSW), PhD (Syd), MMedSci (Clin Epi) (Newc.), FAHMS, FRACP, FAFPHM, FRCP (Lond), FRCP (Edin), FACP, FACG, AGAF
Distinguished Laureate Professor, University of Newcastle and Senior Staff Specialist, John Hunter Hospital, NSW, Australia; Adjunct Professor, Mayo Clinic, Rochester, MN, USA; Adjunct Professor, University of North Carolina, Chapel Hill, NC, USA; Foreign Guest Professor, Karolinska Institutet, Stockholm, Sweden

Simon O'Connor

FRACP, DDU, FCSANZ
Cardiologist, The Canberra Hospital, Canberra; Senior Clinical Lecturer, Australian National University Medical School, Canberra, ACT, Australia

With contributions from
Elise Putt
Alexander Burns
Yamini Yadav

ELSEVIER

ELSEVIER

Elsevier Australia. ACN 001 002 357
(a division of Reed International Books Australia Pty Ltd)
Tower 1, 475 Victoria Avenue, Chatswood, NSW 2067

ISBN: 978-0-7295-4406-1

Notice

Practitioners and researchers must always rely on their own experience and
knowledge in evaluating and using any information, methods, compounds
or experiments described herein. Because of rapid advances in the medical
sciences, in particular, independent verification of diagnoses and drug
dosages should be made. To the fullest extent of the law, no responsibility
is assumed by Elsevier, authors, editors or contributors for any injury and/
or damage to persons or property as a matter of products liability,
negligence or otherwise, or from any use or operation of any methods,
products, instructions, or ideas contained in the material herein.

National Library of Australia Cataloguing-in-Publication Data

NATIONAL
LIBRARY
OF AUSTRALIA

A catalogue record for this
book is available from the
National Library of Australia

Head of Content: Larissa Norrie
Content Project Manager: Shubham Dixit
Edited by Elaine Cochrane
Proofread by Melissa Faulkner
Permissions Editing and Photo Research: Saravanan Murugan
Cover design by Georgette Hall
Index by Straive
Typeset by Aptara
Printed in Singapore by KHL Printing Co Pte Ltd

Last digit is the print number: 9 8 7 6 5 4 3 2 1

Contents

Foreword

Professor Ronald Harden introduced the objective structured clinical examination (OSCE) in the 1970s and since then this has become the cornerstone of clinical competency assessment in medical education. The OSCE format introduced clear objectives, structure and a focus on important clinical topics into medical school examinations and was a landmark innovation in medical education. Before this, the clinical assessments were not structured, topics often depended on the examiner's hobby-horses and there was no blueprint for a fair assessment. The OSCE format has been shown to be very reliable. This, combined with the flexibility of assessing a large number of students across multiple domains of competency, has maintained its popularity all over the world.

The OSCE model is now a very well-researched tool and there are over 2000 publications on the conduct, outcome and benefits of OSCEs in both undergraduate and postgraduate medical education. One of the strengths of the assessment is the ability to provide constructive feedback on student performance. After formative and summative testing, the candidates have an opportunity to fine-tune and improve their performance for future barrier examinations because of the structured feedback. Thus, students expand their knowledge and skills with this assessment each time (hence the value of practising for OSCE examinations too). To gain authenticity, OSCE stations may use role-players (standardised) and real patients, depending on the station. For example, communication skills may be tested by a role-player, whereas a goitre examination will need a real patient. The examiners will mark the candidate on a checklist and at the end they may also provide a global rating of pass (with or without gradations) or fail.

This book on OSCEs, written by two expert medical authors and three recent graduates, will be welcomed by medical students. Professor Nicholas Talley and Dr Simon O'Connor are well known among medical students and postgraduate trainees for their textbooks on clinical examination, revised and published in several editions over the past four decades.

Students are very anxious before any examination, but this book includes many examination tips, including frequently asked questions, to help alleviate any anxiety. For example, what to do if you are asked to go back and examine the patient again or how much you should expose the patient before examining are often very confusing to the examination candidates. The advice in this book is therefore most welcome.

The OSCEs in this book are well structured with possible questions the student can expect, including guidance on the right answers. There are some key theoretical background points included. Useful images, X-rays, ECGs, blood gas values and marking grids are also included. I expect the book will help the examiners who will be organising future OSCEs, too.

I have no hesitation in recommending this book for medical students, medical teachers and medical schools.

Professor Balakrishnan R (Kichu) Nair AM
MBBS, MD (Newcastle), FRACP, FRCPE (Edinburgh), FRCPG (Glasgow), FRCPI (Ireland), FANZSGM, Graduate Dip (ClinEpid)
Professor of Medicine and Associate Dean (Clinical Teaching), School of Medicine and Public Health, University of Newcastle, Australia
Director, Educational Research, Health Education and Training Institute, New South Wales, Australia

Preface

To study the phenomena of disease without books is to sail an uncharted sea, while to study books without patients is not to go to sea at all.

William Osler, 1914

The only method of mastery (of clinical skills) we know of that works is practice and more practice, interacting with as many patients as possible.

Nick Talley & Simon O'Connor 2019. Clinical Examination Essentials, 5th edn. Preface

Clinical skills are the foundation of clinical medicine. Your goal should be to acquire mastery of these skills rather than just aiming to pass examinations, as in the future patients' lives will depend on it.

However, barrier examinations remain a reality for all medical students and are meant to confirm students have reached the required standard to advance. A popular examination format around the world is the objective structured clinical examination (OSCE). These examinations are designed to test your skills in a realistic and reliable format. Core skills tested in OSCEs include the ability to take a history, perform a clinical examination of a system or body part, develop a differential diagnosis and clinical reasoning, interpret tests, perform common procedures, prescribe safely, handle difficult encounters, act professionally, and communicate expertly. As you advance in medical school, OSCEs become more challenging. You should aim to obtain plenty of practice before having to sit your barrier examinations.

We have written this book to help guide you as you prepare for the OSCEs throughout your medical school years. The OSCE stations become progressively harder as you advance through this book, and we've deliberately tried to be challenging to help you prepare most effectively. Please refer to our companion book, *Talley & O'Connor's Clinical Examination* 9th edition, as needed, for more details on history taking, physical examination and differential diagnosis.

The secret to examination success, like success for an Olympic athlete, is practice and more practice. Paraphrasing the American motivational speaker Zig Ziglar, 'You don't need to be amazing to start, but you need to start to be amazing.' Practising in small groups is very helpful and fun as you build your confidence and refine your skills based on others watching you. Take every opportunity to observe and work with master clinicians at the bedside, as experience pays dividends.

Medical school will change you. Learn from patient interactions and senior colleagues. Read widely. Open your mind, observe and explore. Practise the key competencies and refine them based on feedback until your approach is second nature. Once you know how to (and if you really want to master the skills), teach. Enjoy, as the finish line will come soon enough.

We wish you every success!

Nick Talley
Simon O'Connor
Newcastle and Canberra, 2021

Contributors

Alexandra Burns, BSc (Molecular Biology), BMed

Basic Physician Trainee, Hunter New England Health,
Newcastle, New South Wales, Australia

Elise Putt, BMed

Emergency Medicine Senior Resident Medical Officer,
Hunter New England Health,
Newcastle, New South Wales, Australia

Yamini Yadav, BMed, MMed (Pain Mgt)

Conjoint Fellow, School of Medicine and Public Health,
College of Health, Medicine and Wellbeing,
University of Newcastle,
Newcastle, New South Wales, Australia

Reviewers

Andrew Korda, AM MA, MBBS, FRCOG, FRANZCOG

Conjoint Professor of Obstetrics and Gynaecology, Western Sydney University, Sydney, New South Wales, Australia

Peter Pockney, BSc, MBBS, DM, FRCS (Gen Surg), FRACS

Conjoint Senior Lecturer Surgery, University of Newcastle, Newcastle, New South Wales, Australia; NHMRC Centre of Research Excellence in Digestive Health, New South Wales, Australia

Saxon D Smith, MBChB, MHL, PhD, GAICD, FAMA, IFAAD, FACD

The Dermatology and Skin Cancer Centre, St Leonards, New South Wales, Australia; Sydney Adventist Hospital, Wahroonga, New South Wales, Australia

Peter Wark, BMed, PhD, FRACP, FThorSoc

Conjoint Professor, University of Newcastle, Newcastle, New South Wales, Australia; Senior Staff Specialist in Respiratory Sleep and General Medicine, John Hunter Hospital, New Lambton Heights, New South Wales, Australia

The authors and publishers wish to thank Jasmine Wark, BBiomedSc, DipLang, for her expert editorial support.

Introduction to Objective Structured Clinical Examinations (OSCEs)

Medicine is an immensely satisfying career and core clinical skills are the foundation for clinical excellence. You will spend time learning key skills, practising them until they are second nature — and applying them safely and effectively, first under supervision and later on your own. To graduate you will be required to show you have acquired the necessary skills, and objective structured clinical examinations (OSCEs) are the most common assessment format used in medical schools around the world.

Would you want to be qualified but incompetent?

Knowledge can be tested by multiple-choice and short-answer questions, but arguably clinical skills cannot; rather, direct demonstration of competence is needed. Would you let someone drive a car or fly a plane who has only read the instruction book? While students during medical school will be called upon in many informal settings to demonstrate their skills as formative assessments (which do not count towards passing), at various times summative OSCE examinations of increasing difficulty, which do count, will be encountered. These barrier examinations in medicine are set to ensure a basic level of competency has been acquired by students prior to qualification. Do you believe the public would accept doctors graduating who have not met minimum objective standards?

OSCE examination formats

The OSCE is designed to validly assess some or all of the following:

- history-taking skills
- clinical examination skills
- communication skills with patients and families
- data interpretation
- ability to document information or consent
- ability to infer the differential diagnosis
- ability to counsel patients about their disease
- ability to manage a specific medical problem
- technical skills, such as inserting a cannula.

The OSCE consists of multiple stations (anywhere from 6 to 20), and students move from station to station on the same timetable. Each station aims to test a set of skills and you will spend the same time at each station. There may be a real or simulated patient, or no patient at all (with a manikin or machine, or printout or video instead). (See Fig. 1.1).

While the station timing can vary from 6 to 15 minutes, **10 minutes is a common allowance and has been assumed in this book** until the final-year cases. At each changeover, a bell will ring. Different universities and hospitals run their exams differently, but this book sets out common formats. Each station provides information on the rationale and hints on how to excel, as well as an overview of how to tackle the task.

A real patient or an actor may be available to answer questions and enable the examiner to test your interviewing technique and knowledge. Begin by introducing yourself. In most cases the first question will be 'May I ask you some questions?' or 'May I have a look at you?', depending on the written introduction you have been given. If a physical examination or any patient contact is required, make sure you wash your hands at the beginning and when you have finished. Always ask permission before an examination — the patient has a right to refuse. At the end, add: 'Thank you for coming to help in the exams'.

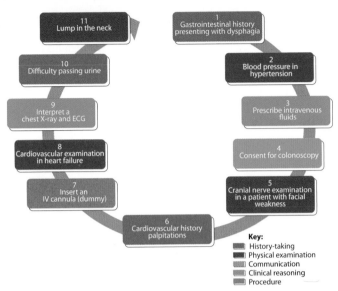

Figure 1.1 Example of an objective structured clinical examination (OSCE) with 11 different stations covering history taking, physical examination, communication and clinical reasoning skills, and procedural skills. (Adapted from Gormley G. Summative OSCEs in undergraduate medical education. *The Ulster Medical Journal* 2011; 80(3):127–32.) (© The Ulster Medical Journal and provided here courtesy of Ulster Medical Society)

The structure of the examination will usually be explained in advance and does usually vary with an increase in complexity as students move into more senior years. Remember to read the introduction and carefully think about the task required at each station, as there are innumerable nuances possible in designing any station.

At the end of the each OSCE we have supplied a marking grid, typical of the type supplied to the examiners, although many different formats are used. This grid may set out standard questions for the examiners to ask and their weighting (by marks). It is not possible to standardise these fully because they depend on the seniority of the students being tested and the key areas that the examiners want students to cover.

Each station is scored separately; the scores are combined to determine the pass level. The pass mark is set prior to the examination for each station and is based on known or expected student performance. In addition to marks for each step, an overall rating may be given for the station (for example, from fail to outstanding on a 5-graded scale). You can fail some stations and still pass overall. Typically, the number of stations that must be passed is also pre-set.

Frequently asked questions

We have set out to answer many of the common questions students ask as they prepare for OSCEs.

WHO WILL BE THERE WHEN I AM AT AN EXAMINING STATION?

There will usually be one examiner but there may be two in later years as this provides better standardisation of assessment, and sometimes an observer — an examiner in training may be present. There may be a real patient with physical signs or symptoms for you to examine or take a history from. In many hospitals, experienced well-briefed actors may be used for history-taking OSCEs (simulated patients who may also provide input into the marks for you).

WILL THERE ALWAYS BE A PATIENT AT THE STATION?

No. At some stations there may be a manikin or model. This may be for you to demonstrate cardiopulmonary resuscitation or perform a simulated rectal or vaginal examination. You could be asked to perform an ECG recording using an ECG machine and a patient or model. Or you could be asked to read a print-out of tests such as spirometry or a chest X-ray.

HOW LONG WILL I HAVE AT EACH STATION?

This will vary from hospital to hospital and usually lengthens as you become more senior. The time will be the same at each station and is usually around 10 minutes. The whole exam will often go for 2 hours.

HOW MUCH TIME WILL THERE BE FOR QUESTIONS FROM THE EXAMINERS?

This will depend on the complexity of the case. In some cases you will spend the whole time with the patient and the examiners will merely watch your technique. This is more likely in history-taking cases. In other cases, they will let you know how long they want you to spend with the patient before asking you to present your findings and answer their questions.

HOW WILL I KNOW IF I AM TAKING TOO LONG AND WON'T HAVE TIME TO FINISH?

The examiners are there to help you and will interrupt if you are too slow. They will generally give you some guidance, such as 'time is running on, perhaps you would like to finish your examination by showing us how you feel for hepatomegaly?' Always take this advice which, however couched, is more of an instruction than a suggestion.

WHAT SORT OF INSTRUCTIONS WILL THE EXAMINERS GIVE ME?

These are usually specific. The examiners want you to take the relevant history or examine the correct part of the patient. It becomes very difficult for them when students get the wrong end of the stick and rush off in the opposite direction. They will almost always redirect you in this case. Follow the instructions to score well!

ARE THE EXAMINERS' INSTRUCTIONS MEANT TO BE A TEST OR AN ATTEMPT TO TRICK ME?

No. The introduction (stem) you are given has been constructed to help you do well. It is very important to read it carefully. It is very common for students to do something quite different from what has been asked because, in their nervous anxiety, they have not considered the introduction. A good example is 'This man has had difficulty walking. Please examine him'. You must begin by asking the patient to walk, not with a lower limb neurological examination on the bed (although this is likely to come later in your evaluation).

WHAT EQUIPMENT WILL I NEED?

Most equipment will be provided at the site, for example neurology pins or tendon hammers, but you should use equipment of your own that you are familiar with. This would normally include a stethoscope and, if you have one, an ophthalmoscope. There will usually be paper for you to make notes on, but you should bring a pen and a spare, and a notebook (blank rather than filled with exam notes). Usually you can't bring in your phone or tablet.

HOW GOOD ARE THE SIMULATED PATIENTS?

The actors are usually very well prepared and know how to respond to your questions. The most difficult interviews with real and simulated patients are those in which you are asked to give the 'patient' or 'relative' bad news or apologise for and explain a medical error. Some actors will convincingly appear angry or upset, and this tests your ability to manage the situation calmly and professionally.

WHAT MISTAKES MIGHT CAUSE A FAILURE IN THE EXAM?

The 'don'ts' are highlighted in Box 1.1. Hurting a patient by a rough or thoughtless technique is a disaster. The examiners are watching for signs of discomfort on the patient's part and will

---

Box 1.1
Know the OSCE: the 'don'ts' list

- Don't skimp on sleep the night before, and don't arrive late.
- Don't forget your pen and favourite stethoscope (most tools otherwise will be supplied).
- Don't forget to read the instructions carefully at each station (and any pre-instructions sent to you).
- Don't forget to be nice and polite.
- Don't forget to address the patient by his or her name and title (as the patient prefers). Introduce yourself, ask permission, say thank you at the end (every time).
- Don't forget to wash your hands* before *and* after examining (to protect you and the patient).
- Don't forget to look at the patient *and* the room (be observant — there may be clues to the problem if only you take a mental step back, take a few slow breaths and observe).
- Don't fail to expose the patient adequately AND … don't forget to protect the patient's modesty (we'll explain later in the book).
- Don't apologise repeatedly (e.g. for exposing the relevant body part). Would such behaviour give you confidence in your health professional?
- Don't worry if the diagnosis (explanation of the problem) is elusive — if asked, provide a sensible differential diagnosis list, relevant to the patient in front of you (e.g. unlikely to be ovarian cancer in a male, unlikely to be dementia in a 20-year-old, etc).
- Don't make anything up, ever.

*Now called hand hygiene.

often ask afterwards if the examination was painful. Simple steps, such as asking the patient to let you know at once if anything is uncomfortable and watching the patient's face during examination of potentially tender areas, make a big difference. You should do this in clinical practice and it's therefore part of the assessment in the examination.

Other risky actions include:

- not asking permission of the patient before beginning the examination or interview
- not washing your hands before and after an examination
- not introducing yourself or not thanking the patient at the end
- appearing openly to doubt what the patient has said.

WHAT DO I DO IF A PATIENT SAYS SOMETHING CLEARLY INCORRECT OR INCONSISTENT OR CONTRADICTS HIM OR HERSELF?

Generally, rephrasing the question and asking again will help clarify the issues and inform the examiners that you have realised there is a problem with the answers. It may be necessary to point out to the patient the inconsistency. For example 'You said a moment ago that you have not got high blood pressure but you are taking some blood pressure tablets. Does that mean your blood pressure has been high in the past?'

HOW OBJECTIVE IS THE MARKING SYSTEM?

The examiners will have a list of criteria you will be expected to meet, and points will be allocated for each. The marking is designed to be as objective as possible. Certain criteria will apply to many cases, such as washing your hands before an examination, introducing yourself to the patient and explaining what you are doing as you go along.

Common criteria used by the examiners include:

- communication skills
- professionalism
- clinical knowledge
- ability to interpret findings
- technical skills

Other criteria will depend on the case, such as whether you remembered to position the patient correctly for the examination.

WILL I PASS A STATION AS LONG AS I AM NICE TO THE PATIENT AND WASH MY HANDS?

No.

WHAT SORTS OF QUESTIONS WILL THE EXAMINERS ASK?

As far as possible, questions will be standardised and asked of each student. They tend to be specific and closed questions. For example, 'What do you think is the most likely cause of this man's shortness of breath?', or 'Do you think this woman has a goitre, now that you have examined her?'

Sometimes a more open-ended question may be asked. This can be more difficult to answer as it may need you to have followed the examiners' train of thought. An example would be 'Now that you have examined this man, are there any questions you would like to ask him if you had the chance?' There may be an obvious question; for example, if the patient has a surgical scar, say that you would like to ask what operation has been performed.

A safe and useful question in a history-taking OSCE is 'What medications are you taking?' The answer can be very helpful in giving clues about chronic illnesses, which will help you in the discussion.

SHOULD I BE ALARMED IF THE EXAMINERS INTERRUPT ME?

No. This usually means they are trying to help you keep to time or to keep you on track.

WHAT DOES IT MEAN IF THE EXAMINERS ASK ME TO GO BACK AND EXAMINE SOMETHING AGAIN?

Again, this means they are trying to be helpful. For example, if they say 'Have another feel in the right upper quadrant of the abdomen', this probably means the liver or kidney is palpable and you have missed it. Generally, if they take you back and you find what you had missed, they will be satisfied with that.

HOW MUCH OF THE PATIENT SHOULD I EXPOSE?

This can be tricky. Ask to expose the relevant region just as you would on the wards. Often the examiners will tell you what you can lift up or remove (and just do that in the exam).

- For the abdominal examination for men and women, it is usually reasonable to expose the abdomen from below the nipples to the knees but with underpants left on. These can be removed or pushed aside if the inguinal region needs to be examined.
- For chest and cardiac examinations, it is reasonable to ask men to remove their shirts. For women, a gown may have been provided that can be decorously parted to allow examination of the precordium. If a woman is wearing a bra you might consider saying to the examiners 'ideally I would like to ask Ms X to take off her bra. Would you like me to do that?' It is then up to them to tell you.
- When testing gait, the legs and thighs should be exposed, meaning removal of clothes to the underwear or tucking up a gown to expose most of the thighs.

Always ask the patient, and by implication the examiners, if it is all right for you to have him or her remove whatever item of clothing is required.

Always make sure a curtain is drawn around the bed. The patient comes first, even in examinations.

SHOULD I TALK TO THE EXAMINERS AS I GO ALONG WITH MY EXAMINATION?

Generally not, but the examiners will usually make it clear if they want you to. For example: 'Tell us what you are doing and what you have found as you perform your examination.'

Summary

Practising for OSCEs will help you identify weak areas to work on and refine your clinical skills. Develop your own systematic approach guided by your tutors and textbooks, and practise to make the routines second nature. Aim to excel, not just pass (see Boxes 1.2 and 1.3). It's about *showing*, **not** knowing (much). *It helps to know some facts, but this is less relevant to passing!* But aim to excel because that's our professional obligation. The work will serve you well not only in examinations but at the bedside where it really matters.

Box 1.2
Hints on passing and excelling

- You must be *safe* to practise, you do *not* have to know everything.
- Examiners at undergraduate level *want to pass you*. (Postgraduate, i.e. post-medical school exams, may be a different story.)
- Know what to expect: refer to the blueprint (if available), understand what OSCEs will be assessed in the exam; for example, knowledge, skills, communication or professional practice. Ask more senior students what they experienced, but be aware of their temptation to tell horror stories.
- Read your instructions: make use of reading time, follow the instructions (e.g. if they ask you to do a focused exam, do it!).
- Be organised: develop your own approach to history taking and physical examination.
- Learn a *systematic* method and practise it until it's second nature.
- Work through the problem if the information is not available.
- Communication: don't use a scattergun approach to questioning; listen to your examiner or patient, apply active listening — and look out for non-verbal cues.
- Have a checklist of strategies to *finish* if running short of time.
- It is better to say, 'I don't know' than to make something up.
- Use the rest station to relax; do *not* agonise about how things have gone.
- Practise, practise, practise … so that the examination can be performed quickly and correctly.
- Join a study group to simulate doing OSCEs. Play the role of candidate, examiner, patient — understanding all of these perspectives will help you to excel.
- Exam difficulty increases as you progress to the more senior years — know what's needed at your level. Your study group and tutors will help here.

Box 1.3
You can't fail your OSCE if you pay attention to ALL of the following

- if you have practised a *systematic approach* — it will shine through in the exams that you have talked to and examined many patients
- if you *wash your hands* on entering and leaving
- if you are *nice*
- if you *don't hurt* the patient
- if you act professionally and look professional (just like on the wards)
- if you introduce yourself and thank the patient (simulated or not) at completion of the task
- if you are *safe* (e.g. you avoid prescribing a drug or fluid that will almost certainly kill a real patient…)
- if you don't make anything up

Early to mid-clinical years

Take a history — chest pain and dyspnoea

Background

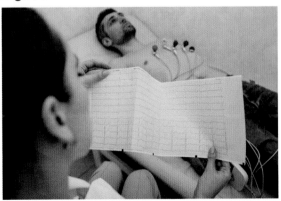

A doctor looking at an ECG in front of a patient

Chest pain is a common presenting complaint. It is not always due to coronary artery disease. Shortness of breath (dyspnoea) often accompanies chest pain due to disease of the heart or lungs.

Introduction

You are a junior medical officer working in the Emergency Department of a large tertiary hospital. Mrs Samantha McIntyre, a 58-year-old female, has presented with a two-day history of chest pain and shortness of breath. Please take a history from her and present her case to the examiner.

Rationale

Chest pain and dyspnoea are two frequent acute presenting symptoms that should trigger you to consider a wide range of differentials. There are a number of serious causes, most importantly an acute coronary syndrome (ACS) or pulmonary embolus, and you should be able to identify patients with a high likelihood of other serious causes.

Method

In approaching all critically ill patients, take a DRS ABCDE approach. First ensure you identify critically unwell patients and prioritise their care:

- **D**anger
- **R**esponse
- **S**end for help
- **A**irway
- **B**reathing
- **C**irculation
- **D**isability
- **E**nvironment

If you have established the patient is not critically unwell, proceed with history and examination.

In a non-exam situation, you would consider other information and investigations you may wish to gather prior to or during history taking and examination, including obtaining an ECG, chest X-ray and relevant blood tests (e.g. troponin). This may be

> **Box 2.1.1**
> **SOCRATES history for pain**
>
> **S**ite — where is the chest pain?
> **O**nset — is it gradual/sudden? What is its frequency and how long does it last? Have you had previous similar episodes
> **C**haracter — is it sharp/dull/burning? For example, in ACS the patient may describe a central chest heaviness. If the patient describes pleuritic pain then consider a pneumonia or a pulmonary embolus
> **R**adiation — acute coronary syndrome pain radiates to the left arm, right arm/shoulder, or both
> **A**ssociated features — key in a chest pain history. Shortness of breath and its nature may indicate a pulmonary embolus (if acute) or pneumonia (gradually worsening). Other symptoms such as cough (pneumonia), fevers (pericarditis, pneumonia), haemoptysis (pulmonary embolus) are all important information to gather
> **T**iming — when did the pain begin?
> **E**xacerbating/relieving factors — is the pain made worse by exertion or relieved by rest?
> **S**everity — does the pain interfere with normal activities or sleep?

relevant to the discussion with the examiners, but focus first on completing the task in the stem.

1. Wash hands and ask if you require personal protective equipment (PPE).
2. Introduce yourself (name, role), obtain consent, and explain confidentiality.
3. Start by assessing the history of the presenting complaint in an open-ended approach, e.g. 'I understand you have been having some shortness of breath. Could you tell me a bit more about that?' Allow the patient (or actor) the chance to talk uninterrupted; they will usually give you some of the important features of their main symptom. Use the SOCRATES layout to cover the rest of the aspects that have not been covered. See Box 2.1.1.
4. Risk factors; practise generating a list of differential diagnoses from the information gathered; Box 2.1.2. At this point, ask specific questions relating to your list, for example:
   - Myocardial infarction: family history, smoking, dyslipidaemia, known coronary artery disease,

Box 2.1.2
Differential diagnosis: acute dyspnoea and chest pain

Acute dyspnoea	Chest pain
Pneumonia	Acute coronary syndrome
Asthma	Pulmonary embolism
Chronic obstructive pulmonary disease	Pneumonia
Pulmonary embolism	Aortic dissection
Myocardial infarction	Musculoskeletal
Congestive cardiac failure	Aortic aneurysm
Pulmonary oedema	Pericarditis
Interstitial pulmonary fibrosis	Myocarditis
Metabolic acidosis	Cancer
Anxiety*	Rib fracture
Anaemia	Oesophageal spasm
Cancer	Anxiety*
	Reflux
	Pneumothorax
	Costochondritis

* Remember that attributing symptoms to anxiety generally requires ruling out other
aetiologies.

hypertension, diabetes mellitus, obesity, age, lack of
exercise, poor diet
- Pulmonary embolism: previous deep vein thrombosis/
pulmonary embolism, symptoms of deep vein
thrombosis, malignancy, medications (e.g. combined
oral contraceptive pill use), recent sedentary period,
family history, recent surgery, clotting disorders
5. Background medical history.
6. Medications.
7. Allergies.
8. Family history.
9. Social history.
10. Hand hygiene.

Information for the patient

This is an example of the type of information that might be
provided to an actor or elicited from a patient, and the level of
detail you would seek to then present to the examiners in the
third-person point of view (not second-person as written
below).

You are Samantha McIntyre, a 58-year-old female presenting to the emergency department of your local hospital.

You have had pain on the left side of your chest for the last 3 days and trouble breathing, especially when walking up stairs. Your symptoms came on gradually. The pain worsens when you take a big breath in or cough, and feels sharp. It is located on the left lower part of the front of your chest. It is 7/10 in severity. You have not coughed up blood.

You have just returned from an overseas trip to the UK, flying home on a long-haul flight one week ago in economy. Following the trip, you noticed your right leg to be swollen and sore for the last three days, leading you to rest in bed. You don't have a cough or sore throat but feel as though you have been having fevers for the past few days. You have not been around anyone who has been sick. You were previously well. You have had all your immunisations including the flu vaccine. You have tried paracetamol and ibuprofen to ease the pain, with little relief.

You have never had pain like this before. You suffer from high cholesterol and osteoarthritis. You have no diagnosis of cancer. You take atorvastatin and paracetamol. You are allergic to penicillin, which causes a rash.

Your mother died of a stroke at age 82 and your father of testicular cancer at 77. Your sister, 55, had a blood clot in her leg during pregnancy. There is no history of heart disease in the family that you know of.

You work as a librarian and live with your husband and cat. You are usually quite active, walking or swimming most days. You eat a healthy diet. You drink occasionally, 1–2 standard drinks once a month. You are an ex-smoker, having quit 10 years ago; you previously smoked 20 cigarettes a day for 20 years. You do not use any other drugs.

SUMMARY

This story is most suggestive of deep venous thrombosis after a long-haul flight and complicating pulmonary embolus. However, other causes, while less likely, need to be considered and excluded, including ACS and pneumonia.

To determine the likelihood of a pulmonary embolus, the Wells score is often used and more senior students may be asked about it. The criteria are:

- Clinical symptoms of deep venous thrombosis (3 points) — in this case yes.
- Other diagnoses less likely (3 points) — in this case yes.
- Immobilisation for 3 or more days or surgery in the past month (1.5 points) — in this case yes.
- Previous deep venous thrombosis or pulmonary embolus (1.5 points) — in this case no.
- Haemoptysis (1 point) — in this case no.
- Known to have cancer (1 point) — in this case no.
- Heart rate >100 beats/minute (1.5 points) — unknown until you examine the patient.

The Wells score is at least 7.5 points: over 6.0 is a high probability of pulmonary embolus.

Present your findings

It is important to clearly summarise your main findings to the examiners. Remember to highlight the presence or absence of any relevant red flags (alarm features from the history, e.g. haemoptysis). For potential causes of chest pain, report the presence or absence of major risk factors (e.g. for coronary artery disease or pulmonary embolus, depending on the case).

Examiners' likely questions

- What is your provisional diagnosis?
- What are your differentials and what makes each more or less likely?
- What are the risk factors for cardiac chest pain?
- What is this patient's Wells score and what does this tell you?
- What further investigations would you want to perform?
- Considering your provisional diagnosis, what would your initial management be?

Marking criteria table

Criteria	Satisfactory	Non-satisfactory
Hand hygiene performed	1	0
Appropriate introduction	1	0
Pain history		
Site	1	0
Onset	1	0
Character	1	0
Radiation	1	0
Associated symptoms	1	0
Temporal sequence	1	0
Exacerbating/relieving factors	1	0
Severity	1	0
Explores further dyspnoea history including		
Paroxysmal nocturnal dyspnoea, orthopnoea	1	0
Exercise tolerance	1	0
Associated symptoms	1	0
Background history	1	0
Medications	1	0
Allergies	1	0
Family history	1	0
Social history	1	0
Cardiac risk factors	1	0
Venous thromboembolism (VTE) risk factors	1	0

Pass mark: 14

Take a history — abdominal pain

Background

Acute abdominal pain is a common presenting complaint. The history is key to a correct diagnosis. Identifying the presence of red flags (alarm symptoms) is important to clinical decision making.

Introduction

You are a junior medical officer working on the surgical ward of a large hospital. You are called to review a patient (Jacob Crawford, 24-year-old male) who was admitted overnight with undifferentiated abdominal pain. He is complaining his pain is getting worse. Please take a history and perform the appropriate examination.

Rationale

Abdominal pain is a common symptom that can be quite distressing for patients. There is a wide range of causes that can often be difficult to differentiate. Strong history taking and examination skills are essential to identify red flag features (e.g. vomiting, weight loss, bleeding) and formulate a list of differential diagnoses. See Box 2.2.1.

Method

In approaching all patients, take a DRS ABCDE approach. First ensure you identify critically unwell patients and prioritise their care.

- **D**anger
- **R**esponse

- **S**end for help
- **A**irway
- **B**reathing
- **C**irculation
- **D**isability
- **E**nvironment

If you have established the patient is not critically unwell, proceed with history and examination.

Box 2.2.1
Differential diagnosis of abdominal pain

Think of these according to the aetiology, i.e. vascular, inflammatory, obstructive, infectious, trauma or metabolic, and according to anatomical location.

Stomach/duodenum
Peptic ulcer disease

Small bowel/colon
Enterocolitis, acute mesenteric ischaemia, ischaemic colitis, inflammatory bowel disease, bowel obstruction, appendicitis, mesenteric adenitis, diverticulitis, constipation

Liver and pancreaticobiliary
Cholangitis, cholecystitis, biliary colic, hepatitis, pancreatitis

Gynaecological
Tubulo-ovarian, e.g. ectopic pregnancy
Endometriosis, pelvic inflammatory disease and ovarian cyst torsion or rupture

Genito-urinary tract
Cystitis, renal or ureteric stones, urinary tract infection, pyelonephritis
Testicular torsion

Vascular
Aortic dissection, ruptured aortic aneurysm

Abdominal wall
Abdominal wall pain, cellulitis, shingles, peritonitis and rib fractures

Metabolic
Diabetic ketoacidosis, hypercalcaemia

1. Wash hands/PPE.
2. Introduce yourself (name, role), obtain consent, and explain confidentiality.
3. Start by assessing the history of the presenting complaint, first in an open-ended approach, then cover the following aspects using the SOCRATES mnemonic (Box 2.2.2).
4. Background medical history, including surgical history.
5. Medications.
6. Allergies.
7. Family history.
8. Social — drug/alcohol/cigarette use, work/education, home situation; assess independence.
9. Summarise, seek questions/concerns.
10. Hand hygiene.

EXAMINATION

1. Positioning — lying flat with head resting on a pillow
2. General examination
3. Peripheries (hands, arms), head, neck and chest examination
4. Abdomen
   a. Inspect
   b. Palpate
   c. Percuss
   d. Auscultate
5. Ask the examiner if you may undertake a hernia examination and rectal examination, or have the results of these examinations.

Consider further examination: lymph nodes, cardiovascular, respiratory, genitourinary systems.

Information for the patient

As explained above, patients who are actors will be given a script to follow so that they can answer the students' questions consistently. This is an example of such a script.

You are a 24-year-old male who has been experiencing abdominal pain for the past 24 hours. You came into hospital with dull lower central abdominal pain associated with nausea and fevers. It came on gradually and doesn't radiate anywhere. It is worse with movement and walking but better with rest and

Box 2.2.2
SOCRATES history for abdominal pain

Site — quadrant/region (see Fig. 2.2.1a, b).
Onset — gradual/sudden, frequency and duration
Character — sharp/dull/burning/colicky
Radiation — or referred pain
Associated features — fevers/nausea/vomiting/urinary symptoms/ bowel symptoms, bloating, appetite, weight change
Timing — when did the pain first begin, any precipitating events (e.g. acute attack of vomiting and diarrhoea suggesting gastroenteritis)
Exacerbating/relieving factors — relieved by defecation (suggests colonic disease)?
Severity — does the pain wake you from sleep?

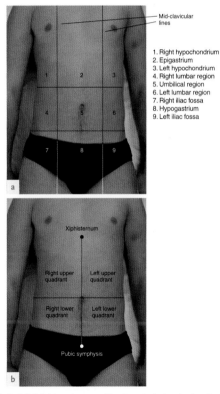

Mid-clavicular lines

1. Right hypochondrium
2. Epigastrium
3. Left hypochondrium
4. Right lumbar region
5. Umbilical region
6. Left lumbar region
7. Right iliac fossa
8. Hypogastrium
9. Left iliac fossa

Xiphisternum

Right upper quadrant — Left upper quadrant
Right lower quadrant — Left lower quadrant

Pubic symphysis

Figure 2.2.1 **(a),(b)** How to specify site of abdominal pain (Talley NJ, O'Connor S. *Talley and O'Connor's Clinical Examination*. Elsevier Australia, 2017.)

lying down with your knees bent. You have just alerted your nurse that the pain is getting worse, despite treatment. The pain has got sharper, it is now in the lower right side of your abdomen and is the worst pain you have ever felt (10/10 severity). You still feel nauseated and have been having chills and shakes.

You were previously well; you have not been around anyone who has been sick and do not take any regular medications. You have been in hospital once before, age 10, following a broken wrist. You suffer from asthma, for which you use a puffer (Salbutamol) when needed. You use this once every few weeks with exercise. You are allergic to latex, which results in itch and a rash. You have had all your immunisations.

You are currently a university student studying teaching. You live with two housemates and consume 1–2 standard drinks most weeknights, up to 10 on weekends. You smoke 5–10 cigarettes daily. You occasionally use marijuana (once per month), and do not use any other drugs. You are currently working at a supermarket and have friends and family nearby. You own no pets.

Your parents are both alive and well. You have a history of heart disease on your father's side and asthma on your mother's side.

Your primary concern is the pain and the fact that the medications you have been given aren't helping.

Please answer the examiner's questions using the above information.

Present your findings

It is important to clearly summarise your findings to the examiners, highlighting the presence or absence of any relevant red flags or risk factors for potential causes of abdominal pain.

Examiners' likely questions

- Please perform an appropriate examination on this patient. (You are likely to be told the findings as the patient may now be asymptomatic or an actor.)

On examination, the patient is taking short, shallow breaths. You find tenderness worst at the McBurney point with rebound tenderness.

- What is your primary diagnosis?
  - The history and examination are most consistent with acute appendicitis.
- What are the differential diagnoses you would consider, and what makes them more or less likely?
  - Acute ileitis from bacterial infection (e.g. *Yersinia*, usually associated with acute diarrhoea). Diverticulitis in the caecum (uncommon but identical clinical features). Meckel diverticulitis (a Meckel diverticulum is a congenital remnant of the omphalomesenteric duct in the small bowel) — uncommon but identical features. Crohn disease (usually there is a history of chronic diarrhoea and abdominal pain, and there may be weight loss or rectal bleeding).
  - In females, a number of gynaecological aetiologies must be considered, including ruptured ovarian cyst and ectopic pregnancy.
- What further investigations would you like to arrange?
  - Tests include a full blood count (look for a high white blood cell count, which will be raised and very high if there is perforation) and imaging (ultrasound or CT scan).
- What is your initial management for this patient?
- Where is McBurney point tenderness?
  - The tenderness in the right iliac fossa is maximal over a point 3.8–5cm along a line from the anterior superior iliac spine to the umbilicus.
- What is the Rovsing sign?
  - Another way to test for right-sided rebound tenderness: press over the left lower quadrant then release quickly — this causes pain in the right iliac fossa.
- What is the psoas sign?
  - This is present with a retrocaecal inflamed appendix. Lay the patient on the left side and attempt to extend the right hip; if painful and resisted, the sign is positive.
- What are the complications of acute appendicitis?
  - A perforated appendix is serious — consider this if there is a high fever (>39.4°C), or signs of generalised peritonitis.

Marking criteria table

Criteria	Satisfactory	Unsatisfactory
Hand hygiene performed	1	0
Appropriate introduction	1	0
Pain history		
Site	1	
Onset	1	0
Character	1	0
Radiation	1	0
Associated symptoms	1	0
Temporal sequence	1	0
Exacerbating/relieving factors	1	0
Severity	1	0
Background history	1	0
Medications	1	0
Allergies	1	0
Family history	1	0
Social history	1	0
Abdominal examination		
General inspection	1	0
Hands, arms	1	0
Face, mouth	1	0
Neck, chest	1	0
Abdomen — inspection	1	0
Abdomen — palpation	1	0
Abdomen — percussion	1	0
Abdomen – auscultation	1	0
Rectal examination, hernia examination requested	1	0
Provisional diagnosis — acute appendicitis	1	0
Reasonable differential diagnosis — at least three identified	1	0
Appropriate investigations requested	1	0
Appropriate initial management suggested	1	0
Correctly identifies McBurney point, Rovsing sign, psoas sign	3	0–2

Pass mark: 20

Take a history — headache

Background

Most headaches have a benign cause, such as a tension headache. While serious underlying causes such as a brain tumour are rare, identifying red flags is critical as this identifies the need to investigate further.

Introduction

A 32-year-old female comes to your GP practice with a 2-month history of headaches. She has not had problems with headaches in the past.

Rationale

Headaches are a common complaint that you will come across in your practice. A good history allows you to differentiate between a primary headache disorder, which is only diagnosed on history, versus a secondary headache condition, which may have a serious underlying cause.

Method

INFORMATION FROM THE PATIENT

My headaches started ~2 months ago. They have progressively worsened over this time. Initially they were a mild dull ache behind the eyes. However, now they are about an 8/10 and are worse in the morning, with a couple of episodes of vomiting when the headache is severe.

They are worse sometimes when I lean forward, but not worse on coughing. I have not had any fevers, rash or neck stiffness. I don't have any weakness or numbness.

I have also noted I have been walking into doors and walls sometimes and noticed my vision can be double when I look certain ways.

I don't have any other medical problems and take no medications. I have used paracetamol and ibuprofen with minimal benefit. I don't drink or smoke alcohol and never use recreational drugs.

1. Wash hands/PPE.
2. Introduce yourself (name, role), obtain consent, and explain confidentiality.
3. Start by assessing the history of the presenting complaint using the SOCRATES history for headache (Box 2.3.1).

Box 2.3.1
SOCRATES history for headache

Site of the pain
- Localised or generalised, unilateral or bilateral
- Unilateral headaches could imply migraine or a trigeminal autonomic cephalalgia (TAC) or temporal arteritis
- Band-like bilateral pain would be consistent with a tension headache

Onset of the pain
- It is important to determine the time course. Was it gradual, sudden or subacute?
- Subarachnoid haemorrhage may present as a sudden onset, very severe headache, often described as 'thunderclap headache'

Character of the pain
- If the patient describes the headache as pounding or throbbing, it could indicate a migrainous headache
- A sharp stabbing pain may be indicative of a TAC, such as a cluster headache or of trigeminal neuralgia
- Sinusitis is often described by patients as a throbbing headache

Radiation
- If the pain radiates to the neck, consider meningitis; if it radiates to the eye, think of acute glaucoma or temporal arteritis

Box 2.3.1
SOCRATES history for headache *continued*

Associated features
This is very important in a headache history.
- *Nausea and vomiting:* this may suggest raised intracranial pressure from a bleed or space-occupying lesion or could be migrainous
- *Visual disturbance:* may be related to a migraine, temporal arteritis, glaucoma or an intracranial lesion. Identifying the 'positive' visual phenomena of a migrainous scintillating scotoma of blurred vision with bright, sparking edges can be useful in differentiation of more sinister visual losses
- *Photophobia:* is suggestive of meningitis or raised intracranial pressure or migraine
- *Neck stiffness:* Meningitis or cervicogenic headache
- *Fever:* an underlying infective process such as meningitis
- *Rash:* most concerning is a non-blanching purpuric rash, suggesting meningococcal meningitis
- *Lacrimation, rhinorrhoea, conjunctival injection or periorbital swelling*: are indicative of TACs such as cluster headache, where they occur only in association with typical, recurrent headache
- *Weight loss:* need to consider malignancy
- *Focal neurological deficits:* consider space-occupying lesion or intracranial bleeding
- *Seizures:* may indicate intracranial bleeding or a space-occupying lesion

Timing
- Ask the patient questions about the duration of headache: how long does it last? has there been a pattern? does it change with the time of day?
- How long has the headache been present?

Exacerbating or relieving factors
- Ask if there are any obvious triggers such as caffeine, other medications or postural change.
- Ask if there are any relieving factors. This is a good opportunity to see if analgesia has been effective.
- Knowing about how a headache changes with posture is important. A headache that is worse on waking in bed in the morning and better once up and around during the day, but worsens with lowering the head below the hips, is suggestive of raised intracranial pressure. A headache that disappears on lying flat but recurs on standing up is suggestive of low intracranial pressure, such as that which would arise from a persistent CSF leak, for example after a lumbar puncture or epidural.

Severity
- Ask the patient to rate the pain, on a scale of 1–10.

Past medical history

It is important to take a thorough medication history, as many medications not only cause headaches but can also be risk factors for serious causes of headaches. For example, oestrogen-containing oral contraceptives are a risk factor for cerebral venous sinus thrombosis.

- Family history (e.g. migraine, stroke)
- Social history — smoking, alcohol use
- Drugs
- Occupation
- Social support

It is always important to screen for red flags of a headache that may indicate need for further imaging or testing.

Present your findings

It is important to clearly summarise your findings to the examiners, highlighting the presence or absence of any relevant red flags (Box 2.3.2) or risk factors for potential causes of secondary headaches.

Box 2.3.2
SNNOOP10 is a reminder of the red flags (danger or alarm features) for headache

Systemic symptoms including fever
Neoplasm history
Neurologic deficit (including decreased consciousness, visual loss)
Onset is sudden or abrupt
Older age (onset after age 50 years)
Pattern change or recent onset of new headache
Positional headache
Precipitated by sneezing, coughing, or exercise
Progressive headache and atypical presentations
Pregnancy or puerperium
Painful eye with autonomic features
Post-traumatic onset of headache
Pathology of the immune system, such as HIV
Painkiller (analgesic) overuse (e.g. medication overuse headache) or new drug at onset of headache
Papilloedema on examination by fundoscopy

Examiners' likely questions

- What examination and investigations would you like to do next?

  The most important next step is to do a complete neurological examination and consider appropriate investigations (Box 2.3.3).

Box 2.3.3
Examination and investigations for headache

- Cranial nerves
- A visual assessment is particularly important, including fundoscopy, ideally after dilating the pupils. Papilloedema is an important sign of a space-occupying lesion
- Upper and lower limb neurological examination for localising signs
- Cardiovascular examination, particularly checking blood pressure
- Investigations are directed by the history and examination
- Imaging is indicated if there are red flags:
  - CT brain (if an emergency, to identify a life-threatening cause)
  - MRI (non-emergency cases, no radiation)

Marking criteria table

Criteria	Satisfactory	Unsatisfactory
Introduction	1	0
Headache characteristics	3	0–2
Red flags	2	0–1
Medications	1	0
Provisional diagnosis	1	0
Differential diagnosis	2	0–1
Next steps	1	0

Pass mark: 7

Wash hands and scrub for theatre

Background

Every doctor needs to know hand washing and must be able to scrub correctly for an operation. Practise the drill so it's second nature.

Introduction

This is a basic skills station. Practise by actually going to theatre to assist and scrubbing in — you will learn a lot (and it's fun), and it'll become second nature.

Rationale

Washing your hands properly before seeing a patient protects the patient, and washing your hands properly after seeing a patient protects you. Refer to Fig. 2.4.1. Scrubbing for theatre protects the patient from life-threatening infections. It matters!

You'll be given an equipment pack. It should be familiar to you if you have practised your technique in preparation. This is a show-and-tell station.

Method

1. You won't usually need to change into scrubs including shoe covers, a theatre cap and surgical mask, but say you would do so to the examiners. Make sure your sleeves are rolled up, jewellery is off (bare below the elbows).
2. Open the sterile theatre gown on a flat clean surface and open the sterile gloves onto the gown without contaminating them.

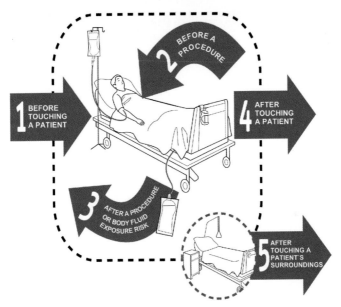

Figure 2.4.1 The '5 Moments for Hand Hygiene' This tool is based on evidence (Reproduced with permission of the World Health Organization.)

3. Turn on the water and wash your hands in three phases.
   * *First wash:* lather with liquid disinfectant including up your arms to just below the elbow. Rinse, starting from your hands moving down to the elbows so the water doesn't re-contaminate your hands.
   * *Second wash:* clean under your fingernails with the nail pick, then use your foot pedal or elbow to dispense soap onto the brush. Scrub from your fingertips to below elbow regions for 30 seconds on each arm. Rinse again.
   * *Third wash:* using the brush, clean your fingernails, each finger and between the digits, palm, back of the hands, and forearms (30 seconds each region). Rinse again.
4. Use the sterile towels to dry (one for each arm).

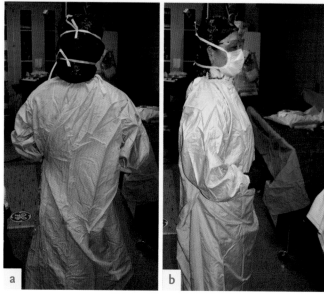

Figure 2.4.2 **(a–b)** It takes practice to dress for theatre without recontaminating yourself (Poole J, Larson LW. *Surgical Implantation of Cardiac Rhythm Devices.* Elsevier Inc., 2018.)

5. Pick up the gown, place your arms through the top before the cuffs, and don the gloves (do not touch the outside) (Fig. 2.4.2). This takes practice to do it without re-contaminating yourself.

T&O'C hint box

Scrubbing for theatre
- You must demonstrate you can maintain sterility.
- Do not rush. Be methodical.

Examiners' likely questions

- Describe your technique of handwashing before seeing a patient in the ward.
  - Remember the six-part standard rubbing technique (Box 2.4.1, Fig. 2.4.3).

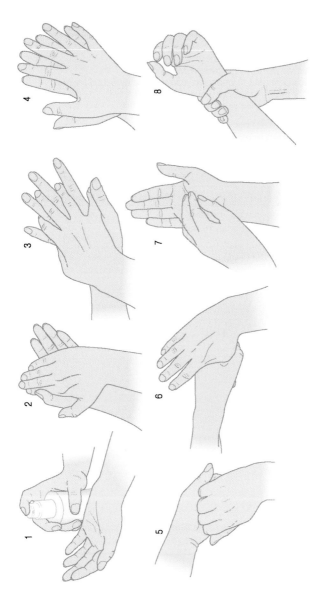

Figure 2.4.3 Correct handwashing technique includes rubbing from the palms to the back of the hands with fingers interlocked (Marsh PD, Lewis MA, Williams D, Martin MV. *Oral Microbiology*. Elsevier Ltd, 2009.)

Box 2.4.1
Standard handwashing rubbing technique

1. Palm to palm
2. Right palm over left fingers and vice versa
3. Palm to palm with fingers interlocked
4. Back of fingers to opposing palms with interlocked fingers
5. Right thumb in left palm and vice versa
6. Right hand in left palm and vice versa.

Marking criteria table

Criteria	Satisfactory	Unsatisfactory
Pre-preparation (scrubs, jewellery)	1	0
Opens gown pack properly/gloves	2	0–1
First wash	1	0
Second wash	1	0
Third wash	1	0
Turns tap on and off without touch	1	0
Dons gown and gloves with sterile technique	2	0–1

Pass mark: 6

Take the blood pressure

Background

Many students have not had much experience in taking blood pressure measurements. Most hospitals use automatic machines. Students, however, are still expected to be able to measure blood pressure manually. There are differences between different sphygmomanometers and it is important to practise with a number of different types. It is embarrassing for both the students and the examiners to hear the crackling Velcro noise of the cuff as it comes apart and falls off the arm. Using a cuff of the right size and putting it on the right way up will prevent this unpleasantness. The usual blood pressure cuff width is 12.5 cm. This is suitable for a normal-sized adult upper arm. However, in obese patients with large arms (up to 30% of the adult population), the normal-sized cuff will overestimate the blood pressure and therefore a large cuff must be used. A range of smaller sizes are available for children. Use of a cuff that is too large results in only a small underestimate of blood pressure.

THE BLOOD PRESSURE

The systolic blood pressure is the peak pressure that occurs in the arteries (and the left ventricle) following ventricular systole; the diastolic blood pressure is the level to which the arterial blood pressure falls during ventricular diastole. Remember, the ventricular pressure continues to fall in diastole but a further drop in the arterial diastolic pressure is prevented by the presence of a competent aortic valve.

TABLE 2.5.1 A classification of blood pressure readings

Category	Systolic (mmHg)	Diastolic (mmHg)
Optimal	<120	<80
Normal	120–129	80–84
High normal	130–139	85–89
Mild hypertension (grade 1)	140–159	90–99
Moderate hypertension (grade 2)	160–179	100–109
Severe	>180	>110

(*2013 ESH/ESC Guidelines for the management of arterial hypertension.* The Task Force for the management of arterial hypertension of the European Society of Hypertension (ESH) and of the European Society of Cardiology (ESC). Reprinted with permission of Oxford University Press.)

HIGH BLOOD PRESSURE

The risk of adverse outcome increases as the blood pressure rises above normal (Table 2.5.1). **Malignant hypertension** is marked hypertension (usually the diastolic is >120 mmHg) with changes on fundoscopy (haemorrhages, exudates and papilloedema; see p. 162).

POSTURAL BLOOD PRESSURE

The blood pressure should be taken routinely with the patient lying and standing (or sitting). A fall of more than 15mmHg in systolic blood pressure or 10 mmHg in diastolic blood pressure on standing is abnormal and is called **postural hypotension**. It may not be associated with symptoms.

CHANGES WITH RESPIRATION: PULSUS PARADOXUS

A **fall in systolic blood** pressure of up to 10 mmHg occurs normally during inspiration. Exaggeration of this response — a fall of more than 10 mmHg — is an important sign called pulsus paradoxus, which may indicate pericardial tamponade (rapid accumulation of fluid in the pericardial space) or severe asthma.

Note: In pulsus paradoxus the change in blood pressure is an exaggerated response of normal (and not a paradoxical response); the paradox is in the difference of peripheral strength of pulse despite no change in praecordial activity, and hence the term is often confusing to many students and doctors.

HIGH BLOOD PRESSURE

High blood pressure is difficult to define (Table 2.5.1). The most helpful definitions of hypertension are based on an estimation of the level associated with an increased risk of vascular disease. If recordings above 140/90 mmHg are considered abnormal, high blood pressure may occur in up to 20% of the adult population. Blood pressure measured by the patient at home, or by a 24-hour monitor, should be up to 10–5 mmHg less than that measured in the office (the so-called 'white coat' hypertension phenomenon).

Introduction

This is more likely to be junior medical student OSCE while senior students might be asked to take the blood pressure and then discuss the diagnosis and complications of hypertension. For junior medical students, the request may just be to take the blood pressure.

Rationale

The ability to measure blood pressure accurately with a manual sphygmomanometer is still important. Some knowledge of different ways of measuring blood pressure, and of how to decide when readings are significantly abnormal, will be expected of you.

Method

1. Introduce yourself and wash your hands. Ask the patient's permission to measure the blood pressure. Make sure there is no arteriovenous fistula present.
2. Ask if the patient has rested for at least 5 minutes, or to wait if not (you won't be allowed but you may obtain a higher than normal reading then). Also ask if the bladder has been emptied (a full bladder might also give you high blood pressure readings).
3. Correctly position the patient so he or she is comfortable (make sure ALL are actioned): legs uncrossed, feet flat on

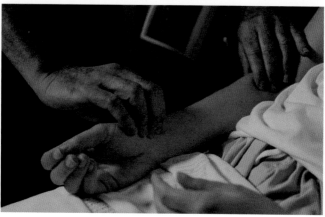

Figure 2.5.1 Taking the radial pulse (Talley NJ, O'Connor S. *Clinical Examination: A systematic guide to physical diagnosis.* Elsevier Australia, 2018.)

the floor, the arms supported, and ask the patient to not talk (or use a mobile phone!). This is again to minimise false positive high blood pressure readings.

4. Choose the right-sized cuff for the patient's size to obtain accurate readings or at least ask to do so (small, medium, large, extra-large).

5. Make sure the arm is bare (do not take the blood pressure over clothes). If it isn't bare, fix it.

6. The cuff is wrapped around the upper arm with the bladder centred over the brachial artery. This is found in the antecubital fossa, one-third of the way over from the medial epicondyle. For an approximate estimation of the systolic blood pressure, the cuff is fully inflated and then deflated slowly (3–4 mmHg per second) until the radial pulse returns (Fig. 2.5.1).

7. Then, for a more accurate estimation of the blood pressure, this manoeuvre is repeated with the diaphragm of the stethoscope placed over the brachial artery, slipped underneath the distal end of the cuff's bladder (Fig. 2.5.2).

8. Five different sounds will be heard as the cuff is slowly released (see Fig. 2.5.3). These are called the Korotkoff sounds. The pressure at which a sound is first heard over

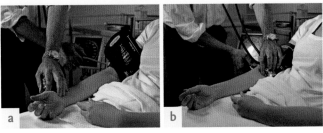

Figure 2.5.2 Measuring the blood pressure, with the patient lying at 45° (Talley NJ, O'Connor S. *Clinical Examination: A systematic guide to physical diagnosis.* Elsevier Australia, 2018.)

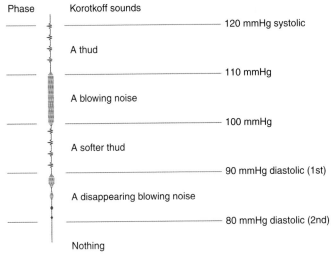

Figure 2.5.3 Systolic pressure is determined by the appearance of the first audible sound, and diastolic pressure is determined by its disappearance (Talley NJ, O'Connor S. *Talley and O'Connor's Clinical Examination.* Elsevier Australia, 2017.)

the artery is the systolic blood pressure (Korotkoff I, or KI). As deflation of the cuff continues, the sound increases in intensity (KII), then decreases (KIII), becomes muffled (KIV) and disappears (KV). Different observers have used KIV and KV to indicate the level of the diastolic pressure. KV is probably the best measure. However, this provides a slight underestimate of the arterial diastolic blood pressure. Although diastolic pressure usually corresponds most closely to KV, in severe aortic regurgitation KIV is a more accurate indication. KV is absent in some normal people and KIV must be used in these cases.

- If the heart is very irregular (most often because of atrial fibrillation), the cuff should be deflated slowly; the point at which most of the cardiac contractions are audible (KI) is taken as the systolic pressure and the point at which most have disappeared (KV) is taken as diastole.
- Aim to record the blood pressure to the nearest 2 mmHg (so deflate at 2 mmHg per second).

9. Occasionally, there will be an auscultatory gap (the sounds disappear just below the systolic pressure and reappear before the diastolic pressure) in healthy people. This can lead to an underestimate of the systolic blood pressure if the cuff is not pumped up high enough.

10. Once finished, ask if you may take the blood pressure in the other arm (usually you won't be allowed). You may be asked why test both arms — clinically, the arm with the *higher* blood pressure is the most relevant and is the arm to be used in future blood pressure monitoring.

11. Ask to take the blood pressure standing after sitting to test for a postural drop. You won't usually be required to do so.

12. **For senior students**, traditionally the blood pressure is not measured using the arm on the side of a previous mastectomy (especially if the axillary nodes have been removed) for fear of further upsetting lymphatic drainage. Modern mastectomies are less extensive than previous 'radical' mastectomies and the risk of causing trouble is very small. Also, blood pressure should not be taken from an arm that has had an arteriovenous fistula inserted for renal dialysis for fear of damaging the fistula and enraging the patient's renal physician and vascular surgeon.

- The systolic blood pressure may normally vary between the arms by up to 10 mmHg; in the legs the blood pressure is normally up to 20 mmHg higher than in the arms unless the patient has coarctation of the aorta (in which case the blood pressure will be much lower in the legs). Measurement of the blood pressure in the legs is more difficult than in the arms. It requires a large cuff that is placed over the mid-thigh; the patient lies prone and the stethoscope is placed in the popliteal fossa, behind the knee.

13. Know how to also use an ambulatory blood pressure device as you may be asked to show the examiners.

Present your findings

It is important in any physical examination OSCE to clearly summarise your relevant positive and negative findings to the examiners. This is more than just stating the blood pressure recording value! One approach is to briefly restate the introduction ('I was asked to take the blood pressure of Mr Smith, a 56-year-old man'), describe the patient positioning and level of comfort ('the patient was sitting comfortably at rest with his legs uncrossed flat on the floor and arms supported'), describe the method ('using a blood pressure cuff suitable for the patient's arm size, I found his palpable systolic blood pressure to be 120 mmHg and on auscultation sitting the blood pressure was 120/80 mmHg with no auscultatory gap'). End with what to do next to complete the evaluation ('I would like next to take the blood pressure in the other arm (*know why if asked*), and then lying and standing to exclude postural hypotension').

Examiners' likely questions

- What would you do if the reading were elevated?
  - Tell the examiners you would like to take it again in about 5 minutes.
- How else might high blood pressure be confirmed or excluded?
  - Suggest home blood pressure readings by the patient but remember that these should be 10 mmHg lower than readings taken in the clinic. The next step would be a 24-hour blood pressure monitor.

Marking criteria table

Criteria	Satisfactory	Unsatisfactory
Introduces self, explains task, obtains consent, washes hands before and after	1	0
Knows how to use blood pressure cuff, uses correct size, positions patient correctly	3	0–2
Takes blood pressure by palpation first (patient sitting)	1	0
Takes blood pressure by auscultatory method (patient sitting)	1	0
Takes blood pressure (or asks to) from the other arm	1	0
Takes blood pressure with patient standing (or asks to)	1	0
Explains Korotkoff sounds	1	0
Obtains a similar reading to the examiners	1	0

Pass mark: 7

Examine the fingernails

Background

Inspecting the fingernails for signs of disease is a routine part of the physical examination of most systems. If you find an abnormality, you need to know what to do next, as described in the station.

Introduction

This 60-year-old man has presented to your outpatients' clinic because of increasing shortness of breath over the last 6 months. He was a heavy smoker until 6 months ago. Please examine his fingernails and go on to further examination if you think that would be relevant.

Rationale

This an important part of the physical examination and you will be expected to recognise significant nail abnormalities and the implications of such as clubbing, splinter haemorrhages or just tar staining. Mention of dyspnoea suggests a cardiac or respiratory problem that might be associated with clubbing.

Method

1. Keep in mind the common nail abnormalities (Table 2.6.1).
2. Introduce yourself and wash your hands. It may be helpful to have the patient sitting and with his hands on a pillow placed in his lap.
3. While arranging this, have a general look at the patient for:
   * dyspnoea
   * cyanosis
   * wasting.

TABLE 2.6.1 Nail signs in systemic disease

Nail sign	Some causes	Example
Clubbing	Lung cancer, cyanotic congenital heart disease, infective endocarditis, inflammatory bowel disease, cirrhosis	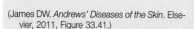

(Zipes DP et al. *Braunwald's Heart Disease: A Textbook of Cardiovascular Medicine*. 7th edn. Philadelphia: Saunders, 2005.)

Koilonychia (spoon-shaped nails)	Iron deficiency anaemia	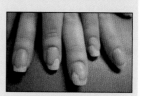

(James DW. *Andrews' Diseases of the Skin*. Elsevier, 2011, Figure 33.41.)

Onycholysis (separation of nail from nail bed)	Psoriasis, infection, hyperthyroidism, trauma	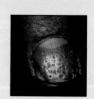

(Bernard A, Cohen MD. *Pediatric Dermatology*. 4th edn. © 2013, Elsevier Limited, Figure 8.67.)

Pitting	Psoriasis, Reiter syndrome	

(Bolognia J et al. *Dermatology* 3rd edn. Elsevier, 2012, Figure 71.4.)

TABLE 2.6.1   Nail signs in systemic disease *continued*

Nail sign	Some causes	Example
Beau lines	Any severe systemic illness that disrupts nail growth, Raynaud disease, pemphigus, trauma	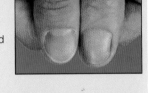

(Habif TP. *Clinical Dermatology: A color guide to diagnosis and therapy*. Elsevier, 2010, Figure 14-13.)

Nail sign	Some causes	Example
Yellow nails	Lymphoedema, pleural effusion, immunodeficiency, bronchiectasis, sinusitis, rheumatoid arthritis, nephrotic syndrome, thyroiditis, tuberculosis, Raynaud disease	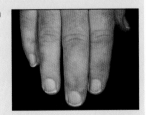

(*American Journal of Medicine* 2010;123(2):125–126, Elsevier, Figure 2.)

Nail sign	Some causes	Example
Terry (white) nails	Cirrhosis, malnutrition	

Callen JP, Jorizzo JL, Bolognia JL, Piette WW, Zone JJ. *Dermatological Signs of Internal Disease*. Elsevier, 2009, Figure 26-5.)

continued

TABLE 2.6.1 Nail signs in systemic disease *continued*

Nail sign	Some causes	Example
Azure lunula (blue nails)	Hepatolenticular degeneration (Wilson disease), silver poisoning	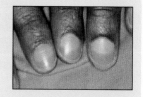

(Naylor EMT, Ruben ES, Robinson-Bostom L, Telang GH, Jellinek NJ. *Journal of the American Academy of Dermatology* 2008; 58(6):1021–1024. © 2008 American Academy of Dermatology, Inc., Figure 1.)

| Half-and-half nails | Chronic kidney disease | 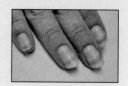 |

(Schwarzenberger K, Werchniak AE, Ko CJ. *General Dermatology*. © 2009, Elsevier Limited, Figure 2-5.)

| Muehrcke lines | Hypoalbuminaemia (any cause) | 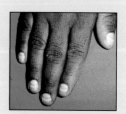 |

(Short N, Shah C. *American Journal of Medicine* 2010; 123(11):991–992. © 2010, Elsevier Inc.)

| Mees lines | Arsenic poisoning, Hodgkin lymphoma, chemotherapy | |

(Chauhan S, D'Cruz S, Singh R, Sachdev A. *The Lancet* 2008;372(9647):1410–1410. © 2008 Elsevier.)

TABLE 2.6.1 Nail signs in systemic disease *continued*

Nail sign	Some causes	Example
Dark longitudinal streaks	Melanoma, benign naevus, chemical staining	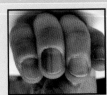

(Piraccini BM, Dika E, Fanti PA. Tips for diagnosis and treatment of nail pigmentation with practical algorithm. *Dermatologic Clinics.* © 2015, Elsevier Inc., Figure 20.)

Nail sign	Some causes	Example
Longitudinal striations	Alopecia areata, vitiligo, atopic dermatitis, psoriasis	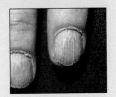

(Paller AS, Mancini AJ. *Hurwitz Clinical Pediatric Dermatology.* Elsevier, Figure 7.54.)

Nail sign	Some causes	Example
Splinter haemorrhages	Infective endocarditis, SLE, rheumatoid arthritis, antiphospholipid syndrome, trauma	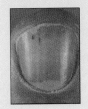

(Forbes CD, Jackson WF. *Color Atlas and Text of Clinical Medicine,* 3rd edn. Elsevier, 2002.)

Nail sign	Some causes	Example
Telangiectasia	Rheumatoid arthritis, SLE, dermatomyositis, scleroderma	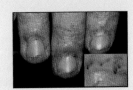

Bolognia JL et al. *Dermatology.* Elsevier, Figure 42.1. Courtesy Julie V Schaffer, MD.)

SLE: systemic lupus erythematosus.

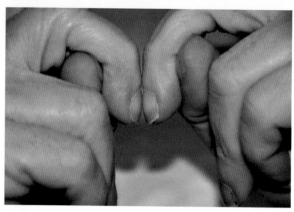

Figure 2.6.1 Schamroth sign (Brown MA, von Mutius EM, Wayne J. Clinical assessment and diagnostic approach to common problems. *Pediatric Respiratory Medicine.* St Louis, MO: Mosby, 1999.)

4. Look at the nails and ask the patient to put his two forefingers together. Look for loss of the trapezoid space normally present (Schamroth sign), which indicates clubbing (Fig. 2.6.1).
5. Look for tar staining, which likely means the patient is a smoker.
6. Look for splinter haemorrhages, which may indicate infective endocarditis.
7. If a breathless patient is clubbed, he may have interstitial lung disease (ILD), bronchiectasis, or carcinoma of the lung.
8. Go on to a formal examination of the respiratory system, looking especially for:
   - fine basal crackles — ILD
   - a pleural effusion or fixed expiratory wheeze — carcinoma of the lung
   - signs of chronic obstructive pulmonary disease (COPD); not in itself associated with clubbing but with smoking.

9. Since clubbing with or without splinter haemorrhages can be a sign of endocarditis, perform a cardiac examination, looking for:

- a murmur of mitral or aortic regurgitation — which can be caused by endocarditis or any other valve lesion, which may be pre-existing but a site for infection.
- signs of heart failure:
    - displaced apex beat
    - S3, caused by severe valvular regurgitation.

Present your findings

- Describe any abnormalities you have noticed on general inspection and say whether you think the patient appears breathless at rest.
- Outline the nail changes you have found and give a brief differential diagnosis for the possible causes of these changes. Fig. 2.6.2 shows some nail changes you may encounter.

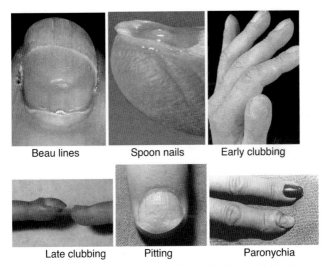

Beau lines   Spoon nails   Early clubbing

Late clubbing   Pitting   Paronychia

Figure 2.6.2 Common nail disorders (Sonia L, Sharma S. *Medical-Surgical Nursing Prep Manual for Undergraduates* vol. I. Elsevier, 2016.)

- Now explain why you have gone on to further examination and what your findings were.

Examiners' likely questions

- Can you put together your nail and general findings?
  - Clubbing + crackles: interstitial lung disease
  - Clubbing + effusion: possible lung carcinoma
  - Tar staining + over-expanded chest, Hoover sign, long forced expiratory time: COPD
  - Splinter haemorrhages with or without clubbing + murmur: infective endocarditis
- What tests might help? You are more likely to be asked what you would look for on the X-ray (Box 2.6.1) than to be shown a chest X-ray until final year, when interpretation might be required.

Box 2.6.1
What to look for in chest X-ray

- Over-expanded lung fields
- Effusion
- Lung mass (Fig 2.6.3)
- Cardiomegaly
- Prosthetic heart valve
- Interstitial changes (honeycombing)

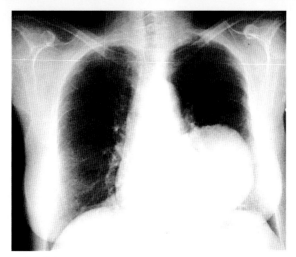

Figure 2.6.3 There is a large solitary mass lesion in the left lower zone. The differential diagnosis is primary or secondary neoplasm, hydatid cyst or large abscess. No air–fluid level is seen within it to indicate cavitation (Talley NJ, O'Connor S. *Talley and O'Connor's Clinical Examination.* Elsevier Australia, 2017.)

Marking criteria table

Criteria	Satisfactory	Unsatisfactory
Introduces self, explains task, obtains consent, washes hands before and after	1	0
Makes a show of examining the nails, looks for Schamroth sign	1	0
Notes any tar staining	1	0
Goes on to examine the lungs: inspection, palpation, percussion, auscultation	3	0–2
Is able to discuss a differential diagnosis	1	0
Knows what to look for on a chest X-ray	1	0
Performs an adequate chest X-ray interpretation	2	0–1

Pass mark: 5

Examine a lump

Background

The finding of a lump often provokes alarm. No matter where the lump is, a systematic approach to the examination will permit you to make an assessment of the likely pathology. Always assess the draining lymph nodes as well.

Introduction

A 47-year-old woman has noticed a lump on her thigh. She first noticed it 3 months ago but is not sure if it has been there for longer. It seems to have been getting bigger. Please examine her and provide a differential diagnosis.

Rationale

Lumps can occur anywhere on the body, but the examination approach is similar in most regions.

Lumps carry a wide differential that varies according to where in the body you find them. The key to a lump examination is to have a systematic approach and describe the lump accurately. This information allows you to determine a reasonable differential diagnosis and subsequent management plan.

Method

1. Introduce yourself, and explain what you would like to do. Wash your hands. Ask permission to proceed.
2. Expose the relevant body part fully where possible (but protect modesty too).

3. Ask if the lump is painful (consider inflammation, or a nerve lesion; cancer is often painless). Do *not* hurt the patient. Be gentle and considerate.
4. Inspect closely — note site, size, shape and contour (well-defined, irregular), and colour (e.g. pigmentation suggests a melanoma). Note any surrounding inflammation (redness, swelling).
5. Palpate for consistency (e.g. hard suggests malignancy, soft a cyst) and tenderness.

> ### T&O'C hint box
>
> Neurofibromas look as if they will feel hard but are in fact very soft to touch.

6. What layer is the lump situated in: skin (moves when skin is moved — sebaceous cyst, epidermoid cyst, papilloma); subcutaneous tissue (skin moves over the lump, e.g. neurofibroma, lipoma); muscle or tendon (contraction reduces lump mobility, especially in the longitudinal axis); nerve (pressure induces pins and needles, mobile in transverse but not longitudinal axis); bone (immobile); or artery (pulsatile).
7. Test for fluctuance (fluid) by palpation (two forefinger technique — watching fingers displaced in both axes when the displacing finger is moved).
8. Test for transillumination (place a torch behind the lump, switch the lights down and look for light shining through the lump).
9. Percussion may tell you if the lump is solid or cystic (but is not very helpful). Auscultate it for a bruit that would indicate it is a vascular structure.
10. Note any evidence of inflammation — hot, red, painful — and if relevant, ask to take the patient's temperature.
11. Look for lumps elsewhere on the skin.
12. Palpate the draining lymph nodes.
13. Ask the patient if they have any questions or concerns. Thank the patient.
14. Wash your hands.

Be ready to offer your summary of the findings and differential diagnosis (see Fig. 2.7.1), plus next steps in management.

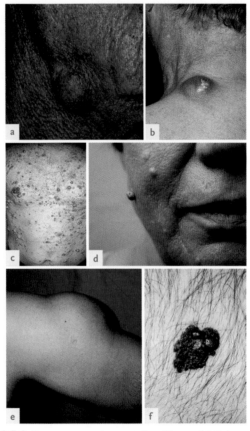

Figure 2.7.1 Some commonly encountered lumps **(a)** Sebaceous cyst **(b)** Epidermoid cyst **(c)** Multiple neurofibromas are present in this individual **(d)** Dermal fibroma **(e)** Lipoma **(f)** Malignant melanoma on arm (Source: **(a)** Giddens JF, Wilson SF. *Health Assessment for Nursing Practice.* Elsevier Inc., 2022. **(b)** Chabner DE. *The Language of Medicine*, 12th edn. Elsevier Inc., 2021. **(c)** Ferri FF. *Ferri's Clinical Advisor 2021: 5 Books in 1.* Elsevier Inc., 2021, **(e)** Shiland BJ. *Medical Assistant: Integumentary, Sensory Systems, Patient Care and Communication — Module A.* Elsevier Inc., 2015, **(f)** Shiland BJ. *Medical Assistant: Integumentary, sensory systems, patient care and communication — Module A.* Elsevier Inc., 2015.)

A lump
- Do not assume the lump is solitary until you have completed your systematic examination.
- Describe each lump with the help of SCoTe: **s**ite, **s**ize, **s**hape; **co**nsistency, **co**lour, **co**ntour; **te**nderness, **te**thering, **te**mperature.
- Ask yourself: what tissue layer? solid or fluid filled?
- Inflammation and malignancy are important causes you don't want to miss. Palpate the draining lymph nodes if you suspect infection or cancer.

Present your findings

- Describe the lump in detail.
- Craft a short differential diagnosis appropriate for the patient's age and sex. If you are not sure what the lump is, try to talk sensibly about likely possibilities depending on the tissue layer involved.
- Remember to comment if inflammation or malignancy is possible.

Examiners' likely questions

- Are you worried this lump might be a cancer? Why, or why not?
- Could this mass be a skin abscess? Why, or why not?
- What would be your next step in management?

Marking criteria table

Criteria	Satisfactory	Unsatisfactory
Introduced/explanation etc.	1	0
Patient set up (exposed body part); washed hands	1	0
Inspection	2	0–1
Palpation	2	0–1
Transilluminates lump	1	0
Draining lymph nodes	2	0–1
Describes differential	2	0–1

Pass mark: 7

Examine a body system (cardiovascular)

Background

The usual cases are cardiac murmurs. While you might be expecting to hear a murmur, remember particularly in the early years a normal patient or actor is often included in such a station. The student is then expected to demonstrate a systematic and comprehensive examination technique and identify normal findings (and what they mean). Never make anything up!

CARDIAC MURMURS

The most likely valve abnormalities you will come across are:

- Pansystolic mitral regurgitation (MR) or mid-systolic aortic stenosis (AS)
- Early diastolic aortic regurgitation (AR)
- Mid-diastolic mitral stenosis (MS)
- Late systolic mitral valve prolapse (MVP).

Depending on the university and your seniority as a medical student, you may be asked just to examine the praecordium (which means by inspection, palpation and auscultation) or to perform a more complete cardiovascular (CVS) examination. The traditional method of performing the CVS examination begins with a general inspection of the patient and goes on to the hands from there. It can, however, begin at the praecordium and, if time is limited, the examiners are more likely to direct you there. Box 2.8.1 sets out the formal CVS examination sequence.

Box 2.8.1
The cardiovascular examination sequence

1. General inspection of the patient
2. Search for the peripheral signs of heart and vascular disease in the arms, face and neck
   - hands and nails
   - radial pulse
   - blood pressure (you may be given the value in an OSCE but be prepared to take it yourself)
   - face
   - neck (jugular venous pressure, JVP)
3. Praecordium
   - inspection
   - palpation
   - auscultation
   - dynamic manoeuvres
4. Back of the chest
   - percussion
   - auscultation
5. Abdomen
   - liver (palpate)
   - spleen (palpate)
6. Legs
   - palpation of the peripheral pulses
   - inspection for oedema
   - examine for signs of arterial and venous disease (if indicated — usually a separate OSCE)

Introduction

The introduction to these cases from the examiner is likely to be:

- This patient has had a murmur detected; please examine him or her.
- This patient has been short of breath. Please examine his or her heart. You may be given a recording of a murmur to comment on. (See Station 21, page 147.)

Rationale

Students are expected to know how to perform a cardiovascular examination. This routine examination should appear practised and smooth.

Method

1. Wash your hands.
2. Make sure the patient is positioned at 45° and that the patient's chest and neck are fully exposed. For a woman, the requirements of modesty dictate that you cover her breasts with a towel or loose garment.
3. While standing back, inspect for obesity, dyspnoea, use of supplementary oxygen and intravenous infusions.
4. Look *at the chest* for scars. These may indicate previous cardiac surgery. Inspect for deformity and look to see if the apex beat is visible. Remember pacemaker and cardioverter-defibrillator boxes may be present.
5. Palpate for the apex beat position. Be seen to count down the correct number of intercostal spaces. The normal position is the fifth intercostal space, 1 cm medial to the midclavicular line. Palpate at the apex for a thrill. A systolic thrill here indicates severe mitral regurgitation. Now feel at the base of the heart for a thrill resulting from severe aortic stenosis.
6. Remember the surface anatomy of the heart (Fig. 2.8.1).

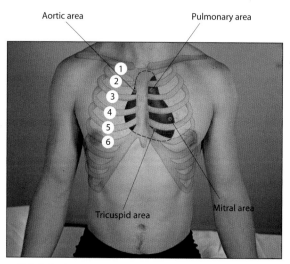

Figure 2.8.1 Surface anatomy of the heart (Talley NJ, O'Connor S. *Talley & O'Connor's Clinical Examination Essentials: An introduction to clinical skills (and how to pass your clinical exams)*. Elsevier Australia, 2020.)

7. Auscultation begins with listening in the mitral area with both the bell and the diaphragm. Spend most time here. Listen for each component of the cardiac cycle separately.

8. Identify the first and second heart sounds and decide whether they are of normal intensity and whether they are split.

9. Now listen for extra heart or prosthetic heart sounds and murmurs.

10. Listen in the axilla to find out if a systolic murmur audible at the apex radiates there (a sign of mitral regurgitation). Repeat the approach at the left sternal edge and then at the base of the heart (aortic and pulmonary areas). Time each part of the cycle with the carotid pulse. Sit the patient up and leaning forward.

11. Listen for the systolic murmur of aortic stenosis and listen over the carotids to find out if the murmur is conducted there. Ask him or her to breathe in and then breathe right out and then stop breathing. Listen here at the left sternal edge for the early diastolic murmur of aortic regurgitation. See Fig. 2.8.5. (Remember: expiration intensifies left-sided murmurs (AR, AS, MR, MS), and inspiration intensifies right-sided murmurs — tricuspid regurgitation (TR).)

12. Feel again at the base of the heart (press firmly onto the chest wall) here for a systolic thrill, usually which indicates severe AS (Fig. 2.8.2).

13. If the examiners indicate there is more time, percuss the bases of the lungs for the dullness of pleural effusion and go on to look at the hands and take the blood pressure. (It is unlikely you will have time to do these things.) You may also ask to examine for enlargement of the liver (e.g. a pulsatile liver in TR) or spleen (may be enlarged in infective endocarditis).

14. Wash your hands again.

Present your findings

● It is often best to begin by thanking them for asking you to examine Mr (or Ms) X (even if you do not mean it). Then repeat the introduction '…, who has had problems with breathlessness'.

- If there is an introduction suggesting a symptom, comment on this, for example the patient's age, body habitus (if relevant) and whether he or she looks breathless or not.
- Describe any abnormal findings (e.g. the presence of scars and apex beat).
- Then describe the murmur, its loudness (out of 6), timing (systolic or diastolic), position of maximum intensity and character (e.g. ejection, pan systolic, early diastolic).

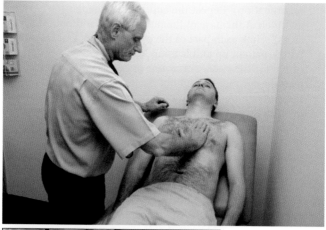

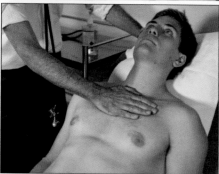

Figure 2.8.2 Palpating the base of the heart for palpable murmurs (thrills) — push firmly (Talley NJ, O'Connor S. *Talley & O'Connor's Clinical Examination Essentials: An introduction to clinical skills (and how to pass your clinical exams)*. Elsevier Australia, 2020.)

- Take a big breath and hazard a diagnosis and your impression of the severity of the lesion (mild, moderate or severe).
- Explain how you think this is consistent with the patient's symptoms as given to you in the introduction.
- Say what features made you decide on its severity or otherwise (e.g. a long early diastolic murmur and displaced apex beat suggest severe aortic regurgitation).
- Have a list in your mind of the most common causes.

Examiners' likely questions

- For junior medical students, examiners may only ask if the murmur is systolic or diastolic or both, and where it was loudest. They will ask if there were any associated signs such as thrills or heaves.
- For more senior students, they will want to know the likely diagnosis and a list of differentials. They may go on to ask:
  - What are the likely causes of this lesion?
  - What symptoms would suggest the lesion is severe?
  - What tests might be useful?
  - ECG and chest X-ray are usually first line, followed by echocardiography.

Marking criteria table		
Criteria	Satisfactory	Unsatisfactory
Introduces self, explains task, obtains consent, washes hands before and after	1	0
Makes a general inspection of the patient	1	0
Examines the praecordium for scars etc.	1	0
Feels for the apex beat	1	0
Feels for thrills and a parasternal impulse	2	0–1
Auscultates at apex and at the base of the heart	1	0
Detects a murmur	1	0
Is able to say whether it is systolic or diastolic	1	0

Pass mark: 5

Examine a body system (respiratory)

Background

The usual cases here are:
- chronic obstructive pulmonary disease (COPD)
- a pleural effusion
- interstitial lung disease (ILD)
- chronic productive cough (often bronchiectasis).

Introduction

This is likely to be 'Please examine this patient with dyspnoea' or 'with a cough'.

Rationale

This is another important and routine examination. You should know the main steps and be able to perform them elegantly.

Method

The examiners may direct you to the chest examination, but if not and if you are practised and quick, you should probably start (after your general inspection) with the hands. See Fig. 2.9.1.

1. Wash your hands.
2. Ask the patient to undress to the waist and sit over the side of the bed.
3. While standing back to make your usual inspection, ask whether sputum is available for you to look at. A large volume of purulent sputum is an important clue to

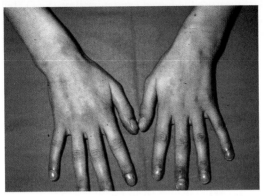

Figure 2.9.1 COPD peripheral cyanosis (Shiland BJ. *Medical Terminology & Anatomy for Coding.* Elsevier Inc., 2021.)

bronchiectasis. Haemoptysis suggests lung carcinoma or pulmonary infection.

4. Look for dyspnoea (the work of breathing appears to be increased) and count the respiratory rate. Note the use of the accessory muscles of respiration and any intercostal in-drawing of the lower ribs anteriorly (a sign of emphysema). General cachexia should also be noted.

5. Pick up the patient's hands. Note clubbing (see Table 2.6.1), peripheral cyanosis, nicotine (actually, tar) staining. Look for wasting of the small muscles of the hands and weakness of finger abduction (which may be caused by a lower trunk brachial plexus lesion from apical lung carcinoma involvement).

6. Go on to the face. Look closely at the eyes for ptosis and constriction of the pupils (Horner syndrome). Inspect the tongue for central cyanosis.

7. Estimate the respiratory rate. Generally a decision about whether it is normal or increased is enough. There is not usually enough time to count it.

8. Palpate the position of the trachea.

9. Ask the patient to cough and note whether this is a loose cough, a dry cough.

10. Next measure the forced expiratory time (FET). Tell the patient to take a maximal inspiration and blow out as rapidly and completely as possible. Note audible wheeze. Prolongation of expiration beyond 3 seconds is evidence of chronic airflow limitation.

T&O'C hint box

Always ask the patient to cough.

The next step is to examine the chest.

11. Inspect the back. Look for kyphoscoliosis (Fig. 2.9.2). Look for thoracotomy scars and prominent veins. Also note any skin changes from radiotherapy.
12. Palpate the cervical nodes from behind.

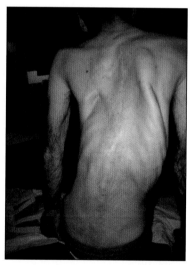

Figure 2.9.2 Very severe kyphosis and scoliosis spinal deformations at an adult age, causing major back pain and contributing to the onset of restrictive respiratory insufficiency (Laffont I, Tiffreau JM, Yelnik V, Herisson A, Pelissier C. Aging and sequelae of poliomyelitis. *Annals of Physical and Rehabilitation Medicine* 2009; 53(1):24–33.)

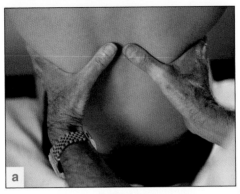

Expiration

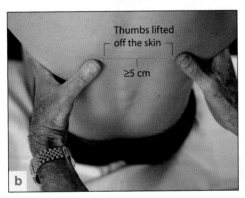

Thumbs lifted
off the skin
≥5 cm

Inspiration

Figure 2.9.3 Testing chest expansion: normal findings **(a)** 'Breathe right out.' **(b)** 'Breathe in as far as you can' (Talley NJ, O'Connor S. *Talley & O'Connor's Clinical Examination Essentials: An introduction to clinical skills (and how to pass your clinical exams)*. Elsevier Australia, 2020.)

13. Then examine for expansion (Fig. 2.9.3). First, upper lobe expansion is best seen by looking over the patient's shoulders at clavicular movement during moderate respiration. The affected side will show a delay or decreased movement. Then examine lower lobe expansion by palpation. Note asymmetry and reduction of movement.

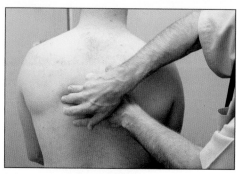

Figure 2.9.4 Percussing the back (Talley NJ, O'Connor S. *Talley & O'Connor's Clinical Examination Essentials: An introduction to clinical skills (and how to pass your clinical exams).* Elsevier Australia, 2020.)

14. Ask the patient to bring his elbows together in front of him to move the scapulae out of the way. Then percuss the back of the chest and include both axillae (Fig. 2.9.4). Do not miss a pleural effusion (stony dullness).

15. Auscultate the chest, remembering the list of things you are looking for is not exhaustive. Note breath sounds (whether bronchial or vesicular) and their intensity (normal or reduced). Listen for adventitial sounds (crackles and wheezes). See Fig. 2.9.5. The differential diagnosis depends on whether your findings are symmetrical or not, and comment on symmetry. You may rarely hear a pleural friction rub.

16. Return to the front of the chest. Inspect again for chest deformity, symmetry of chest wall movement, distended veins, radiotherapy changes and scars. Palpate the supraclavicular nodes carefully. Proceed with percussion and auscultation as before. Listen high up in the axillae too. Before leaving the chest, feel the axillary nodes and breasts.

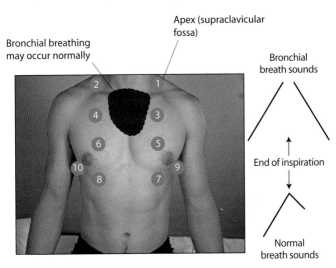

Figure 2.9.5 Where to auscultate, 1–10 (Talley NJ, O'Connor S. *Talley & O'Connor's Clinical Examination Essentials: An introduction to clinical skills (and how to pass your clinical exams).* Elsevier Australia, 2020.)

T&O'C hint box

If COPD seems likely, test for Hoover sign. Place your hands along the costal margins with your thumbs close to the xiphisternum. Normally inspiration causes your thumbs to separate, but the overinflated chest of the COPD patient cannot expand any further and so the diaphragm pulls the ribs and your thumbs closer together. See Fig. 2.9.6.

Present your findings

- Start with a general statement about the patient's breathlessness, cyanosis and comfort or otherwise.
- Outline the positive findings (e.g. clubbing and fine inspiratory crackles) and your differential diagnosis.

- Hazard an opinion about the severity. (In general, the more breathless the patient at rest or during manoeuvres required by the examination, the more severe the condition.)
- If the introduction mentioned a cough, describe the patient's cough (dry or loose) and what features you have found on examination to explain it, for example coarse (bronchiectasis) or fine (interstitial lung disease) crackles.

T&O'C hint box

Remember that the common respiratory OSCE cases are:
- idiopathic pulmonary fibrosis (dry cough, crackles and clubbing). The fine inspiratory crackles are loudest at the bases and very distinctive. The further up the chest they are audible, the more severe the disease
- bronchiectasis (loose cough, full sputum mug, coarse crackles and wheezes, clubbing)
- COPD (overinflated chest, possible cyanosis, pursed lips breathing, reduced breath sounds and wheezes, Hoover sign)
- pleural effusion (stony dullness, bronchial breathing on top, needle marks from previous aspirations)
- Investigations to ask for include:a chest X-ray:
- interstitial markings — interstitial lung disease, for example fibrosis
- overinflated chest — COPD
- thickened bronchi and tram tracking — bronchiectasis
- opacity at the base — pleural effusion
- mass — carcinoma or abscess
  It is unlikely you would be asked to read a CT scan, but knowing their indications is important: ILD, bronchiectasis, carcinoma.
  Know the basic spirometry findings for these conditions.

Examiners' likely questions

- What are the likely causes of this patient's cough (breathlessness)?
- What questions would you like to ask the patient?
  Have you been a smoker?
  How much phlegm do you cough up?
  What is your work? (occupational exposure to dust currently or in the past, etc.)

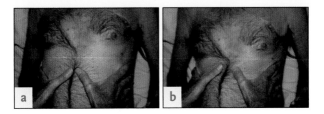

Figure 2.9.6 Testing for Hoover sign: **(a)** Hoover sign positive inspiration **(b)** Hoover sign positive expiration (Talley NJ, O'Connor S. *Talley & O'Connor's Clinical Examination Essentials: An introduction to clinical skills (and how to pass your clinical exams).* Elsevier Australia, 2020.)

What medications do you take? (angiotensin converting enzyme (ACE)-inhibitor cough, use of bronchodilators and antibiotics)

- What investigations might be helpful?
  Always ask for simple tests first — chest X-ray and spirometry (see Station 76) before CT scan.
- Be able to outline the likely information these tests will provide — see Figs 2.9.7–2.9.11.

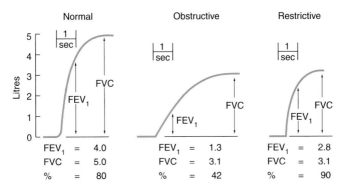

Figure 2.9.7 Spirometry tracings (Talley NJ, O'Connor S. *Talley and O'Connor's Clinical Examination.* Elsevier Australia, 2017.)

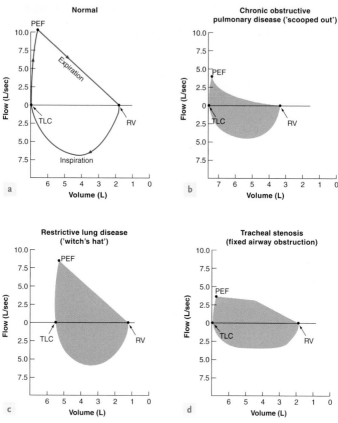

Figure 2.9.8 Flow volume curves. Look at the shape of the loop in each case **(a)–(d)**. A normal flow volume curve is convex and symmetrical. In COPD, all flow routes are reduced and there is prolonged expiration (creating a 'scooped out' shape). In restrictive lung disease (e.g. pulmonary fibrosis), the loop is narrow but the shape normal (like a witch's hat). In fixed airway obstruction (e.g. tracheal stenosis), the loops look flattened as both expiration and inspiration are limited. PEF = peak expiratory flow; TLC = total lung capacity; RV = residual volume (Talley NJ, O'Connor S. *Talley and O'Connor's Clinical Examination*. Elsevier Australia, 2017.)

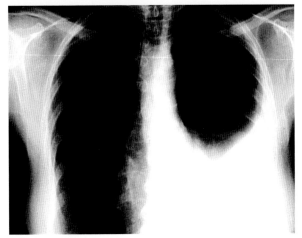

Figure 2.9.9 Pleural effusion. The upper margin of the effusion is curved ('meniscus sign'). The left hemidiaphragm is not seen because there is no adjacent aerated lung for contrast. The heart shows some deviation to the right. It is unlikely that this is caused by an effusion of this size; it is probably related to the lower thoracic scoliosis (Talley NJ, O'Connor S. *Talley and O'Connor's Clinical Examination*. Elsevier Australia, 2017.)

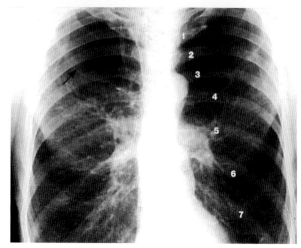

Figure 2.9.10 Emphysema. The lungs are overinflated with low, flat hemidiaphragms. The level of the hemidiaphragms is well below the anterior aspects of the sixth ribs. The diaphragm normally projects over the sixth rib anteriorly and the tenth intercostal space posteriorly. Count the ribs anteriorly (1–6). There is increased translucency of both upper zones with loss of the vascular markings due to bulla formation (arrow). This increased translucency is not due to overexposure. The hila are prominent because of the enlarged central pulmonary arteries. In contrast, the smaller peripheral pulmonary arteries (the lung markings) are decreased in size and number. This is due to actual destruction, displacement around bullae and decreased perfusion through emphysematous areas (Talley NJ, O'Connor S. *Talley and O'Connor's Clinical Examination*. Elsevier Australia, 2017.)

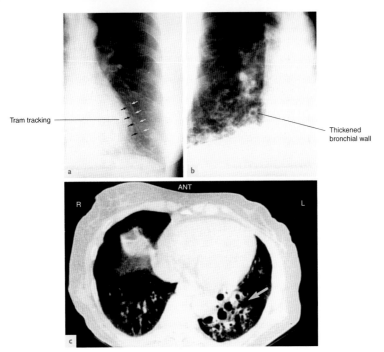

Tram tracking

Thickened bronchial wall

Figure 2.9.11 Bronchiectasis **(a)**, **(b)** X-ray **(c)** CT scan; arrow points to dilated bronchioles (Mettler FA. *Essentials of Radiology*. 2nd edn. Philadelphia: Saunders, 2005.)

Marking criteria table

Criteria	Satisfactory	Unsatisfactory
Introduces self, explains task, obtains consent, washes hands before and after	1	0
Makes a general inspection, asks patient to cough	2	0–1
Notes supplemental oxygen	1	0
Notes increased respiratory rate	1	0
Notes cyanosis	1	0
Notes over-expanded chest	1	0
Looks for peripheral signs of lung disease	2	0–1
Performs adequate chest examination front and back	3	0–2
Describes positive findings and important negatives	3	0–2
Hazards a differential diagnosis	2	0–1

Pass mark: 10
Note many OSCEs would break this type of case up into separate OSCEs.

Examine a body system (abdomen)

Background

If the station requires an abdominal examination, either it will be normal or you will likely find evidence of an enlarged organ, usually a liver and/or spleen.

Remember, while the common abnormalities in this examination are hepatomegaly, often with splenomegaly in cirrhosis with portal hypertension (in which case you should also find other signs of chronic liver disease such as ascites), you may also be shown a case of polycystic kidneys (associated with hypertension but not signs of chronic liver disease). The differential diagnosis of hepatosplenomegaly includes haematological malignancy.

Introduction

The introduction can include a number of scenarios, such as:

- This man has noticed abdominal distension. Please examine him.
- This woman has become jaundiced. Please examine her.
- This man has been found to have an abdominal mass. Please examine him.

Rationale

Although the gastrointestinal system is less important than the heart and probably than the lungs, students are expected to know how to perform a competent examination and find important signs. See Figs 2.10.1 and 2.10.2.

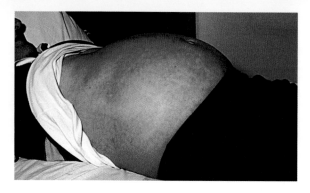

Figure 2.10.1 Abdomen distended with ascites (patient supine): umbilicus points downwards, unlike in cases of distension due to a pelvic mass (Courtesy of Dr A Watson, Infectious Diseases Department, The Canberra Hospital.)

Method

1. Wash your hands.
2. Position the patient correctly, with one pillow for the head and complete exposure of the abdomen.
3. Briefly look at the patient's general appearance and inspect particularly for signs of chronic liver disease (jaundice, wasting, scratch marks, confusion) and less commonly renal disease (sallow appearance, scratch marks, fistula in arm or dialysis catheter in abdomen).
4. Inspect the abdomen from the side, squatting to the patient's level. Large masses may be visible. Ask the patient to take slow, deep breaths — an enlarged liver or spleen may be seen to move downwards during inspiration. Stand up and look for scars, distension, prominent veins, striae, bruising and pigmentation.
5. Ask first whether any particular area is tender (to avoid causing pain and also to obtain a clue to the site of possible pathology).

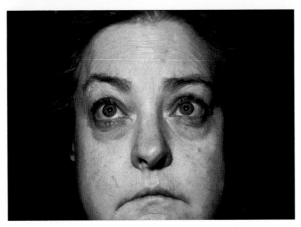

Figure 2.10.2 Scleral icterus (jaundice) (Talley NJ, O'Connor S. *Talley and O'Connor's Clinical Examination*. Elsevier Australia, 2017.)

6. Palpate lightly in each quadrant. Spend time assessing the abdomen intelligently for localised tenderness and any masses. Do *not* hurt the patient (if you want to pass; actually, don't hurt him or her regardless) — watch the patient's face and be gentle.

7. Next palpate more deeply in each quadrant and then feel specifically for hepatomegaly and splenomegaly.
   - A palpable liver may be a result of enlargement or ptosis. If there is hepatomegaly, confirm with percussion and estimate the span (normal span is approximately 12.5 cm).
   - The same procedure is followed for splenomegaly (use a two-handed technique). Percussion is useful to exclude splenomegaly (over the lowest intercostal space in the left anterior axillary line; if dull in full inspiration, suspect splenomegaly and palpate again). Always roll the patient on to the right side and palpate again if no spleen is palpable. Be seen to watch the patient's face intermittently for signs that the examination is uncomfortable.

8. Carefully feel for the kidneys bimanually. Remember that any left-sided mass may arise from a number of sites.

9. Percuss for ascites as a routine. If the abdomen is resonant out to the flanks on percussion, do not bother to roll the patient over (as you can't assess shifting dullness — there isn't any!). Otherwise, look for shifting dullness. The technique is usually performed by percussing away from your side of the bed until you reach a dull note, then rolling the patient towards you and waiting at least a short time before percussing again for resonance.

10. If you have time, auscultate briefly over the liver, spleen and renal areas. Listen for bruits, rubs and a venous hum. Note the presence of bowel sounds. An arterial systolic bruit over the liver is usually caused by either hepatocellular carcinoma or acute alcoholic hepatitis. A friction rub audible over the liver may be caused by tumour or recent liver biopsy; splenic rubs indicate infarction. Auscultation is less useful than palpation in the abdominal examination.

If there is still time:

T&O'C hint box

The usual distinguishing features of a spleen compared with a kidney are as follows.
1. The spleen has no palpable upper border. (You can't get above it.)
2. The spleen has a notch.
3. The spleen moves inferomedially on respiration.
4. There is usually no resonance over an enlarged spleen whereas the kidney can be resonant due to overlying bowel.
5. The spleen is not bimanually palpable (i.e. not ballottable).
6. A friction rub may occasionally be heard over the spleen.

---

11. Palpate anteriorly for supraclavicular nodes, then sit the patient forwards and feel posteriorly for the other cervical nodes. Look at the back for sacral oedema and spider naevi.

12. Look at the face next. Note any scleral abnormality (jaundice, anaemia). Xanthelasma are may be seen in patients with advanced primary biliary cirrhosis (rare).

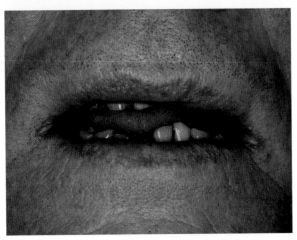

Figure 2.10.3 Angular stomatitis (Sproat C, Burke G, McGurk M. *Essential Human Disease for Dentists.* London: Churchill Livingstone, 2006.)

Inspect the mouth with a torch and spatula for angular stomatitis (Fig. 2.10.3), ulceration (Fig. 2.10.4) and atrophic glossitis. Smell the breath for fetor hepaticus.

13. Look at the arms for bruising and spider naevi, signs of chronic liver disease. Next examine the hands. Ask the patient to extend his arms and hands and look for evidence of hepatic flap. Look also at the nails for clubbing and white nails (leukonychia) and note any palmar erythema and Dupuytren contractures (the latter are associated with alcohol or trauma, or familial) (Fig. 2.10.5).

Present your findings

- Try to connect the physical abnormalities with the introduction. After a general statement about the patient such as:

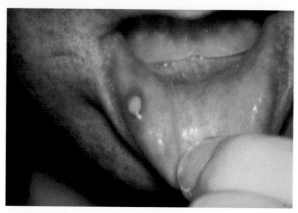

Figure 2.10.4 Aphthous ulcer (McDonald FS (Ed.). *Mayo Clinic Images in Internal Medicine*, with permission. © Mayo Clinic Scientic Press and CRC Press. Reproduced by permission of Taylor and Francis Group, LLC, a division of Informa plc.)

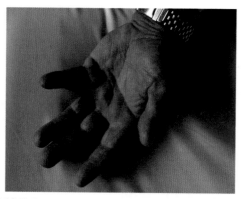

Figure 2.10.5 Dupuytren contracture of the hand (Talley NJ, O'Connor S. *Talley & O'Connor's Examination Medicine*. Elsevier Australia, 2020.)

'Thanks for asking me to examine this man who has presented with an abdominal mass. He is an overweight middle-aged man who looks jaundiced.'

- Outline your findings, starting with those related to the introduction.

'He has an enlarged liver which extends 4 cm below the costal margin.'

- Go on then to describe what you have found and what important abnormalities are not present.

Examiners' likely questions

The examiners' questions will be directed at using your findings to make a differential diagnosis and there may be time for them to ask what investigations would be helpful.

- If there are abdominal masses, is this hepatosplenomegaly or polycystic kidney disease?
- If there is hepatosplenomegaly, are there signs of portal hypertension or peripheral stigmata of chronic liver disease?
- Are there enlarged lymph nodes, suggesting a haematological cause or other malignancy?

Consider the important causes of hepatomegaly and of hepatosplenomegaly and the characteristic features (Boxes 2.10.1, 2.10.2).

If there is time you may be asked about appropriate investigations (Box 2.10.3).

Box 2.10.1
Hepatomegaly

Massive
- Metastases
- Alcoholic liver disease with fatty infiltration
- Myeloproliferative disease
- Right heart failure
- Hepatocellular carcinoma

Moderate
- The above causes
- Haemochromatosis
- Haematological disease — chronic myeloid leukaemia, lymphoma
- Fatty liver — obesity, diabetes mellitus

Mild
- The above causes
- Hepatitis (viral, drugs)
- Cirrhosis
- Biliary obstruction

Firm and irregular liver
- Cirrhosis
- Metastatic disease

Tender liver
- Hepatitis
- Rapid liver enlargement — right heart failure, Budd–Chiari syndrome
- Hepatocellular carcinoma

Pulsatile liver
- Tricuspid regurgitation
- Hepatocellular carcinoma
- Vascular abnormalities

Box 2.10.2
Common causes of hepatosplenomegaly

Chronic liver disease with portal hypertension
Haematological disease
- myeloproliferative disease
- lymphoma
- leukaemia

Infection
- acute viral hepatitis
- glandular fever
- cytomegalovirus infection

Box 2.10.3
Investigations

For probable liver disease
- Liver function tests (including coagulation studies)
- Abdominal ultrasound
- Abdominal CT scan

For polycystic kidney disease
- Abdominal ultrasound
- Renal function tests (creatinine, eGFR, urinalysis for proteinuria)
- Possible CT scan to search for cerebral aneurysms

For haematological disease
- Full blood count
- Abdominal ultrasound
- Bone marrow aspiration

Marking criteria table for gastrointestinal system examination of a patient with cirrhosis

Criteria	Satisfactory	Unsatisfactory
Introduces self, explains task, obtains consent, washes hands before and after	1	0
Makes a general inspection	1	0
Examines the abdomen competently: inspection, palpation, percussion, auscultation	4	0–3
Identifies an enlarged liver	1	0
Identifies an enlarged spleen	1	0
Correctly identifies no ascites	1	0
Examines for the peripheral signs of gastrointestinal disease: hands and arms	2	0–1
Can provide a differential diagnosis not based on fantasy	2	0–1
Can suggest sensible investigations	3	0–2

Pass mark: 10

Examine a body system (upper cranial nerves)

Background

To examine the cranial nerves, you need to remember the basic anatomy and have mastered the specific tests for each nerve. Practice makes perfect in neurology.

Introduction

In junior years, students may be asked to examine a person without abnormal cranial nerves so that they can demonstrate the routine of this examination. In senior years, a patient with abnormalities is more likely to be seen.

Common introductions to upper cranial nerve (II, III, IV, and VI) OSCEs include:

- This man has had problems with diplopia. Please examine his eyes. (Suggests III, IV, VI cranial nerve abnormality or ocular myopathy)
- This man has had some loss of vision. Please examine his eyes. (Suggests retinal or optic disc problem or field loss)

Rationale

This is a difficult examination. The examiners expect a systematic approach (or systematic attempt) during the examination and the detection of gross changes. The OSCE is often even more targeted, for example 'Examine this man's eye movements', 'Examine the fundi' (in a patient with dilated pupils), 'Look at the pupils and comment on the abnormalities'. Junior students will only be expected to have an idea of what is involved in cranial nerve examination. More senior students may be asked to have a go at the diagnosis and differential diagnosis.

Method

Have the patient sit over the edge of the bed facing you and look for:

- any craniotomy scars (often well disguised by hair)
- skin lesions that may give clues, for example neurofibromata (Fig. 2.11.1).
- acromegaly features (pituitary adenoma)
- facial asymmetry
- obvious ptosis, proptosis, skew deviation of the eyes or pupil inequality
- characteristic facies of myasthenia gravis (bilateral ptosis) (Fig. 2.11.2) or myotonic dystrophy (frontal balding, triangular facies).

SECOND (OPTIC) NERVE

- Test visual acuity (with the patient's spectacles on, because refractive errors are not cranial nerve abnormalities) using a visual acuity chart.
- Test each eye separately, covering the other eye with a small card.
- Examine the visual fields by confrontation using a red-tipped hat-pin, making sure your head is level with the patient's head. Explain before each step what it is you want the patient to do. Test each eye separately. If the patient has such poor acuity that a hat-pin is difficult to use, map the fields with your fingers. When you are testing the patient's right eye, he or she should look straight into your left eye. The patient's head should be at arm's length and he or she should cover the eye not being tested with a hand. Bring the hat-pin from the four main directions diagonally towards the centre of the field of vision.
- Next, map out the blind spot by asking about disappearance of the hat-pin lateral to the centre of the field of vision of each eye. Only a gross enlargement may be detectable by comparison with your own blind spot.
- Consult your memory of Fig. 2.11.3 and Box 2.11.1 to work out the defect and the nature of the lesion.

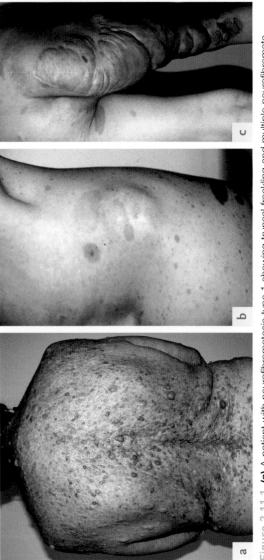

Figure 2.11.1 **(a)** A patient with neurofibromatosis type 1 showing truncal freckling and multiple neurofibromata. **(b)** Café-au-lait spots on the chest of a child, axillary freckling and a subcutaneous plexiform neurofibroma below and lateral to the left nipple. **(c)** A large and unsightly plexiform neurofibroma affecting the right buttock and leg (Ellard S, Cleaver R, Turnpenny PD. *Emery's Elements of Medical Genetics and Genomics*, 16th edn. Elsevier, 2020.)

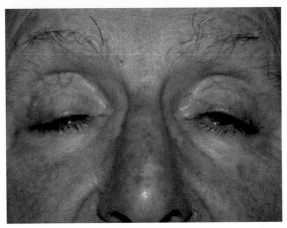

Figure 2.11.2 Myasthenia gravis patient with bilateral ptosis (Liu GT, Volpe NJ, Galetta SL. *Neuro-ophthalmology: Diagnosis and management*, 2nd edn. Elsevier, 2010.)

1. Tunnel vision: concentric diminution (e.g. glaucoma, papilloedema)	◐ ◑
2. Enlarged blind spot: optic nerve head enlargement	◌ ◌
3. Central scotomata: optic nerve head to chiasmal lesion (e.g. demyelination, toxic, vascular, nutritional)	◌ ◐
4. Unilateral field loss: optic nerve lesion (e.g. vascular, tumour)	● ◌
5. Bitemporal hemianopia: optic chiasma lesion (e.g. pituitary tumour, sella meningioma)	◐ ◑
6. Homonymous hemianopia: optic tract to occipital cortex, lesion at any point (e.g. vascular, tumour). *Note:* Incomplete lesion results in macular (central) vision sparing	◐ ◐
7. Upper quadrant homonymous hemianopia: temporal lobe lesion (e.g. vascular, tumour)	◓ ◓
8. Lower quadrant homonymous hemianopia: parietal lobe lesion	◒ ◒

Figure 2.11.3 Visual field defects associated with lesions of the visual system (Talley NJ, O'Connor S. *Talley and O'Connor's Examination Medicine*. Elsevier Australia, 2020.)

Box 2.11.1
How to analyse your findings

Pupil abnormalities

Causes of constriction
- Horner syndrome (Box 2.11.3)
- Argyll Robertson pupil
- Pontine lesion (often bilateral, but reactive to light)
- Narcotics
- Pilocarpine drops
- Old age

Causes of dilatation
- Mydriatics, atropine poisoning or cocaine
- Third nerve lesion
- Adie pupil (subtle slow reaction to accommodation and a more pronounced impaired direct and consensual reaction to light. It is due to a lesion in the efferent parasympathetic pathway.)
- Iridectomy, lens implant, iritis
- Post-trauma, deep coma, cerebral death
- Congenital

Visual field defects
Have ready a mental list of the common causes of the abnormalities shown in Fig. 2.11.3.

Causes of papilloedema
- Space-occupying lesion (causing raised intracranial pressure) or a retro-orbital mass
- Benign intracranial hypertension (pseudotumour cerebri, associated with small ventricles):
  - idiopathic
  - contraceptive pill
  - Addison disease
  - drugs — nitrofurantoin, tetracycline, vitamin A, steroids
  - head trauma
- Hypertension (grade IV)
- Central retinal vein thrombosis

Causes of optic atrophy
- Chronic papilloedema or optic neuritis
- Optic nerve pressure or division
- Glaucoma
- Ischaemia

Causes of cataract
- Old age (senile cataract)

Box 2.11.1
How to analyse your findings *continued*

- Endocrine — diabetes mellitus, steroids
- Hereditary or congenital — dystrophia myotonica, Refsum disease
- Ocular disease — glaucoma
- Irradiation
- Trauma

Causes of ptosis

With normal pupils
- senile ptosis (common)
- myotonic dystrophy
- thyrotoxic myopathy
- myasthenia gravis
- fatigue.

With constricted pupils
- Horner syndrome

With dilated pupils
- third nerve lesion

- Look into the fundi. Students will be expected to detect gross changes. In this case, optic atrophy (Fig. 2.11.4) or hypertensive or diabetic changes are the most likely findings.

THIRD (OCULOMOTOR), FOURTH (TROCHLEAR) AND SIXTH (ABDUCENS) NERVES

- Look at the pupils. Note the shape, relative sizes and any associated ptosis. Use your pocket torch and shine the light from the side to gauge the reaction to light on both sides. Practise assessing the direct (contraction of pupil into which light is shone) and consensual (reaction of other pupil) responses rapidly.
- Look for the Marcus Gunn phenomenon (afferent pupillary defect). Tell the patient 'I am going to test your pupils. Please look into the distance (at an object).' Move the torch from the side (about 45°), close to the patient quickly in an arc, below the line of site, from pupil to pupil. The affected

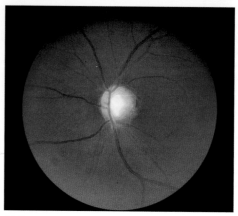

Figure 2.11.4 Diffuse optic atrophy in a 41-year-old woman with neuromyelitis optica after a severe attack that left her with no light perception (Talley NJ, O'Connor S. *Talley and O'Connor's Examination Medicine*. Elsevier Australia, 2020.)

pupil will paradoxically dilate after a short time when the torch is moved from a normal eye to one with optic atrophy or decreased visual acuity from other causes. The test will be abnormal even when visual loss is relatively mild.

- Test accommodation by asking the patient to look into the distance and then at your red hat-pin placed about 15 cm from his or her nose.
- Assess eye movements with both eyes first (Fig 2.11.5). Ask the patient to look voluntarily and quickly from left to right and then to follow the red hat-pin in each direction — right and left lateral gaze, plus up and down in the central position. Look for failure of movement and nystagmus.
- Ask about diplopia (double vision) when the eyes are in each position. For complex lesions, assess each eye separately. Move the patient's head if he or she is unable to follow movements. Beware of strabismus.

T&O'C hint box

Subtle nystagmus is normal at the extremes of gaze (Box 2.11.2.)

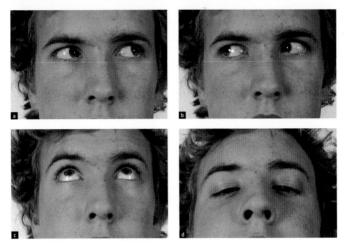

Figure 2.11.5 Cranial nerves III, IV and VI: Normal voluntary eye movements. **(a)** 'Look to the left.' **(b)** 'Look to the right.' **(c)** 'Look up.' **(d)** 'Look down' (Talley NJ, O'Connor S. *Clinical Examination: A systematic guide to physical diagnosis.* Elsevier Australia, 2018.)

T&O'C hint box

Upward gaze is normally limited in elderly patients.

Box 2.11.2
Causes of nystagmus

Horizontal:
- Vestibular lesion (Note: chronic lesions cause nystagmus to the side of the lesion — fast component.)
- Cerebellar lesion (Note: unilateral disease causes nystagmus to the side of the lesion.)

Vertical:
- Brain stem lesion
- Toxic, e.g. alcohol

THIRD (OCULOMOTOR) NERVE

Clinical features of a third nerve palsy

- Complete ptosis (partial ptosis may occur with an incomplete lesion)

- Divergent strabismus (eye 'down and out')
- Dilated pupil unreactive to direct or consensual light and unreactive to accommodation if the parasympathetic fibres that surround the third cranial nerve are damaged. Remember that your sympathetic nerve supply to the eye comes from the sympathetic chain surrounding the carotid artery.

Aetiology
Central
- Vascular (e.g. brain stem infarction)
- Tumour
- Trauma

Peripheral
- Compressive lesions:
    - aneurysm (usually on the posterior communicating artery)
    - tumour causing raised intracranial pressure (dilated pupil occurs early)
    - nasopharyngeal carcinoma
- Infarction — diabetes mellitus, arteritis (pupil is usually spared)
- Trauma

SIXTH (ABDUCENS) NERVE

Clinical features of a sixth nerve palsy
- Failure of lateral movement
- Affected eye is deviated inwards in severe lesions
- Diplopia — maximal on looking to the affected side; the images are horizontal and parallel to each other; the outermost image is from the affected eye and disappears on covering this eye (this image is also usually more blurred).

Aetiology
Bilateral
- Trauma (head injury)
- Raised intracranial pressure as the sixth cranial nerve has the longest intracranial path and therefore is most vulnerable to pressure damage

- Mononeuritis multiplex

Unilateral

Central
- Vascular
- Tumour
- Wernicke encephalopathy

Peripheral
- Diabetes, other vascular lesions
- Trauma
- Raised intracranial pressure

Box 2.11.3
Examination for Horner syndrome

If you suspect Horner syndrome because the pupils are unequal, or there is unilateral ptosis, examine as follows
1. Test for a difference in sweating over each brow with the back of your finger (even though your brow is usually sweatier than the patient's); this occurs only when the lesion is proximal to the carotid bifurcation. Absence of sweating differences does not exclude the diagnosis of Horner syndrome.
2. Ask the patient to speak and note any hoarseness (which may be caused by recurrent laryngeal nerve palsy from a chest lesion or a cranial nerve lesion).
3. Look at the hands for clubbing. Test finger abduction to screen for a lower trunk brachial plexus (C8, T1) lesion.
4. If there are signs of hoarseness or a lower trunk brachial plexus lesion, consider a carcinoma of the lung.
5. Examine the neck for lymphadenopathy.
    When asked, remember the common causes (Box 2.11.4).

Box 2.11.4
Common causes of Horner syndrome

Carcinoma of the lung apex (usually squamous cell carcinoma)
Neck — thyroid malignancy, trauma
Carotid arterial lesion — carotid aneurysm or dissection
Brain stem lesion — vascular disease, tumour
Retro-orbital lesion

Present your findings

- Perhaps begin by saying which cranial nerves were abnormal or if you felt the problem was something else, for example a myopathy.
- Were the changes unilateral or bilateral, sensory or motor or both?
- If you can, hazard a differential diagnosis.

Examiners' likely questions

They will probably begin by asking you to repeat your positive findings and explain how these fit with the relevant cranial nerves.

- What possible causes are there for these changes?
  - Consult the various lists above but try to mention only the more likely possibilities.

Marking criteria table

Criteria	Satisfactory	Unsatisfactory
Introduces self, explains task, obtains consent, washes hands	1	0
Appears to have performed the examination before	1	0
Inspects for unequal pupils, scars, ptosis etc.	3	0–2
Confines examination to nerves II, III, IV, VI	1	0
Tests acuity	2	0–1
Tests eye movements	2	0–1
Tests visual fields correctly	2	0–1
Asks to examine the fundi	1	0
Is able to say which nerves are responsible for which eye movements	1	0
Presents findings coherently	1	0
Has a go at differential diagnosis (senior students)	1	0

Pass mark = 9 (junior student) or 10 (senior student)

Examine a body system (lower cranial nerves)

Background

Remember to refresh your knowledge of the anatomy. Facial nerve palsy is one of the most common abnormalities. Remember the difference between upper versus lower motor neuron findings as discussed below.

Introduction

- This man has noticed numbness in the face. Please examine his cranial nerves, starting with the 5th.
- This woman has noticed some facial asymmetry. Please examine her cranial nerves.
- This man has had difficulty with his speech. Please examine him. (Consider dysarthria — lower cranial nerve lesion, cerebellar speech, dysphasia from a stroke.)

  Doing it all would make this too long an OSCE unless all is normal. If abnormalities are actually present (usually for more senior students) you are more likely to be directed to a particular nerve or group.

  The sixth nerve is not included in this assessment.

Rationale

Here again a systematic examination and ability to detect fairly gross changes is expected. It will be obvious to the examiners which students have practised this examination and which ones have not (Box 2.12.1).

Box 2.12.1
Facts about the lower cranial nerves to have ready for the examiners

Fifth (trigeminal) nerve palsy

Aetiology
- Central (pons, medulla and upper cervical cord)
  - Vascular
  - Tumour
  - Multiple sclerosis
  - Peripheral (posterior fossa)
  - Aneurysm
  - Tumour
- Trigeminal ganglion (petrous temporal bone)
  - Meningioma
  - Fracture of the middle fossa
- Cavernous sinus (associated third, fourth and sixth nerve palsies)
  - Aneurysm
  - Thrombosis
  - Tumour

Seventh (facial) nerve palsy

Aetiology
Know the difference between an upper versus lower motor neuron lesion.
- Upper motor neuron lesion (supranuclear)
  - Vascular
  - Tumour
- Lower motor neuron lesion
1. Pontine (often associated with nerves V, VI)
   - Vascular
   - Tumour
   - Multiple sclerosis
2. Posterior fossa
   - Tumour
3. Petrous temporal bone
   - Bell palsy
   - Ramsay Hunt syndrome
   - Otitis media
   - Fracture
4. Parotid
   - Tumour
   - Sarcoidosis

Box 2.12.1
Facts about the lower cranial nerves to have ready for the examiners   *continued*

Eighth (acoustic) nerve

Causes of deafness
- Nerve (sensorineural) deafness
  - Degeneration (e.g. presbycusis)
  - Trauma (e.g. high noise exposure, fracture of the petrous temporal bone)
  - Toxic (e.g. aspirin, alcohol, streptomycin)
  - Infection (e.g. congenital rubella syndrome)
  - Tumour
  - Brain stem lesions
  - Vascular disease of the internal auditory artery
- Conductive deafness
  - Wax
  - Otitis media
  - Otosclerosis
  - Paget disease of bone

Ninth (glossopharyngeal) and tenth (vagus) nerve palsy

Aetiology
- Central
  - Vascular (e.g. lateral medullary infarction owing to vertebral or posterior inferior cerebellar artery disease)
  - Tumour
  - Motor neuron disease (vagus nerve only)
- Peripheral — posterior fossa
  - Aneurysm
  - Tumour
  - Chronic meningitis
  - Guillain-Barré syndrome (vagus nerve only)

Twelfth (hypoglossal) nerve palsy

Aetiology
- Upper motor neuron lesion
- Vascular
- Motor neuron disease
- Tumour
- Multiple sclerosis

Causes of multiple cranial nerve palsies
First establish that you are not dealing with a myopathy: the combined presence of ptosis along with weakness of the jaw, facial,

continued

Box 2.12.1
Facts about the lower cranial nerves to have ready for the examiners *continued*

pharyngeal and tongue muscles in the absence of sensory signs is likely due to a myopathy rather than a combined III, V, VII and IX to XII nerve palsies.

Causes to consider
- Chronic meningitis (e.g. carcinoma, tuberculosis, and sarcoidosis)
- Guillain-Barré Miller-Fisher variant syndrome (spares nerves I, II and VIII)
- Brain stem lesions — these are usually as a result of vascular disease causing crossed sensory or motor paralysis (i.e. cranial nerve signs on one side and contralateral long tract signs); patients with brain stem gliomas may have similar signs and may live for many years
- Trauma
- Lesion of the base of the skull (e.g. Paget disease, large meningioma, metastasis)
- Rarely, mononeuritis multiplex (e.g. diabetes mellitus)

Method

FIFTH (TRIGEMINAL) NERVE

Common introduction: 'The patient has noticed numbness in his face. Please examine the cranial nerves.'

1. Inspect for obvious abnormalities, for example a herpes zoster rash.

T&O'C hint box

Corneal reflex: when there is an ipsilateral seventh nerve palsy, only the contralateral eye will blink — sensation is preserved (nerve VII is the motor component).

2. Test facial sensation in the three divisions (fifth nerve): ophthalmic, maxillary and mandibular. Use a pin first to assess pain. Map out any area of sensory loss from dull to sharp and check for any loss on the posterior part of the head (C2) and neck (C3). Light touch must be tested also, as there may be some sensory dissociation.

3. Examine the motor division by asking the patient to clench his or her teeth (feeling the masseter muscles) and open the mouth; the pterygoid muscles will not allow you to force it closed if the nerve is intact. A unilateral lesion causes the jaw to deviate towards the weak (affected) side.

4. Ask permission to test the corneal reflexes (this may not be given but know how to!). Make sure you touch the cornea (not the conjunctiva) gently with a piece of cotton wool. Come in from the side and do this only once on each side. If the nerve pathways are intact, the patient will blink both eyes. Ask whether he or she can actually feel the touch (the fifth cranial nerve is the sensory component; the motor component is innervated by the seventh nerve).

5. Test the jaw jerk (with the mouth just open, the finger over the jaw is tapped with a tendon hammer). An increased jaw jerk occurs in pseudobulbar palsy.

SEVENTH NERVE

Common introduction: 'The patient has noticed weakness in his face. Please examine the cranial nerves.'

1. Look for facial asymmetry and then test the muscles of facial expression. Ask the patient to look up and wrinkle the forehead. Look for loss of wrinkling and feel the muscle strength by pushing down on each side. This is preserved in an upper motor neuron lesion because of the bilateral cortical representation of these muscles.

2. Next ask the patient to tightly shut the eyes — compare how deeply the eyelashes are buried on the two sides and then try to open each eye. Ask the patient to grin and compare the nasolabial grooves.

3. If a lower motor neuron lesion is detected, quickly check for ear and palatal vesicles of herpes zoster of the geniculate ganglion — the Ramsay Hunt syndrome. Examining for taste on the anterior two-thirds of the tongue is not required.

EIGHTH NERVE

Common introduction: 'This woman has noticed some hearing loss. Please examine her cranial nerves.'

1. Whisper a number softly about 0.5 m away from each ear and ask the patient to repeat the number.

2. Perform Rinne and Weber tests with a 256 Hz tuning fork.
3. If indicated, ask for an auriscope (wax is the most common cause of conductive deafness).

NINTH AND TENTH NERVES

Common introduction: 'This man has noticed a hoarse voice. Please examine his lower cranial nerves.'

- Look at the palate and note any uvular displacement. Ask the patient to say 'aaah' and look for asymmetrical movement of the soft palate. With a unilateral tenth nerve lesion, the uvula is drawn towards the unaffected (normal) side.
- Testing the gag reflex is traditional but adds little to the examination. If the palate moves normally and the patient can feel the spatula, the same information is obtained (the ninth nerve is the sensory component and the tenth nerve the motor component): touch the back of the pharynx on each side. Remember to ask the patient whether he or she feels the spatula each time. You may not attain top marks if the patient vomits all over the examiners. If the spatula is used correctly, the patient will gag only if the reflex is hyperactive.
- Ask the patient to speak (to assess hoarseness) and to cough (listen for a bovine cough, which may occur with a recurrent laryngeal nerve lesion).

ELEVENTH NERVE

Common introduction: 'This woman has noticed some muscle wasting in her neck. Please examine her.'

1. Ask the patient to shrug the shoulders and then feel the trapezius bulk and push the shoulders down.
2. Then instruct the patient to turn his or her head against resistance (your hand) and also feel the muscle bulk of the sternomastoids for sternocleidomastoid wasting.

TWELFTH NERVE

Common introduction: 'This woman has had some difficulty with speech and swallowing. Please examine her lower cranial nerves and tongue.'

- As instructed, examine the lower cranial nerves systematically.

- While examining the mouth, inspect the tongue for wasting and fasciculation (best seen with the tongue not protruded; it may be unilateral or bilateral).

T&O'C hint box

Take time to inspect the tongue. Fasciculations and wasting are easily missed but are very important in the diagnosis of a lower motor neuron twelfth nerve palsy.

Present your findings

- As with the upper cranial nerves, perhaps begin by saying which cranial nerves were abnormal or if you felt the problem was something else, for example a myopathy.
- Were the changes unilateral or bilateral, sensory or motor or both?
- If you can, hazard a differential diagnosis.

Examiners' likely questions

- Can you summarise for us your positive findings?
    - Don't be alarmed; this question is to help you clarify your findings, not an indication that you have everything wrong.
- Do you think this is a cranial nerve problem or something else?
    - Consider myopathy.
- What tests might help?
    - If there is time to discuss investigations, a CT scan or MRI is the usual way of looking for the causes of cranial nerve abnormalities. You would not be expected to read these unless there was a very obvious abnormality. Specific tests, for example for myasthenia gravis, may be relevant.

Marking criteria table

Criteria	Satisfactory	Unsatisfactory
Introduces self, explains task, obtains consent, washes hands	1	0
Makes a general inspection	1	0
Examines the correct cranial nerves	1	0
Asks to perform corneal reflex	1	0
Fifth nerve sensory	1	0
Fifth nerve motor	1	0
Seventh nerve: tests the muscles of facial expression	1	0
Tests hearing, Weber and Rinne tests	2	0–1
Tests nerves nine and ten; asks before testing gag reflex, warns patient	3	0–2
Tests eleventh nerve	1	0
Tests twelfth nerve	1	0
Summarises findings	1	0

Pass mark: 8

Examine a body system (arms neurologically)

Background

Patients can present with neurological findings in the upper limb. It carries a broad differential which can be grouped into central or peripheral cause. Central causes include a cerebral vascular accident or cerebral mass (benign, malignant or infection), multiple sclerosis and spinal cord lesion. A peripheral cause can be a result of a plexus injury, a peripheral nerve or myotome. The neurological examination allows you to systematically examine and sort through your differential diagnosis.

Introduction

The introduction will often make it clear that this is a neurological rather than a rheumatological case.

Common introductions include:

- This man has noticed weakness in his arms. Please examine him.
- This woman has had difficulty combing her hair. Please examine her upper limbs neurologically.

Rationale

The examiners expect students to be able to perform a neurological examination of the upper limbs. You must be able to assess for weakness and distinguish upper and lower motor neuron signs. Types of sensory changes (usually quite gross) must be distinguished from each other; for example, peripheral neuropathy, peripheral nerve or nerve root or occasionally cortical. The examiners will soon know if you have been practising. As with most parts of the neurological examination, junior students will be often expected to demonstrate the examination in a normal person and expected to havea grasp of the general technique. Later on, real patients with neurological abnormalities (usually not subtle) are likely to be presented in the station.

Method

As always stand back and look at the whole patient briefly. Note particularly evidence of a myopathic face, Parkinsonian features or flexion of the elbow on one side, suggesting an upper motor neuron lesion and probable stroke.

MOTOR SYSTEM

Inspect first for wasting (both proximally and distally) and fasciculations. Do not forget to include the shoulder girdle in your inspection.

1. Ask the patient to hold both his hands out with the arms extended and close his eyes.
2. Look for drifting of one or both arms. There are only three causes for this drift:
   - upper motor neuron weakness (usually downwards owing to muscle weakness)
   - cerebellar lesion (usually upwards owing to hypotonia)
   - posterior column loss (any direction, owing to joint position sense loss).
3. Look for any tremor.
4. Feel the muscle bulk next, both proximally and distally, and note any muscle tenderness. In the presence of wasting (Fig. 2.13.1 and Fig. 2.13.2) and weakness, fasciculation indicates lower motor neuron degeneration.
5. Test tone at the wrists and elbows by moving the joints at varying velocities.
6. Assess and grade the power (Boxes 2.13.1, 2.13.2).
7. Test for an ulnar lesion (loss of finger abduction and adduction) and a median nerve lesion (loss of thumb abduction.
8. Examine the reflexes:
   - biceps (C5, C6) — biceps muscle
   - triceps (C7, C8) — triceps muscle

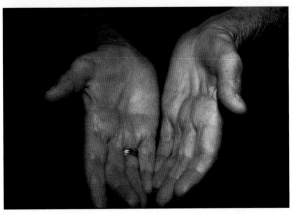

Figure 2.13.1 Wasting of the small muscles of the hand (Talley NJ, O'Connor S. *Talley and O'Connor's Clinical Examination*. Elsevier Australia, 2017.)

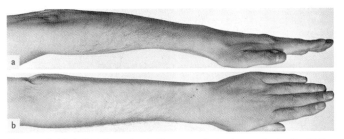

Figure 2.13.2 Distal wasting in the upper limbs in a patient with DM1 muscular dystrophy (Miller DC, Lane RJM, Hochberg FH, Perkin GD, Patel MC. *Atlas of Clinical Neurology*, 3rd edn. Elsevier Inc., 2010.)

Box 2.13.1
Assessing power

Shoulder
- Abduction (C5, C6): tell the patient to abduct the arm with the elbow flexed and not to let you push it down.
- Adduction (C6–C8): tell the patient to adduct the arm with the elbow flexed and not to let you push it up.

Elbow
- Flexion (C5, C6): tell the patient to bend the elbow and pull so as not to let you straighten it.
- Extension (C7, C8): tell the patient to bend the elbow and push so as not to let you bend it.

Wrist
- Flexion (C6, C7): tell the patient to bend the wrist and not to let you straighten it.
- Extension (C7, C8): tell the patient to straighten the wrist and not to let you bend it.

Fingers
- Extension (C7, C8): tell the patient to straighten the fingers and not to let you push them down.
- Flexion (C7, C8): tell the patient to squeeze two of your fingers.
- Abduction (C8, T1): tell the patient to spread out the fingers and not to let you push them together.

Box 2.13.2
Grading muscle power (British Medical Research Council)

0. Complete paralysis
1. Flicker of contraction
2. Movement with *no* gravity
3. Movement with gravity only (any resistance stops movement)
4. Movement with gravity plus some resistance
5. Normal power

This grading is weighted towards severe weakness (grades 0–3 are all severe). A more sensible scale would be the following:
- Complete paralysis
- Severe weakness
- Moderate weakness
- Mild weakness
- Normal.

- supinator (C5, C6) — brachioradialis muscle (elbow flexion)
- inverted supinator jerk — when tapping the lower end of the radius, elbow extension and finger flexion are the only response; if associated with an absent biceps and exaggerated triceps jerk, this indicates an intraspinal lesion compressing the spinal cord and nerve roots at C5, C6.

9. Assess coordination with finger–nose testing and look for dysdiadochokinesis and rebound.

Motor weakness can be caused by an upper motor neuron lesion, lower motor neuron lesion, neuromuscular junction disorder or myopathy. If there is evidence of a lower motor neuron lesion, consider:

- anterior horn cell
- nerve root and brachial plexus lesions
- peripheral nerve lesions
- motor peripheral neuropathy.

SENSORY SYSTEM

Examine the sensory system after motor testing because this can be time-consuming (and confusing, even when assessed by experts). See Fig. 2.13.3. The OSCE will often specify if this part of the examination is needed.

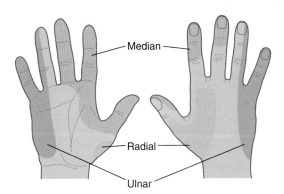

Figure 2.13.3 Average loss of pain sensation (pinprick) with lesions of the major nerves of the upper limbs (Talley NJ, O'Connor S. *Talley and O'Connor's Clinical Examination*. Elsevier Australia, 2017.)

- First test the spinothalamic pathway (pain and temperature). Use a new blunt neurology pin.
  - Demonstrate to the patient the sharpness of the pin on the anterior chest wall or forehead.
  - Then ask him to close his eyes and tell you if the sensation is sharp or dull. Start proximally and test each dermatome (so know them).
- As you are assessing, try to fit any sensory loss into dermatomal (cord or nerve root lesion), peripheral nerve, peripheral neuropathy (glove) or hemisensory (cortical or cord) distribution. Also remember that 'cape' sensory loss (neck, shoulders and arms) suggests syringomyelia, whereas 'shield' sensory loss (front of the chest) may occur with syphilis.
- It is not usually necessary to test temperature perception in the examination if you have tested pain sensation. However, some neurologists test perception of cold using the metal of a tuning fork and find this more accurate than testing with a pin prick.
- Next test the posterior column pathway (vibration and proprioception). Use a 128 Hz tuning fork (not 256Hz) to assess vibration sense. Place this when vibrating on the ulnar head at the wrist when the patient has his eyes closed and ask whether it can be felt. If so, ask the patient to tell you when the vibration ceases and then stop the vibration. If the patient has deficient sensation, test at the elbow, then the shoulder. Test both arms.
- Examine proprioception first with the distal interpharangeal (DIP) joint of the index finger. When the patient has the eyes open, grasp the distal phalanx from the sides and move it up and down to demonstrate, then ask him to close the eyes and repeat the manoeuvres. Normally, movement through even a few degrees is detectable and the patient can tell whether it is up or down. If there is an abnormality, proceed to test the wrist and elbows similarly.

> **T&O'C hint box**
>
> Proprioceptive loss may be subtle. A normal person can detect movement and usually direction changes of 1 or 2°. Begin with small joint movements.

- Test light touch with cotton wool. Touch the skin lightly in each dermatome. Do NOT stroke.
- Feel for thickened nerves — ulnar at the elbow, median at the wrist and radial at the wrist — and feel the axillae if there is evidence of a plexus lesion. Do not forget to mention any scars that may be present.

The examiners will want you to be able to say whether the findings of weakness are typical of a lower or upper motor neuron lesion (Box 2.13.3).

Have a go at the site of the lesion and at a short differential diagnosis. See Box 2.13.4.

Present your findings

- The key is to decide if this an upper motor or lower motor neuron lesion and then attempt to identify where the lesion is.
- Begin with general observational findings, for example wasting, posture (flexion deformity, hemiplegia, symmetrical or asymmetrical changes), presence of fasciculations, presence of wheelchair, wheelie walker etc.

Box 2.13.3
Features of upper and lower motor neuron lesions

You will always be asked to say whether weakness is due to an upper or a lower motor neuron lesion.

Signs of a lower motor neuron lesion	Signs of an upper motor neuron lesion
• Weakness • Wasting • Hypotonicity • Decreased or absent reflexes • Fasciculation (prominent in anterior horn cell diseases unless far advanced)	• Weakness in an 'upper motor neuron pattern'; all muscle groups are weak, but may be more marked in upper limb abductor and extensor muscles — shoulder abduction, elbow and wrist extensors — and lower limb flexor muscles — hip flexion, knee flexion, ankle dorsiflexion • Spasticity • Clonus • Increased reflexes and extensor plantar response

Box 2.13.4
Important facts to know about peripheral neuropathy

This may be sensory (glove and stocking, given these areas are supplied by the longest nerve tracts), with or without motor involvement.

Causes of peripheral neuropathy
These can be roughly divided into diabetes mellitus 30%, hereditary 30%, and idiopathic 30%, all others 10%.
• Drugs and toxins — isoniazid, vincristine, phenytoin, nitrofurantoin, cisplatin, amiodarone, heavy metals
• Alcohol (with or without vitamin B_1 deficiency); amyloidosis
• Metabolic — diabetes mellitus, uraemia, hypothyroidism, porphyria and infiltrative processes such as amyloidosis
• Immune-mediated — Guillain-Barré syndrome
• Tumour — paraneoplastic or compressive neuropathy such as with lung carcinoma
• Vitamin B_{12} or B_1 deficiency or B_6 excess
• Idiopathic
• Connective tissue diseases or vasculitis — systemic lupus erythematosus, polyarteritis nodosa
• Hereditary.

- Next describe muscle power and reflexes. Be aware of inconsistency — if this is present, outline which features are in keeping with an upper or a lower motor neuron weakness.
- Discuss your sensory findings and try to fit them with peripheral, nerve, nerve (glove and stockings), nerve root or cerebral problems (whole body including face). When these are very difficult to assess you may get away with describing them as 'patchy' changes.

Examiners' likely questions

- If you have been too reluctant to say, they will ask if the muscle weakness was upper or lower motor neuron in type and what pattern the sensory changes showed.
- Can you say what the likely lesion is?
- Can you outline a differential diagnosis?

Marking criteria table

Criteria	Satisfactory	Unsatisfactory
Introduces self, explains task, obtains consent, washes hands	1	0
Makes a general inspection and positions patient before launching into examination	1	0
Feels or notes muscle bulk and symmetry	1	0
Tests tone	2	0–1
Tests power	2	0–1
Tests reflexes	3	0–2
Tests coordination	2	0–1
Tests various sensory modalities	2	0–1
Summarises findings	1	0
Looks as though he or she has done this examination many times before (proficient)	2	0–1

Pass mark: 9

Examine a body system (legs neurologically)

Background

As with the rest of neurological assessment, the more advanced you are in your course the more that will be expected of you (bad luck). In the early years of your course you are likely to encounter a normal person on whom to demonstrate your examination skills.

Introduction

Common introductions include:

- Please demonstrate a neurological examination of the lower limbs on this man, who has not noticed any problem (code for a normal person).
- This man has had difficulty walking. Please examine his lower limbs.
- This man has become unsteady when walking. Please examine him.

> ### T &O'C hint box
>
> If the stem mentions walking, **always** ask if you can get the patient to walk.

Rationale

This examination is an opportunity for the examiners to see that you know how to perform the required neurological examination but also that you can test function (walking).

Method

1. Make a general inspection. Notice any wasting, or fasciculations. Run your hand along the shin to feel for obvious wasting. Are there any walking aids? Look around the room for a walking stick or frame and special shoes. Is a urinary catheter present (spinal cord disease)?

2. If the patient can walk, ask them to walk across the room, turn around and walk back. If they look to be in difficulty, offer to help. Look for obvious weakness or an obviously abnormal gait (hemiplegic — one leg swings outwards; high stepping — peripheral neuropathy; wide based and staggering — cerebellar disease; shuffling, small steps — Parkinson syndrome).

   - Ask the patient to try heel-to-toe walking (for cerebellar disease) and then try standing and then walking on toes and heels (for an S1 or L4/L5 lesion, respectively).
   - Ask them to squat and stand (for proximal myopathy).
   - Assess station (Romberg test) for loss of proprioception. Note if the unsteadiness increases with eye closure.

T&O'C hint box

Specific testing of gait should help you decide whether there is an ataxic or high stepping gait (cerebellar or proprioceptive problems) or muscle weakness (proximal or distal, or both).

   - Look for pes cavus — a sign that the muscle weakness is not recent (Fig. 2.14.1).
   - Look for upper limb wasting.

Next examine the patient on the bed.

3. Have the patient lie in bed with the legs entirely exposed. Place a towel over the groin.

4. Look at the patient's back for scars.

5. Look for muscle wasting and fasciculation or tremor. Feel the muscle bulk of the quadriceps and run your hand up each shin, feeling for wasting of the anterior tibial muscles.

6. Test tone at the knees and ankles.

7. Test clonus at this time. Warn the patient first. Push the patella sharply downwards. Sustained rhythmical contractions indicate an upper motor neuron lesion. Also test the ankle by sharply dorsiflexing the foot with the knee bent and the thigh externally rotated. Always test both sides.

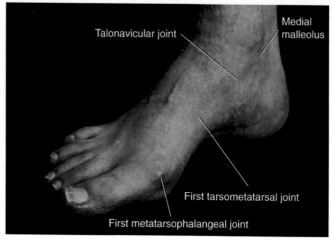

Figure 2.14.1 The right foot of a man with idiopathic pes cavus (Neumann DA. *Kinesiology of the Musculoskeletal System: Foundations for rehabilitation*, 2nd edn. Elsevier Inc., 2010.)

8. Assess power next (Box 2.14.1).
9. Elicit the reflexes:
   - Knee (L3, L4) — quadriceps muscle
   - Ankle (S1, S2) — calf muscle
   - Plantar response (S1).
10. Test coordination with the heel–shin test, toe–finger test and tapping of the feet.
11. Examine the sensory system as for the upper limbs: pin prick, then vibration and proprioception, and then light touch.
    - If there is a peripheral sensory loss, attempt to establish a sensory level on the abdomen.

Box 2.14.1
Assessing power

Hip
- Flexion (L2, L3): ask the patient to lift up his straight leg and not let you push it down (having placed your hand above his knee)
- Extension (L5, S1, and S2): ask him to keep his leg down and not let you pull it up
- Abduction (L4, L5, and S1): ask him to abduct his legs and not let you push them together
- Adduction (L2, L3, and L4): ask him to keep his legs adducted and not let you pull them apart

Knee
- Flexion (L5, S1): ask him to bend his knee and not let you straighten it
- Extension (L3, L4): with the knee slightly bent, ask him to straighten the knee and not let you bend it.

Ankle
- Plantar flexion (S1): ask him to push his foot down and not let you pull it up
- Dorsiflexion (L4, L5): ask him to bring his foot up and not let you push it down
- Eversion (L5, S1): ask him to evert his foot against resistance; loss of this may also indicate a common peroneal (lateral popliteal) nerve palsy
- Inversion (L5): ask him to invert his plantar flexed foot against resistance.

Present your findings

- Does the gait appear normal or wide based (suggests cerebellar disease and ataxia) or limited by pain (antalgic) (suggests hip or knee arthritis) or hemiplegic with circumduction of the leg (suggests an upper motor neuron lesion) or Parkinsonian (small steps, and hurried (festination) alternating with freezing).
- Explain how the rest of the examination might explain the patient's gait (if that was the introductory problem).

Examiners' likely questions

● If you have been too reluctant to say, they will ask if the muscle weakness was upper or lower motor neuron in type and what pattern the sensory changes showed.

● Can you say what the likely lesion is?

● Can you outline a differential diagnosis?

Marking criteria table

Criteria	Satisfactory	Unsatisfactory
Introduces self, explains task, obtains consent, washes hands before and after	1	0
Exposes patient's legs before general inspection	1	0
Asks patient to walk	1	0
Asks patient to squat and stand	1	0
Asks patient to stand on heels and then toes	1	0
Tests for Romberg sign	1	0
Tests tone	1	0
Tests power	2	0–1
Tests reflexes	2	0–1
Tests coordination	2	0–1
Tests various sensory modalities	2	0–1
Summarises findings	1	0
Appears to have done this examination before	1	0
Has a go at answering examiners' questions	1	0

Pass mark: 10

Examine the neck (thyroid)

Background

Thyroid disease can affect many parts of the body. Students need to know what the major manifestations of hypo- and hyperthyroidism are. The thyroid itself may or may not be clinically abnormal in these patients. The gland may be visible in thin normal people. A normal person may be used so that the technique of the examination of the gland and for the signs of thyroid disease throughout the body can be demonstrated by the eager student.

Introduction

- Please examine this woman's thyroid. She has noticed loss of weight and has a tremor.
- This 40-year-old woman has noticed some discomfort in her neck. Please examine her.
- This woman has hypothyroidism. Please examine her.

Rationale

These introductions suggest the examiners want a thyroid examination with or without an examination for signs of thyrotoxicosis or myxoedema. A glass of water placed next to the patient may be a clue that a thyroid examination is required. See Figs 2.15.1 and 2.15.2.

Method

1. Wash hands as usual.
2. Take time first to look at the face for signs of thyrotoxicosis or myxoedema.

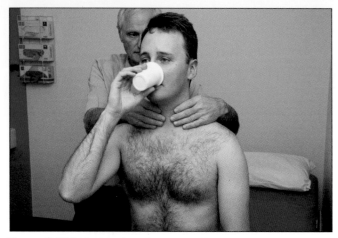

Figure 2.15.1 Examination of the thyroid (Talley NJ, O'Connor S. *Talley & O'Connor's Clinical Examination Essentials: An introduction to clinical skills (and how to pass your clinical exams)*. Elsevier Australia, 2020.)

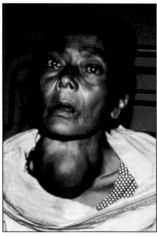

Figure 2.15.2 Endemic goitre. This condition, caused by iodine deficiency, is extremely common in isolated mountainous regions. The thyroid may reach enormous size yet the symptoms are minimal and the patient is usually euthyroid (Raftery A, Lim E, Östör A. *Churchill's Pocketbook of Differential Diagnosis*. Elsevier, 2014, Figure 25.)

3. With the patient sitting up and the neck fully exposed, inspect for scars, swelling and prominent veins.

4. Look at the front and the sides. Ask her to swallow a sip of water and look for thyroid enlargement.

5. Observe whether the thyroid moves up with swallowing.

6. Ask if the neck is tender (a clue to subacute thyroiditis) and note any hoarseness of the voice (which may be caused by recurrent laryngeal nerve palsy).

7. Palpate gently from behind, with the neck flexed, feeling for any thyroid mass. Most people will need reassurance that you are not trying to choke them. Use one hand to steady the gland and the index and middle fingers of the other to feel. Note the shape, consistency and distribution of the thyroid enlargement. If a nodule is palpable, determine whether this is single or part of a multinodular goitre.

8. Decide whether you can palpate the lower border of the gland (to exclude retrosternal extension) and whether there is a thrill. Feel from behind for cervical lymphadenopathy.

9. Next, palpate the gland from in front and note the tracheal position.

10. Percuss over the upper part of the manubrium from one side to the other, right across the bone, and note any change from resonant to dull (a sign of retrosternal extension).

11. Auscultate over the thyroid gland for bruits (a sign of active thyrotoxicosis).

12. Perform the Pemberton sign. Ask the patient to lift her arms over her head. Look for suffusion of the face, elevation of the jugular venous pressure and inspiratory stridor. Any retrosternal mass may cause these changes.

13. Look to see if there is evidence of a goitre and obvious eye disease (indicating the presence of thyrotoxicosis).

14. Examine the pulse rate and blood pressure.

15. Proceed to the face. Assess for thyrotoxicosis. Examine the eyes for exophthalmos by noting the presence of sclera below the cornea when the patient is looking straight ahead.

16. Note lid retraction by looking for the presence of sclera above the cornea.

17. Then test for lid lag by asking the patient to follow your finger descending at a moderate rate.

18. Now examine the conjunctiva for chemosis (Fig. 2.15.3).

19. Test eye movements for ophthalmoplegia. In thyrotoxicosis, the inferior oblique muscle power is lost first, then convergence is affected, followed by the other muscles. Ask to examine the fundi because optic atrophy can occur late. Then look from behind, over the patient's forehead, when she is looking forward, for proptosis.

20. Examine the patient's outstretched hands for tremor. It is worthwhile placing a sheet of paper over the dorsal aspects of the fingers. Note any palmar erythema. Feel for warmth and sweating. Feel the radial pulse for sinus tachycardia, atrial fibrillation or a collapsing pulse.

21. Test for proximal myopathy in the arms and tap the arm reflexes for briskness.

22. If there is time, proceed to the legs and look for skin manifestations: pretibial myxoedema — bilateral firm, elevated dermal nodules and plaques that can be pink, brown or skin-coloured and that are caused by

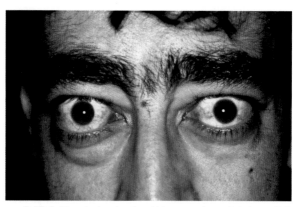

Figure 2.15.3 Thyrotoxicosis: thyroid stare and exophthalmos (Talley NJ, O'Connor S. *Talley and O'Connor's Clinical Examination*. Elsevier Australia, 2017.)

mucopolysaccharide accumulation — and vitiligo. Test for proximal myopathy and hyperreflexia in the legs.

23. Ask to examine the chest for evidence of gynaecomastia (in men) and the heart for an ejection systolic murmur and signs of congestive cardiac failure.

Have a similar system memorised for likely hypothyroidism (often *no* goitre).

- Hands
  - coarse, cool dry skin
  - cold dry palms
  - puffiness of the wrists
  - bradycardia
- Face
  - loss of eyebrow hair
  - periorbital swelling
  - slow speech
- Legs
  - hung up reflexes (delayed relaxation)
  - non-pitting oedema

Present your findings

- Did the patient appear obviously hypo- or hyperthyroid?
- Was the gland visible or palpable? Did it move up when the patient swallowed?
- Was it tender?
- What did the gland feel like?
- Did it extend below the supraclavicular notch?
- Was there a bruit audible?
- Was the Pemberton sign positive?
- Were there specific signs of thyrotoxicosis or myxoedema? List them, including the eye signs.

Examiners' likely questions

- Was there a goitre? How big was it?
- What was its consistency (smooth or multinodular)?

- Was the patient euthyroid? You should already have told them that but they may want you to go through his positive and negative findings, for example no tremor, reflexes normal etc.

Marking criteria table

Criteria	Satisfactory	Unsatisfactory
Introduces self, explains task, obtains consent, washes hands before and after	1	0
Positions patient and exposes neck	1	0
Inspects visible gland, scars and as patient sips water	1	0
Asks about tenderness	1	0
Palpates gently from behind	1	0
Feels and percusses for lower border	1	0
Looks for signs of hyperthyroidism, including tremor and eye signs	3	0–2
Presents a coherent list of findings	2	0–1

Pass mark: 7

Examine the neck lymph nodes

Background

Lymph nodes are often found and can be reactive in responsive to infection or can represent a lymphoma. A good examination can guide appropriate investigation and management.

Introduction

- This woman has found a lump in her neck. Please examine her lymph nodes.
- Please examine this woman's supraclavicular lymph nodes.

Rationale

The introduction will suggest whether this is a real patient or a normal volunteer. Either way the examination technique can be assessed, or the causes of lymphadenopathy discussed. Poor technique is easily uncovered in this OSCE. Practice in examining properly will prevent the embarrassment of not being able to find something the examiners have told you is there.

Method

1. Wash your hands.
2. Ask the patient to remove her shirt and sit up over the edge of the bed.

3. Stand back to look for wasting or obvious scars in the neck or elsewhere that might indicate biopsy or surgical removal. Look for abdominal distension — ascites or organomegaly.

4. Examine the cervical (including the supraclavicular) nodes with the patient in this position. Keep in mind the characteristics of different lymph node abnormalities (Box 2.16.1).

5. Ask if you may examine other lymph node groups. Move on to the axillary lymph nodes first. Then examine the epitrochlear nodes (Figs 2.16.1–2.16.3).

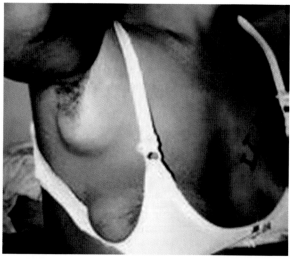

Figure 2.16.1 Enlarged axillary nodes (Courtesy of Dr A Watson, Infectious Diseases Department, The Canberra Hospital.)

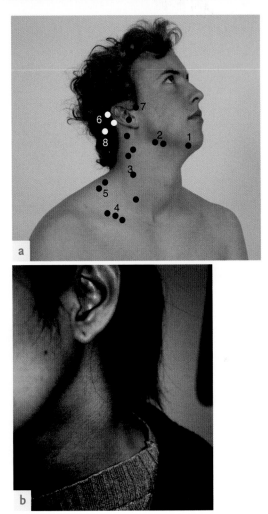

Figure 2.16.2 **(a)** Cervical and supraclavicular lymph nodes.
1 = submental; 2 = submandibular; 3 = jugular chain (posterior cervical
and anterior or deep cervical); 4 = supraclavicular; 5 = posterior triangle;
6 = postauricular; 7 = preauricular; 8 = occipital. **(b)** Cervical
lymphadenopathy. **(c)** Submandibular lymphadenopathy (**(b)** and **(c)** Courtesy
of Dr A Watson, Infectious Diseases Department, The Canberra Hospital.)

continued

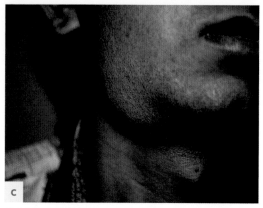

Figure 2.16.2 *(continued)*

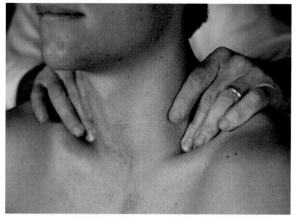

Figure 2.16.3 'Shrug your shoulders for me' — feeling for the supraclavicular lymph nodes (Talley NJ, O'Connor S. *Talley and O'Connor's Clinical Examination*. Elsevier Australia, 2017.)

6. Next lay the patient flat and expose the abdomen. Palpate for inguinal nodes, for splenomegaly and for hepatomegaly.

Box 2.16.1
Characteristics of lymph nodes

During palpation of lymph nodes the following features must be considered.

Site
Palpable nodes may be localised to one region (e.g. local infection, early lymphoma) or generalised (e.g. late lymphoma).

Palpable lymph node areas are:
- Epitrochlear
- Axillary
- Cervical and occipital
- Supraclavicular
- Paraaortic (rarely palpable)
- Inguinal
- Popliteal

Size
Large nodes are usually abnormal (greater than 1cm).

Consistency
Hard nodes suggest carcinoma deposits; soft nodes may be normal; and rubbery nodes may be due to lymphoma.

Tenderness
This implies infection or acute inflammation.

Fixation
Nodes that are fixed to underlying structures are more likely to be infiltrated by carcinoma than mobile nodes.

Overlying skin
Inflammation of the overlying skin suggests infection, and tethering to the overlying skin suggests carcinoma.

Affected nodes — potential aetiology
- *Inguinal nodes:* infection of lower limb, sexually transmitted disease, abdominal or pelvic malignancy, immunisations
- *Axillary nodes:* infections of the upper limb, carcinoma of the breast, disseminated malignancy, immunisations
- *Epitrochlear nodes:* infection of the arm, lymphoma, sarcoidosis
- *Left supraclavicular nodes:* metastatic malignancy from the chest, abdomen (especially stomach — Troisier sign) or pelvis
- *Right supraclavicular nodes:* malignancy from the chest or oesophagus

7. If a group of nodes is abnormal, consider their area of drainage and ask to examine that region.

Present your findings

- Describe the size and characteristics of any palpable nodes, especially whether they are likely to be malignant (fixed to underlying structures and painless), inflammatory (tender) or benign (small and non-tender).
- Outline the presence or absence or other node groups.
- Mention other abnormalities — splenomegaly or other organ enlargement.

Examiners' likely questions

- What is the pattern of the lymphadenopathy?
    - Outline what groups are involved.
- What is the differential diagnosis?
    - Consider infection, lymphoma, and other malignancy (Box 2.16.2).
- Where else might you examine?
    - Ask to look in more detail for head and neck and lung malignancies.

**Box 2.16.2
Causes of lymphadenopathy**

Generalised lymphadenopathy
- Lymphoma (rubbery and firm)
- Leukaemia (e.g. chronic lymphocytic leukaemia, acute lymphocytic leukaemia)
- Infections:
    - viral (e.g. infectious mononucleosis, cytomegalovirus, HIV)
    - bacterial (e.g. tuberculosis, brucellosis, syphilis)
    - protozoal (e.g. toxoplasmosis)
- Connective tissue diseases (e.g. rheumatoid arthritis, systemic lupus erythematosus)
- Infiltration (e.g. sarcoid)
- Drugs (e.g. phenytoin [pseudolymphoma])

Localised lymphadenopathy
- Local acute or chronic infection
- Metastases
- Lymphoma, especially Hodgkin disease

Marking criteria table

Criteria	Satisfactory	Unsatisfactory
Introduces self, explains task, obtains consent, washes hands before and after	1	0
Positions patient in approved manner	1	0
Inspects for visible nodes	1	0
Palpates appropriate groups of nodes	3	0–2
Palpates other relevant organs (spleen, liver)	2	0–1
Describes findings accurately	2	0–1
Discusses differential diagnosis	2	0–1

Pass mark: 6

Basic cardiac life support

Background

Everyone who works in a hospital is expected to be able to provide basic life support and to know how to help when the resuscitation team arrives.

Introduction

You have been called to see a patient in the ward whom the nursing staff have been concerned is deteriorating. When you arrive, the patient unconscious. Describe what you would do and demonstrate where necessary on the manikin here.

Rationale

Most hospitals expect all their staff to be able to begin basic life support. Senior medical students and medical staff should be able to perform competent advanced life support.

Method

D	CHECK FOR DANGER
	Look quickly around the room for obstacles, broken or fallen glass etc.
R	**CHECK FOR RESPONSIVENESS**
	Call the patient and ask 'Are you all right?' Touch and the shake the patient if there is no response.
S	**SEND FOR HELP**
	Options include calling for help from the closest hospital staff, pressing a 'MET call' button or ringing the emergency switchboard number, depending on the situation and presence or not of other staff.

| A | **OPEN AIRWAY** |

Look to see if the patient's airway is open and not obstructed. Put on some gloves quickly if they are available and open the patient's mouth. Clear any obvious obstructions (food, vomitus, false teeth). Extend the neck and pull the jaw forward if the airway still seems obstructed. Demonstrate this on the manikin.

| B | **NORMAL BREATHING?** |

Check for normal breathing. Listen for air movement and watch for effective chest movements.

| C | **START CPR** |

You will be expected to demonstrate an effective technique. This involves the use of two hands over the central sternum and compression of the chest by a third of its depth. Usually 90 compressions a minute is recommended. If you are still alone with the patient, do not interrupt chest compression to ventilate the patient. If help has arrived, one person should ventilate using a mask and bag. Thirty compressions should be followed by 2 breaths.

The technique for bag-and-mask ventilation requires practice. The mask must be held airtight over the mouth. The jaw should be drawn forward to open the airway.

| D | **ATTACH DEFIBRILLATOR (AED)** |

BLS training would usually mean using an automatic defibrillator. If more people are available, the combined monitoring and defibrillator pads should be attached with minimal interruption to CPR. These are peel-off adhesive pads. They may not stick well if the patient is very hairy and must either be placed on the least hairy appropriate place or an attempt made at a rapid shaving. The pads usually have diagrams showing where they should be placed — usually over the sternum and on the left lateral chest or posteriorly on the thorax if that is practical. These devices are designed to be easy to operate and there should be a clear 'on' button. An ECG should come up on the screen. It may be necessary to pause CPR for a stable tracing to be obtained. The device will interpret the tracing and ask permission to give a shock (for ventricular fibrillation or ventricular tachycardia). It will warn everyone to stand clear. Issue this order clearly and loudly.

Look at the monitor to see if normal rhythm and at the patient to see if responsiveness have been restored. If not, recommence CPR.

Present your findings

It is important to clearly summarise your findings to the examiners. Here state the patient status at the initial encounter, resuscitation steps undertaken, outcome (was a call made to cease, or did the pulse and breathing return?) and next steps.

Examiners' likely questions

- How would you manage resuscitation if a patient is already on a cardiac monitor and is seen to develop ventricular fibrillation?
    - These patients should have immediate DC cardioversion with 200 joules if a defibrillator is available. They should not have this delayed by commencement of CPR.
- How would you decide when to stop unsuccessful resuscitation?
    - A patient who has a terminal illness and who has not-for-resuscitation orders should not have CPR. Sometimes this directive is not immediately known to the resuscitation team. When help has arrived, enquiries about the patient's underlying illness, prognosis and resuscitation directives must be obtained from the ward staff. This can obviously help in deciding to cease resuscitation attempts. Otherwise, the decision to stop resuscitation attempts is a difficult one but survival after more than 30 minutes of CPR is uncommon and neurological injury is likely even in survivors.

Marking criteria table

Criteria	Satisfactory	Unsatisfactory
Can outline initial approach to patient and surroundings	1	0
Checks for responsiveness	1	0
Knows how to call for help	1	0
Opens airway (demonstrates)	1	0
Checks breathing	1	0
Can demonstrate adequate chest compression	1	0
Can demonstrate adequate CPR	1	0
Can demonstrate use of AED	1	0
Knows how to assess for return of responsiveness	2	0–1
Knows to ask about resuscitation orders	1	0

Pass mark: 7

Intermediate clinical years

Take a history — cardiovascular risk factors

Background

You may have a real patient with risk factors or an actor given a script of answers. Assessment of a patient's cardiovascular risk factors and advice about them should be a routine part of health maintenance.

Introduction

Question this patient about her risk factors for cardiovascular disease.

Rationale

This OSCE is a test of your ability to make a rapid assessment of cardiovascular risk. The examiners will expect you to ask only relevant questions and to direct the patient tactfully away from long rambling stories about a great uncle's possible stroke. Senior students will need to put the risk factors in context to assess overall risk.

Method

Introduce yourself and say that you would like to ask some questions about the patient's medical history. Ask the patient the following:

1. How old are you? (Risk increases with age.)
2. Do you have a previous history of cardiovascular disease? (Previous ischaemic heart disease is the strongest risk factor.) (Check for history of angina, myocardial infactions, cerebrovascular and peripheral vascular disease. If present, you will be expected to elicit details.)
3. Do you know your cholesterol level? Has it been treated with medication?
4. Have you been diagnosed with high blood pressure? When? How often is your blood pressure monitored and by whom?
5. Are you being treated for this with medications? Has the blood pressure returned to normal? (Remember that hyperlipidaemia is a more important risk factor for ischaemic heart disease and hypertension is a more important risk factor for stroke.)
6. Do you have diabetes? If so, for how long? Are you taking insulin? (Risk increases with duration of the disease and when patients are taking insulin.)
7. Do you smoke? If so, for how long? How many? (Risk of myocardial infarction declines to that of non-smokers after one year and risk of angina declines to that of non-smokers after 10 years.)
8. Do you have a family history of cardiovascular disease? If so, who was affected and at what age? (Only first degree relatives — siblings and parents — with premature (generally under 60 years of age) coronary disease indicate an increase in a person's risk.)
9. Have you had problems with your kidney function? (Chronic kidney disease and especially dialysis increases cardiovascular risk dramatically.)

10. Have you had problems with arthritis? What type?
(Chronic inflammatory disease such as rheumatoid
arthritis is associated with increased cardiovascular risk.)

Present your findings

Synthesise and present your findings. Summarise the positive
risk factors roughly in order of importance or, even better,
according to whether they are modifiable or not in this particular patient.

Examiners' likely questions

- Can you comment on this woman's overall cardiovascular
  risk?
  - Here it is important to stress the importance of overall
    risk. A combination of risk factors makes each factor
    more important and more likely to need treatment.
- Do you think more should be done to improve her risk?
  - Point out that there are some absolute indications for
    drug treatment; for example, severe hypertension or
    very high total cholesterol levels, for example a total
    cholesterol of 9 mmol/L, is an indication for drug
    treatment for a woman with no other significant risk
    factors. Explain that patients who have already had an
    ischaemic event need aggressive control of all their risk
    factors, for example aiming at a total cholesterol level of
    less than 4 mmol/L and LDL cholesterol level of 1.8 or
    less.
- How would you explain this to the patient?
  - You can refer to cardiovascular risk factor tables, which
    can help quantify the effect of multiple risk factors and
    help explain to a patient the need for treatment.

Marking criteria table

Criteria	Satisfactory	Unsatisfactory
Introduces self, explains task, obtains consent	1	0
Asks about previous history of ischaemic heart disease, stroke etc.	1	0
Obtains details of the relevant disease	1	0
Asks about cholesterol level	1	0
Asks about hypertension	1	0
Asks about diabetes mellitus	1	0
Asks about smoking history	1 Any; 2 current, past	0–1
Asks about family history	1 Any; 2 first-degree, premature	0–1
Can describe risk factors in order of importance	2	0–1
Synthesises risk	2	0–1

Pass mark: 8

19

Take a history — obesity

Background

Talking to patients about their weight is a very common part of medical consultations. A practical and sympathetic approach to the problem will be expected of students.

Introduction

This 50-year-old woman has had problems with her weight for many years. Her sister has recently been treated for a myocardial infarction and she is concerned about her weight as a contributor to her own risk. Please take a history from her about this.

Alternative introductions include assessment of an obese patient for surgical and anaesthetic risk.

Rationale

This increasingly common chronic disease is associated with several medical problems.

Obesity is defined as a BMI (body mass/height squared) of 30 or more, and about one-third of adults are obese.

Method

1. Introduce yourself. Say that you would like to ask some questions about the patient's health and weight.
2. General questions about the weight. Some tactful first questions would be: Have you had problems with your weight for a long time or only fairly recently? Do you know what your weight is at the moment?

> **Box 3.19.1**
> **Medications associated with weight gain**
>
> Hypoglycaemics — insulin, sulphonylureas, thiazolidinediones
> Antipsychotics (atypical) — clozapine, risperidone,
> Corticosteroids
> Anticonvulsants — carbamazepine, valproate
> Antidepressants — tricyclic antidepressants, some selective
> serotonin antagonists, mirtazapine

Then:
- Has your weight gone up and down over the years?
  What is the heaviest you have been? And the lightest?
  What do you think has caused these changes?
- Is there a history of weight problems in your family? Is
  there a history of diabetes in your family?
- Have you been on any medications that may have
  contributed to your gaining weight? (Ask about those in
  Box 3.19.1.)
- Are you active? What sort of exercise do you do? How
  often and for how long each time?
- Tell me about your diet? Have you ever kept a food
  diary? (Keep this general or time will disappear.)
- Do you see your weight as a problem for your health or
  not really? What do you think might be done about it?
- Have you tried to lose weight in the past? What sorts of
  thing have you done? Have you had any success with
  these attempts to lose weight?
- Have you felt depressed about your weight?
- Has anyone mentioned bariatric surgery to you as a
  possible treatment? Do you know what this involves?
- Have you had diabetes diagnosed when you were
  pregnant?

3. Ask about problems associated with obesity and their effect
   on ability to exercise and on normal activities.
   - Have you had arthritis? Where has it affected you? Does
     it stop you doing activities? What treatment has been
     suggested — drugs, joint replacement?
   - Have you been diagnosed with diabetes? How long ago?
     Did you lose weight when it was first diagnosed? Have
     there been any complications of the diabetes — eye
     problems, nerve problems (peripheral neuropathy),

strokes or heart problems? What treatment have you been taking for it? Have you needed insulin? Do you know what your HbA1c is?

– Ask about her cardiovascular disease and risk factors (hyperlipidaemia, smoking, and hypertension). How old was your sister when she had her heart attack?

– Have you been diagnosed with sleep apnoea or been told you snore badly? Have you used a sleep apnoea mask? Has it helped you feel less sleepy during the day?

– Have you been told you have a fatty liver? Have you had attacks of abdominal pain caused by gallstones?

– Does your weight and arthritis make it difficult for you to do activities of daily living? (Give examples, such as exercise, bathing, getting out of the house.)

– Are you able to manage shopping and cooking? Can you get fresh fruit and vegetables or do you manage on take-away? (Shopping for fresh food and ability to cook are important for a healthy diet.)

– Have you been able to work? What do you do? Are you able to get out to see friends?

Present your findings

- Outline the age of onset of obesity and the history of weight gain and attempts to lose weight.
- List the important complications of the patient's obesity.
- Suggest changes to medications if this seems possible.
- Summarise her cardiovascular risk factors.
- Give your understanding of the patient's mood and the effect of the problem on her life. Suggest that her concerns about her cardiovascular risk might make this a good time for her to try again with a weight loss program.

Examiners' likely questions

- Do you think weight loss would help with her diabetes?
  - If the body mass index has not been provided to you, ask for it. Remember severe obesity is a BMI $\geq 40\,\text{kg/m}^2$. At high risk are those with a BMI of $35\,\text{kg/m}^2$ or higher, especially if they have comorbid disease such as diabetes mellitus.

- – In type 2 diabetes, substantial loss of weight will often return glucose tolerance to normal. Say that in these circumstances you would explain the great benefits to her health of not being diabetic. Otherwise, if the diabetes is longstanding, blood sugar control and some complications of diabetes will be improved by weight loss.
- How would you help her lose weight?
  - – There may be no sure way of achieving this. If numerous attempts with the help of dietitians and exercise classes have failed, it may be best to say that realistically the chances of success are small. Nevertheless you need to have a strategy to address the problem.
  - – A combination of diet (the type based on patient preference), exercise (30 minutes or more at least 5 days a week tailored to the patient's ability) and behavioural modification such as a food diary and controlling stimuli that trigger eating, is most helpful. An exercise program that takes into account problems like arthritis (e.g. swimming or aqua-aerobics) should be discussed. Suggesting she use a step counter, or an exercise app might encourage regular exercise.
  - – Reduce food intake. Reduction of food intake by 2000 to 4000 kilojoules a day will cause 400–500 g of weight loss a week.
  - – Drug therapy is of limited value and can be expensive.
    - ■ Fat absorption inhibitors (e.g. orlistat) have a modest benefit — 8 kg in a year in a placebo-controlled study
    - ■ Sympathomimetic appetite suppressants tend to work only when being taken continuously and have side effects including hypertension and arrhythmias
    - ■ One new effective option is a glucagon-like peptide agonist (GLP-1 agonist).
- Would you recommend bariatric surgery to her?
  - – Bariatric surgery is only indicated if other treatment has failed *and* the BMI (in an adult or adolescent) is 40 kg/m^2 or over, or 35 kg/m^2 or over *and* there is one serious comorbidity.

- This is an opportunity to discuss the risks and benefits of this surgery. Serious attempts at changing her diet and an exercise program must have been tried. You need to assess her surgical risk and her understanding of the way the operation works. Emphasise that she must be willing to continue with careful control of her diet after surgery. Bariatric surgery can achieve up to 40% weight loss 12–18 months post procedure.

Marking criteria table

Criteria	Satisfactory	Unsatisfactory
Introduces self, explains task, obtains consent	1	0
Asks matter-of-fact questions about the patient's current weight and history of weight gain	2	0–1
Asks about relevant medications	1	0
Establishes the history of attempts at weight loss	1	0
Asks patient about current diet	1	0
Assesses patient's insight into the problem	1	0
Asks about complications of obesity, notably diabetes mellitus, osteoarthritis, cardiovascular disesae	2	0–1
Discusses future weight loss strategies, including bariatric surgery	2	0–1
Talks about how realistic the patient's approach to the problem is	1	0

Pass mark: 7

Obesity examination

Background

The increasingly common occurrence of obesity means that many patients who present with medical problems are obese. Their weight will have a direct or indirect effect on the problem and treatment.

Introduction

Please examine this man. He has had some complications related to having been overweight for many years.

Rationale

This is a test of your knowledge of the particular physical problems obesity can cause. You should also assess for rare secondary causes of obesity (e.g. Cushing syndrome, usually due to exogenous steroid prescription).

Method

1. Introduce yourself, wash your hands, obtain consent and ask the patient to undress to his underwear. Get him to put on a hospital gown.
2. Ask if you may weigh and measure the height of the patient so that you can calculate the BMI (body weight/height squared). There may be scales and a height measure attached to the wall, or the examiners may give you these measurements.
3. Measure waist circumference at the level of the iliac crest. (>88 cm for women or 105 cm for men is associated with increased risk of diabetes, hyperlipidaemia, hypertension and heart disease, independent of BMI.)

4. Take the blood pressure. Use a large enough cuff — remember that too small a cuff may burst off the patient's arm (embarrassing) or overestimate the blood pressure.

5. Look for peripheral oedema (distinguish this from adipose tissue by attempting to indent the area gently), varicose veins and venous ulcers.

6. Note central obesity. Look for other signs of Cushing syndrome (purple striae, moon face, proximal muscle weakness).

7. Inspect the neck for a goitre (hypothyroidism — if suspected, search for other signs). Also look for acne and hirsutism on the face in a woman (polycystic ovary syndrome).

8. Look for deformity or signs of osteoarthritis in large weight-bearing joints (most often obvious in the knees).

9. Ask the patient to sit in a chair and then get up and walk. Note need for walking aids because of arthritis or obesity itself. Severe obesity interferes with normal activities.

10. Ask for a urinalysis (for sugar) or blood sugar (or HbA1c) result. If diabetic, ask to examine for the possible complications of diabetes, including peripheral vascular disease and neuropathy in the legs, and eye complications (fundoscopy for diabetic retinopathy) (usually there won't be time!).

Present your findings

- Start with the actual weight, waist measurements and BMI. Tell the examiners what normal measurements would be.
- Comment on the presence of absence of myxoedema or signs of Cushing syndrome.
- Give them the blood pressure reading.
- Describe any findings of diabetic complications.
- Mention any venous changes in the legs or signs of osteoarthritis in weight-bearing joints.
- Describe the patient's mobility.

Examiners' likely questions

- How severe do you think the patient's problem is?
  - Remind the examiners of the patient's BMI compared with normal and describe the patient's limitations when he attempts to get up and walk.

- What might be done?
  As in Station 19; suggest management strategies — much depends on patient's insight and motivation.
  - Dietary advice, exercise and behavioural therapy are the backbone of management
  - A food diary can help patients appreciate their food intake accurately
  - Exercise program — tailored to limitations such as arthritis (water aerobics)
  - Ways of encouraging exercise — pedometer, fitness watch, gymnasium program
  - Remember that exercise alone has modest effects on weight loss but can help maintain weight loss
  - Remember that no particular weight loss diet has been shown to be better than any other, but enthusiasm for a particular diet may be valuable.
- Can any medications be changed?
  - Drug treatment for weight loss has generally been disappointing (see Station 19)
- What about surgery?
  - Usually reserved for those with BMI ≥40 or those with BMI ≥35 and one or more comorbidities of obesity (e.g. diabetes mellitus)
  - Must have an acceptable surgical and anaesthetic risk
  - Must be enthusiastic and understand that long-term results still depend on changes to diet and exercise. Usually patients are required to demonstrate this by achieving some preoperative weight loss
  - Can be dramatically effective and has been shown to reduce complications of obesity.

T&O'C hint box

A common manageable weight reduction goal to suggest is 10% of current body weight over 6 months at a rate of 0.5–1 kg a week.

Marking criteria table

Criteria	Satisfactory	Unsatisfactory
Introduces self, explains task, obtains consent, washes hands before and after	1	0
Weighs patient	1	0
Measures waist circumference	1	0
Calculates or asks for BMI (and knows what this means)	2	0–1
Notes fat distribution	1	0
Measures blood pressure	1	0
Assesses mobility	1	0
Knows the complications of obesity, including diabetic complications	2	0–1
Knows rare secondary causes of obesity (e.g. Cushing syndrome)	1	0

Pass mark: 7

Cardiac disease examination

Background

The usual finding is a cardiac murmur.

The most likely valve abnormalities you will come across are:

- mitral regurgitation (Fig. 3.21.1)
- aortic stenosis (Fig. 3.21.2)
- aortic regurgitation (or both aortic stenosis and aortic regurgitation).

Depending on the university and your seniority as a medical student, you may be asked just to examine the heart or praecordium or to perform a cardiovascular (CVS) examination. The traditional CVS examination begins with a general inspection of the patient and goes on to the hands from there. It can, however,

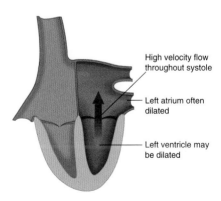

High velocity flow
throughout systole

Left atrium often
dilated

Left ventricle may
be dilated

Figure 3.21.1 Mitral regurgitation: anatomy (Talley NJ, O'Connor S. *Talley and O'Connor's Clinical Examination*. Elsevier Australia, 2017.)

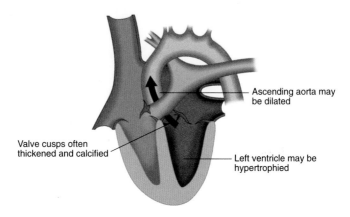

Ascending aorta may
be dilated

Valve cusps often
thickened and calcified

Left ventricle may be
hypertrophied

Figure 3.21.2 Aortic stenosis: anatomy (Talley NJ, O'Connor S. *Talley and O'Connor's Clinical Examination*. Elsevier Australia, 2017.)

begin at the praecordium, and if time is limited the examiners are more likely to direct you there. Box 3.21.1 sets out the formal CVS examination sequence.

T&O'C hint box

You must learn basic chest X-ray interpretation
- how to measure for cardiomegaly
- the borders of major cardiac structures — left ventricle, right ventricle, left atrium, left atrial appendage, aortic root, aortic knuckle, left and right pulmonary arteries
- the location of the mitral and aortic valves

T&O'C hint box

A loud systolic murmur, rarely with a thrill, may be present in patients with severe aortic regurgitation without any organic aortic stenosis being associated. The peripheral signs of aortic regurgitation are the clue that this is the real lesion in this situation (Fig. 3.21.3).

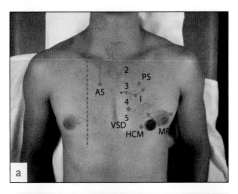

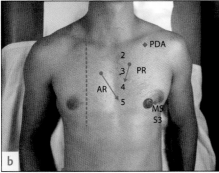

(2–5 refer to intercostal spaces; dotted line = midclavicular line)

(a) Systolic murmurs:

AS = aortic stenosis
MR = mitral regurgitation
HCM = hypertrophic cardiomyopathy
PS = pulmonary stenosis
VSD = ventricular septal defect
I = innocent

(b) Diastolic murmurs and sounds:

AR = aortic regurgitation
MS = mitral stenosis
S3 = third heart sound
PR = pulmonary regurgitation
PDA = patent ductus arteriosus (continuous murmur)

Figure 3.21.3 Radiation and sites of maximum intensity of heart sounds and murmurs. The midclavicular line (on the right) is shown for illustrative purposes (Talley NJ, O'Connor S. *Talley & O'Connor's Clinical Examination Essentials: An introduction to clinical skills (and how to pass your clinical exams).* Elsevier Australia, 2020.)

> **Box 3.21.1**
> **The cardiovascular examination sequence**
>
> 1. A general inspection of the patient
> 2. A search for the peripheral signs of heart and vascular disease in the arms, face and neck
>   - hands and nails
>   - radial pulse
>   - blood pressure
>   - face
>   - neck
> 3. The praecordium
>   - inspection
>   - palpation
>   - auscultation
>   - dynamic manoeuvres
> 4. The back
>   - percussion
>   - auscultation
> 5. The abdomen
>   - the liver
>   - ascites
>   - the spleen
> 6. The legs
>   - palpation of the peripheral pulses
>   - inspection for oedema and signs of arterial and venous disease

Introduction

The introduction to these cases from the examiner is likely to be:

- This patient has had a murmur detected. Please examine him or her.
- This patient has been short of breath. Please examine his or her heart.

Rationale

Students are expected to know how to perform a cardiovascular examination. This routine examination should appear practised and smooth. You will be expected to be able to hear and diagnose clear examples of common valve abnormalities.

Method

1. Wash your hands. Obtain consent. Explain what you are going to do.
2. Make sure the patient is positioned at 45° and that the patient's chest and neck are fully exposed. For a woman, the requirements of modesty dictate that you cover her breasts with a towel or loose garment.
3. While standing back, inspect! Look for dyspnoea, use of supplementary oxygen and intravenous infusions. (Most students waste a lot of time here. Remember this should take 30 seconds although there is a lot to report on.)
4. Look *at the chest* for scars. These may indicate previous cardiac surgery. Inspect for deformity and look to see if the apex beat is visible. Do not forget about pacemaker and cardioverter-defibrillator boxes.
5. Palpate for the apex beat position. Be seen to count down the correct number of intercostal spaces. The normal position is the fifth intercostal space, 1 cm medial to the midclavicular line. Palpate at the apex for a thrill. A systolic thrill here indicates severe mitral regurgitation (Box 3.21.2). Now feel at the base of the heart for a thrill resulting from severe aortic stenosis.
6. Remember the surface anatomy of the heart (Fig. 2.8.1).
7. Auscultation begins with listening in the mitral area with both the bell and the diaphragm. Spend most time here. Listen for each component of the cardiac cycle separately.
8. Identify the first and second heart sounds and decide whether they are of normal intensity and whether they are split.
9. Now listen for extra heart or prosthetic heart sounds and murmurs.
10. Listen in the axilla to find out if a systolic murmur audible at the apex radiates there (a sign of mitral regurgitation). Repeat the approach at the left sternal edge and then at the base of the heart (aortic and pulmonary areas). Time each part of the cycle with the carotid pulse. Sit the patient up and leaning forward.
11. Listen for the systolic murmur of aortic stenosis and listen over the carotids to find out if the murmur is conducted there. Ask him or her to breathe in and then breathe right

Box 3.21.2
Mitral regurgitation

Causes — chronic
Degenerative disease
Mitral valve prolapse
Rheumatic (men more often than women) — rarely is mitral
    regurgitation the only murmur present
Papillary muscle dysfunction, due to left ventricular failure, ischaemia

Causes — acute
Infective endocarditis (perforation of anterior leaflet), rupture of a
    myxomatous cord
Myocardial infarction (chordae rupture or papillary muscle
    dysfunction)

Clinical signs of severity
Enlarged left ventricle (displaced apex beat)
Murmur is loud, thrill is present
Third heart sound (not always present)
Soft first heart sound
Left ventricular failure

Results of investigations

ECG
P mitrale (broad P wave)
Atrial fibrillation
Q waves indicating previous ischaemia

Chest X-ray
Large (sometimes gigantic) left atrium
Increased left ventricular size
Mitral annular calcification

Echocardiography
This will give information about the possible aetiology, the severity,
and any associated valve or structural abnormalities:
Thickened leaflets — rheumatic aetiology
Prolapsing leaflet(s)
Left atrial size (a sign of chronicity and severity)
Left ventricular size and function
Doppler detection of the regurgitant jet in the left atrium
Calcification of the mitral annulus — common in elderly people

out and then stop breathing. Listen here at the left sternal edge for the early diastolic murmur of aortic regurgitation (Box 3.21.3).

12. Feel again at the base of the heart (press firmly onto the chest wall — see Fig. 2.8.6b) for a systolic thrill which indicates severe aortic stenosis (Box 3.21.4).

Box 3.21.3
Aortic regurgitation

Causes

Valvular
Rheumatic (rarely the only murmur in this case)
Congenital (e.g. bicuspid valve)
Seronegative arthropathy, especially ankylosing spondylitis

Aortic root dilatation
Marfan syndrome
Dissecting aneurysm
Old age

Clinical signs of severity
Collapsing pulse
Wide pulse pressure
Length of the *decrescendo* diastolic murmur
Third heart sound (left ventricular)
Left ventricular failure

Results of investigations

ECG
Left ventricular hypertrophy (deep S wave in V1, tall R wave in V5–V6. (Sum of S wave in V1+ R wave in V5 = 35 small squares (mm))

Chest X-ray
Left ventricular dilatation
Aortic root dilatation or aneurysm (see Fig. 3.21.4)
Valve calcification

Echocardiography
Left ventricular dimensions (severe dilatation can occur) and function
Doppler estimation of size of regurgitant jet
Aortic root dimensions
Valve cusp thickening or prolapse

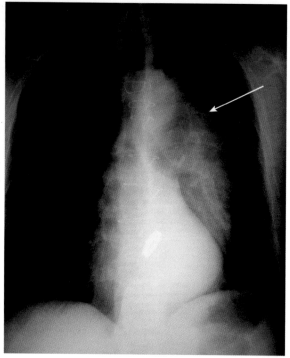

Figure 3.21.4 Massive dilatation of the thoracic aorta (arrow) is seen in this patient with Marfan syndrome and aortic regurgitation (Figure reproduced courtesy of The Canberra Hospital.)

13. If the examiners indicate there is more time, percuss the bases of the lungs for the dullness of pleural effusion and go on to look at the hands and take the blood pressure. (It is unlikely you will have time to do these things.)

14. Wash your hands.

Present your findings

- It is often best to begin by thanking them for asking you to examine Mr/Ms X (even if you do not mean it). Then repeat the introduction: 'Mr or Ms X, who has had problems with breathlessness'.

Box 3.21.4
Aortic stenosis

Valve area 1.5–2.0 cm^2. Significant stenosis at <1 cm^2. In critical aortic stenosis, less than 0.7 cm^2/m^2 or a mean valve gradient >40 mmHg. See Fig. 3.21.2.

Causes
Degenerative senile calcific aortic stenosis (the most common cause in the elderly)
Rheumatic (rarely isolated)
Calcific bicuspid valve

Clinical signs of severity
Plateau pulse
Aortic thrill (very important sign of severe stenosis)
Length, harshness and lateness of the peak of the systolic murmur
Fourth heart sound (S4).
Paradoxical splitting of the second heart sound (delayed left ventricular ejection and aortic valve closure)
Left ventricular failure (a late sign — right ventricular failure is preterminal)

Results of investigations

ECG
Left ventricular hypertrophy (systolic overload)

Chest X-ray
Left ventricular hypertrophy
Valve calcification

Echocardiography
Doppler estimation of gradient
Valve cusp mobility
Left ventricular hypertrophy
Left ventricular dysfunction

- If there is an introduction suggesting a symptom, comment on this, for example whether the patient looks breathless of not.
- Then make a general observation about the patient's age, body habitus (if relevant) and whether he or she looks breathless or not.
- Describe any abnormal findings (e.g. the presence of scars and apex beat).

- Then describe the murmur, its loudness (out of 6), timing (systolic or diastolic), position of maximum intensity and character (e.g. ejection, pan systolic, early diastolic).
- Take a big breath and hazard a diagnosis and your impression of the severity of the lesion (mild, moderate or severe). One simple discriminator of severity is to note if the murmur is/is not associated with signs of decompensated heart failure at rest.
- Explain how you think this is consistent with the patient's symptoms as given to you in the introduction.
- Say what features made you decide on its severity or otherwise (e.g. a long early diastolic murmur and displaced apex beat suggest severe aortic regurgitation).
- Have a list in your mind of the common causes.

Examiners' likely questions

- For junior medical students, examiners may only ask if the murmur is systolic or diastolic or both, and where it was loudest. (See Station 8, page 56.) They will ask if there were any associated signs such as thrills or heaves.
- For more senior students, they will want to know the likely diagnosis and a list of differentials.
- They may go on to ask:
  - What the likely causes of this lesion?
  - What symptoms would suggest the lesion is severe?

T&O'C hint box

If things are going well, the examiners may ask what investigations you would like to see — consider a chest X-ray.
  You will need to have a rough idea how each of the investigations you suggest might help (Figs 3.21.5, 3.21.6).

T&O'C hint box

Severe valvular heart disease, of almost any sort, usually causes dyspnoea. Aortic stenosis can cause exertional chest tightness and dyspnoea and if very severe, exertional syncope.

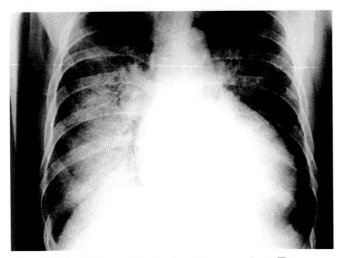

Figure 3.21.5 Cardiomegaly in alveolar pulmonary oedema (The Canberra Hospital X-Ray Library, reproduced with permission.)

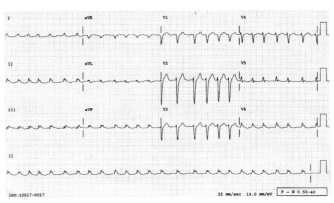

Figure 3.21.6 Atrial fibrillation, which can occur in a patient with mitral stenosis (Talley NJ, O'Connor S. *Talley and O'Connor's Examination Medicine*. Elsevier Australia, 2020.)

T&O'C hint box

A loud systolic murmur, rarely with a thrill, may be present in patients with severe aortic regurgitation without any organic aortic stenosis being associated. The peripheral signs of aortic regurgitation are the clue that this is the real lesion in this situation.

T&O'C hint box

You must learn basic chest X-ray interpretation:

- how to measure for cardiomegaly (cardiothoracic ratio)
- the borders of major cardiac structures — left ventricle, right ventricle, left atrium, left atrial appendage, aortic root, aortic knuckle, left and right pulmonary arteries
- the location of the mitral and aortic valves (see Figs 3.21.7 a and b)

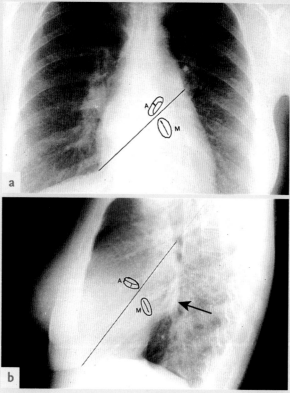

Figure 3.21.7 Location of the mitral (M) and aortic (A) valves (The Canberra Hospital X-Ray Library, reproduced with permission.)

Marking criteria table

Criteria	Satisfactory	Unsatisfactory
Introduces self, explains task, obtains consent, washes hands before and after	1	0
Makes a general inspection of the patient	1	0
Examines the praecordium for scars	1	0
Feels for the apex beat	1	0
Feels for thrills and a parasternal impulse	2	0–1
Auscultates at apex and at the base of the heart	1	0
Detects a murmur	1	0
Is able to say whether the murmur is systolic or diastolic	1	0
Makes an attempt at a diagnosis	1	0
Makes an attempt at diagnosing the severity of the lesion	1	0
Is able to suggest helpful investigations	1	0
Makes an attempt at chest X-ray interpretation	1	0

Pass mark: 6

Background

Hypertension is prevalent throughout the community. Often it is idiopathic but it is important not to miss a secondary cause that requires prompt investigation and management.

Introduction

This 30-year-old man has hypertension. Please examine him.

Rationale

Senior students might be asked to examine a hypertensive patient and then comment on possible causes, further investigations and need for treatment. Students should be able to take the blood pressure and have an idea about possible causes and complications of hypertension.

Method

1. Stand back and inspect the patient. Look for evidence of systemic disease such as Cushing syndrome or acromegaly (see Box 3.22.1). Examine for cushingoid features (moon face, central obesity).
   If one of these is present, modify your examination appropriately.

2. Next, wash your hands then confirm that the blood pressure is elevated. Mention that you would like to allow the patient to rest if they have just arrived (for at least

> ### Box 3.22.1
> ### Causes of hypertension
>
> Essential (most common cause)
> Secondary
> 1. Renal disease
>   - Renovascular disease (renal artery atherosclerosis, fibromuscular disease, aneurysm, vasculitis)
>   - Diffuse renal disease
> 2. Endocrine
>   - Conn syndrome (primary aldosteronism), Cushing syndrome (especially steroid treatment)
>   - 17- and 11-beta-hydroxylase defects
>   - Phaeochromocytoma
>   - Acromegaly
>   - Myxoedema
>   - Contraceptive pill
> 3. Coarctation of the aorta
> 4. Other
>   - Polycythaemia rubra vera
>   - Toxaemia of pregnancy
>   - Neurogenic (increased intracranial pressure, lead poisoning, acute intermittent porphyria)
>   - Hypercalcaemia
>   - Alcohol
>   - Sleep apnoea

Note: Alcohol consumption and obesity are associated with essential hypertension.

5 minutes) and empty their bladder. Ask if they have drunk coffee or smoked cigarettes beforehand.

3. Position the patient correctly — the patient should be sitting comfortably with legs uncrossed, feet flat on the floor, the bare arm supported, not talking or otherwise distracted.

4. Make sure you measure blood pressure in both arms with the correct cuff size (small, medium, large, extra-large). Measure by palpation then auscultation.

5. Examine the patient both lying and standing.

6. Feel the radial pulse and very carefully feel for radio femoral delay (coarctation of the aorta — an important but rare cause of hypertension in young people).

7. Ask to examine the fundi for hypertensive changes (see Table 3.22.1). Describe what you see when presenting, rather than just giving a grade (Fig. 3.22.1).

TABLE 3.22.1 Fundoscopy changes in hypertension

Grade	Changes
Grade 1	Silver wiring
Grade 2	Above change plus arteriovenous nipping
Grade 3	Above changes plus haemorrhages (characteristically flame-shaped) and exudates: soft exudates, also called cotton wool spots, owing to ischaemia; hard exudates owing to lipid residues from leaky vessels
Grade 4	Above changes plus papilloedema

8. Ask if you may examine the rest of the cardiovascular system, looking especially for left ventricular failure and coarctation of the aorta. Usually a fourth heart sound is present in severe hypertension.

9. The abdomen should be examined for renal masses, adrenal masses and an abdominal aneurysm. Auscultate for renal bruits (as a result of fibromuscular dysplasia or atheroma). These may have a diastolic component. Listen first just to the right or left of the midline above the umbilicus. Then sit the patient up and listen in the flanks. (A systolic–diastolic bruit in the costovertebral area suggests a renal arteriovenous fistula.)

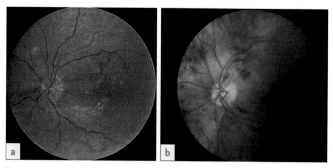

Figure 3.22.1 **(a)** Hypertensive retinopathy grade 3. Note the flame-shaped haemorrhages and cotton wool spots. **(b)** Hypertensive retinopathy grade 4. Note AV nipping, silver wiring and papilloedema. (Talley N, O'Connor S. *Clinical examination*, 7th edn. Figs 7.4, 7.5. Elsevier Australia, 2013, with permission. Courtesy of Dr Chris Kennedy and Prof. Ian Constable. Copyright Lion's Eye Institute, Perth).

10. At the end, ask for the results of urine analysis (proteinuria and haematuria due to glomerular renal disease, either nephritic or nephrotic syndrome).
11. Previous strokes, secondary to hypertension, may cause other physical signs.

Present your findings

- The blood pressure sitting or lying, by palpation and auscultation
- The blood pressure standing, if permitted
- The presence or absence of radio-femoral delay in a young person
- Signs of other abnormalities such as Cushing syndrome or obesity
- Fundoscopy findings — if you have been allowed to look at the fundi.

Examiners' likely questions

- Is the blood pressure normal?
  - See Table 3.22.2.
- Is there a significant postural change?
  - Postural hypotension is a common effect of antihypertensive drugs, diabetic autonomic neuropathy,

TABLE 3.22.2	A classification of blood pressure readings	
Category	Systolic (mmHg)	Diastolic (mmHg)
Optimal	<120	<80
Normal	120–129	80–84
High normal	130–139	85–89
Mild hypertension (grade 1)	140–159	90–99
Moderate hypertension (grade 2)	160–179	100–109
Severe hypertension (grade 3)	>180	>110

(2013 ESH/ESC Guidelines for the management of arterial hypertension. The Task Force for the management of arterial hypertension of the European Society of Hypertension (ESH) and of the European Society of Cardiology (ESC). Reprinted with permission of Oxford University Press.)

alpha-blockers used for prostatic enlargement and rarely a result of Addison disease.

- What measures other than an increase in medication might help reduce this patient's blood pressure?
  - Loss of weight, exercise, salt and alcohol restriction.
- How else might high blood pressure be confirmed?
  - Home blood pressure monitoring, 24-hour blood pressure monitoring. The confident student might go on to talk about the controversy to do with the use of automatic blood pressure measurement in the clinic with a machine programmed to take the blood pressure after the patient has been left alone in the room for 5–10 minutes. These readings are usually lower than those taken by a clinician and have been used in recent blood pressure trials.
- What are the principles of drug treatment of hypertension?
  - You need to know some details of the various classes of antihypertensive medication, the common side effects and indications, such as beta-blockers for hypertensive patients with angina. The approach to drug treatment is changing from the use of a single agent at increasing doses until blood pressure control is achieved or the maximum dose reached to the use of lower doses of drugs in combination.

Marking criteria table

Criteria	Satisfactory	Unsatisfactory
Introduces self, explains task, obtains consent, washes hands before and after	1	0
Makes a general inspection	1	0
Positions patient correctly	2	0–1
Takes blood pressure competently	2	0–1
Is able to comment on the readings and on what would be considered normal or optimal	2	0–1
Knows reasons blood pressure measurement may be inaccurate (e.g. white-coat hypertension)	1	0
Is able to discuss the important complications of hypertension	2	0–1
Is able to say what further examination might be useful	1	0
Is able to discuss home blood pressure monitoring and automatic blood pressure recordings	2	0–1
Knows what non-drug measures may help reduce blood pressure	1	0
Has some thoughts on appropriate initial drug treatment	1	0

Pass mark: 9

Background

Myocardial infarction is a life-threatening disease. Patients who have gone home after having an infarct can be physically and emotionally affected. They may have had difficulty understanding all the advice given to them in hospital. The follow-up appointments for these patients are very important, not just for assessment of cardiac complications or problems but also for monitoring treatment and the patient's mental state.

Introduction

This man was discharged from hospital 3 months ago after an admission for an acute myocardial infarction. Please take a history from him.

Rationale

Management of patients following an infarct can be complicated. They are often prescribed numerous medications and adherence can be a problem. Regular review and explanation about the importance of treatment make a difference to the long-term outcomes in these patients. The examiners will expect you to be able to discuss these issues with the patient and with them. The stem above is broad; the OSCE is likely to be much more directed to permit the assessment to be completed in time, but here we broadly cover the key components.

Method

1. Introduce yourself and explain that you would like to ask some questions about his recent heart attack. Begin with general biographical information that will be important for managing the patient: age, occupation and who is at home. Then ask questions about the infarct itself.

   - Can you tell me what happened when you had your heart attack?
     Let the patient tell you in his own words but, if he has not told you, ask about:
     - the symptoms
     - time it took to get to hospital
     - whether urgent angiography and angioplasty was performed, and how quickly.
   - Do you know if stents were inserted in your arteries — how many?
   - Have you been started on new medications and, if so, do you know what?
   - Were you told if other arteries had blockages that might need treatment?
   - Did they say how much or how little damage there was to your heart?

2. Now ask how things have been since discharge.

   - Have you had any more chest pain or discomfort? If yes, ask about the details.
   - Are you back to normal activities and work?
   - If not, what has been holding you back? For example, more chest pain, dyspnoea, lack of confidence?
   - Have you been to a cardiac rehabilitation course? Has that been helpful?
   - Have you been back to see your cardiologist?
   - Have you had an echocardiogram to look at your heart's function — in hospital or as an outpatient?
   - Have you felt depressed about things or optimistic about the future? (Depression is common after this life-threatening illness.)
   - How have you been managing at work? Has your employer been understanding?

3. Now ask about risk factors.

   - Are you diabetic? For how long? How has your blood sugar control been? Do you know your HbA1c?

- Do you know what your cholesterol level has been? Has it been tested since your heart attack? Have you been told a target cholesterol level?
- Have you been a smoker? How many a day? Have you managed to stop? What have you been using to try to help you stop?
- Have you had high blood pressure? Was this being treated?

4. Now ask about medications.
   - Do you know what medications you are taking?
   - Can you tell me what they are for? (Go through the list with the patient and ask about each drug.)
5. What tablets are you taking?
   - All infarct patients are routinely discharged on:
     - two antiplatelet drugs (aspirin and clopidogrel, ticagrelor or prasugrel)
     - a cholesterol-lowering statin
     - an angiotensin converting enzyme (ACE) inhibitor or angiotensin receptor (AR) blocker and a beta-blocker
     - if there has been significant left ventricular dysfunction, a loop diuretic and spironolactone or eplerenone may have been added.
   - Has it been difficult for you to manage all these tablets? (a way of asking about adherence)
   - Do you think any of the tablets has been causing side effects?

Present your findings

- Outline your understanding of the severity of this infarct and the prognosis.
- Tell the examiners what understanding the patient seems to have about what has happened and the purpose of his medications and likely adherence.
- Give your impression of the patient's mood and how well he is coping emotionally and financially.

Examiners' likely questions

- Are there any test results you would like to look at?
  - Ask to see the patient's electrocardiogram (ECG).

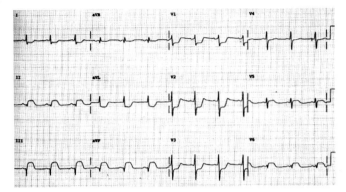

Figure 3.23.1 Acute inferior infarct. Note ST segment elevation and Q waves in leads II, III and aVF (Figure reproduced courtesy of The Canberra Hospital.)

- – Ask for the cholesterol level including the total (TC) and the LDL fraction. The target is a TC of less than 4 mmol/L and an LDL of less than 1.8 mmol/L
- Examiners' comment: 'This is the patient's ECG at the time of his admission to hospital (Fig. 3.23.1). What do you see here?'
    - – ST segment elevation in leads II, III and aVF with reciprocal ST depression in V2. This ECG shows an acute inferior infarct.
- Examiners' comment: 'This is the patient's current ECG.' (Fig. 3.23.2)
    - – In this ECG there are Q waves in leads II, III and aVF with T wave inversion or flattening. This is diagnostic of a completed inferior infarct.
- What might be done to help this man stop smoking?
    - – Most students go on about how difficult this is, but it's better to give your answer in bullet points to impress the examiners:
        - ■ First assess his motivation: is he contemplating stopping, has he already tried, and what has worked before

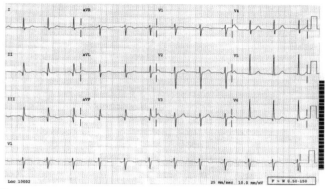

Figure 3.23.2 Old inferior infact. Q waves are present in the anterior leads (Figure reproduced courtesy of The Canberra Hospital.)

- Obtain an understanding of other aspects of his social history, including other substance misuse, and whether anyone else smokes at home
- Provide brief counselling that includes information on the risks of continuing to smoke and stressing that the benefits begin shortly after quitting
- Mention follow-up discussions, and if needed the use of drug and alcohol services and pharmacotherapy (nicotine replacement).

- What would you tell the patient about possible side effects with the prescribed medications?
  - It is important to be frank with patients about possible side effects but to avoid suggesting them.
  - Mention in particular:
    - increased risk of bleeding and bruising with dual antiplatelet drugs
    - a feeling of breathlessness or difficulty taking a satisfying breath with ticagrelor
    - a dry cough with angiotensin converting enzyme (ACE) inhibitors
    - wheezing with beta-blockers.

- Say that trials have shown that myositis occurs only rarely with statin use but that many patients attribute aches and pains to them.

Marking criteria table

Criteria	Satisfactory	Unsatisfactory
Introduces self, explains task, obtains consent	1	0
Asks patient for details of the presenting symptoms	1	0
Asks about treatment received in a logical way, prompts patient where needed	1	0
Asks about risk factors	1	0
Asks about current medication	1	0
Assesses patient's understanding and insight into his illness	2	0–1
Asks about side effects of treatment	1	0
Is able to discuss appropriate follow-up	1	0
Makes an assessment of the psychological effect of the illness	2	0–1
Interprets ECGs adequately	2	0–1

Pass mark: 9

24

Peripheral oedema examination

Background

The assumption that all peripheral oedema is due to heart failure is common but in fact the minority of these patients have heart failure. Many unnecessary tests and much angst will be avoided if this is kept in mind.

Introduction

This man has peripheral oedema. Please assess him.

Rationale

Peripheral oedema is common and has a number of possible causes. The likely cause may be obvious if a proper examination is performed.

Method

1. First, stand back and look at the patient. Obtain consent.
2. While washing your hands, consider the causes of oedema (Box 3.24.1) and which causes are more common.
3. Ask if you may uncover the legs to at least the mid-thighs. Palpate for pitting. Press gently with your thumb over the tibias and note pitting (Fig. 3.24.1). This manoeuvre can be painful for patients if performed thoughtlessly. Meanwhile, keep in mind the important causes of oedema.
4. Note whether the oedema is localised or generalised and whether it is gravitational or not. For ambulant patients, this means it is in the lower legs, but patients who are bed-bound may have it around the sacrum.

Box 3.24.1
Causes of oedema

1. Drugs — calcium channel blockers
2. Cardiac — congestive cardiac failure, cor pulmonale, constrictive pericarditis
3. Venous disease — deep vein thrombosis, varicose veins
4. Renal — nephrotic syndrome
5. Hepatic — cirrhosis
6. Malabsorption or starvation
7. Protein-losing enteropathy
8. Lymphoedema
9. Myxoedema

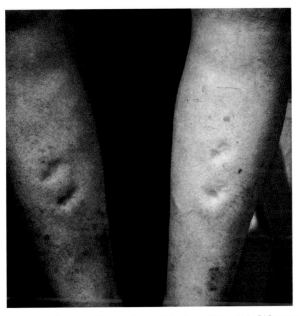

Figure 3.24.1 Severe pitting oedema of the legs (Talley NJ, O'Connor S. *Talley and O'Connor's Clinical Examination*. Elsevier Australia, 2017.)

5. Look for signs of wasting and cachexia (possible evidence of hypoalbuminaemia as a cause of oedema).
6. Signs of myxoedema may be present (non-pitting swelling).

PITTING LOWER LIMB OEDEMA

See Fig. 3.24.1.

7. Define the extent of the oedema (go up to the abdomen if needed, palpating for pitting).
8. Look for signs of deep-vein thrombisis (DVT): 2 cm difference in calf swelling, prominent superficial veins and increased warmth have minor diagnostic value; Homan's sign is unhelpful.
9. Note the presence of varicose veins (a common cause of mild peripheral oedema) and the presence of vein-harvesting scars (for coronary artery surgery or varicose vein treatment).
10. Look for venous staining of the skin above the ankles. Haemosiderin deposition in the skin occurs as a result of increased venous pressure and is an important sign of venous disease (Fig. 3.24.2).
11. Look for venous ulcers (usually on the medial aspect of the leg above the malleolus); scaling and erythema of the skin (venous eczema) may be present (Fig. 3.24.3).
12. Feel the inguinal nodes. Obvious severe lymphadenopathy suggests lymphatic obstruction as the cause of the oedema. (It is non-pitting.)
13. Go to the abdomen and look for abdominal wall oedema (a sign of severe oedema), prominent abdominal wall veins (inferior vena cava obstruction), ascites, any abdominal masses and evidence of liver disease.
14. A pulsatile liver (tricuspid regurgitation) or malignant involvement should be particularly examined for.
15. Next examine the jugular venous pressure (JVP). Large V waves mean tricuspid regurgitation and possible right heart failure as the cause of the oedema.
16. Look for signs of heart failure — displaced apex beat, third heart sound, basal crackles in the lungs.

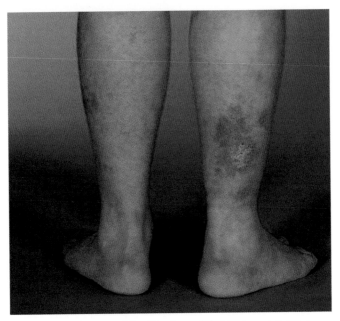

Figure 3.24.2 Venous staining (Courtesy of Dr A Watson, Infectious Diseases Department, The Canberra Hospital.)

17. A patient with signs of chronic obstructive pulmonary disease (COPD) — over-expanded chest, dyspnoea, use of accessory muscles of respiration and cyanosis — may have right heart failure (cor pulmonale) as the cause of oedema.

18. Ask the patient to sit up and examine the sacral area for oedema by attempting to indent the skin gently with your thumb.

19. Finally, examine for delayed ankle jerks (to exclude hypothyroidism) and look at the urine analysis. (Albuminuria may mean nephrotic syndrome and hypoalbuminaemia are the cause of the oedema.)

20. Ask if you may examine the genitals with severe oedema (usually with nephrotic syndrome).

Remember that vasodilating drugs used for hypertension or angina are a very common cause of oedema.

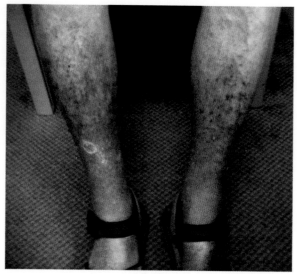

Figure 3.24.3 Venous eczema, with evidence of haemosiderin pigmentation and superficial varicosities (Blyth KG, Jones JB, Scott HR. *Davidson's Foundations of Clinical Practice.* Elsevier Ltd, 2009.)

NON-PITTING LOWER LIMB OEDEMA

21. Feel for lymphadenopathy. Examine for an enlarged liver. Look for radiotherapy marks.
22. Examine for signs of hypothyroidism (myxoedema)

Present your findings

- The extent of the oedema
- Whether it is pitting or not
- The presence or absence of signs of venous disease
- Any signs of cachexia or heart failure
- An ulcer or tinea (interdigital) as this can cause life-threatening infections in lymphoedema.

Examiners' likely questions

- What is the most likely cause of this oedema?
    - This depends if it's pitting (Box 3.24.1) or non-pitting. Mention the important causes of non-pitting oedema,

including lymphoedema (from malignant infiltration, radiotherapy, congenital disease, filariasis, Milroy disease) and myxoedema.

- What questions would you like to ask the patient?
  - Do you take any blood pressure tablets? (calcium antagonists)
  - Have you had problems with varicose veins?
  - Does the swelling get worse as the day goes on? (typical of pitting oedema)
  - Have you been treated with supporting stockings or with fluid tablets (diuretics)?
- How would you investigate this patient?
  - Obvious venous disease may require no investigation.
  - If there are signs of heart failure, suggest cardiac investigations — chest X-ray, ECG, echocardiogram.
  - If there is cachexia or non-gravitational generalised oedema, suggest liver function tests and serum albumin and urinary protein measurements.

Marking criteria table

Criteria	Satisfactory	Unsatisfactory
Introduces self, explains task, obtains consent, washes hands before and after	1	0
Makes general assessment of the patient	1	0
Inspects legs and gently tests for pitting oedema	2	0–1
Notes associated skin changes	1	0
Notes varicose veins	1	0
Examines inguinal nodes	1	0
Looks for evidence of right heart failure	2	0–1
Is able to discuss possible causes on the basis of the examination findings	2	0–1

Pass mark: 6

Perform an electrocardiogram

Background

An electrocardiogram (ECG) is an essential investigation that can be performed at the bedside. It provides vital information about the electrical activity of the heart, which in turn gives information about pathology affecting the heart.

Introduction

Mrs Tunbridge is a 70-year-old woman who recently had a myocardial infarction and has presented with chest pain and breathlessness. You have been requested to conduct an ECG. Please proceed.

Rationale

The examiners want you to be able to show them that you know how an ECG is recorded.

Method

1. You need to be able to show them:
   - how to explain to the patient what you are doing, after obtaining consent
   - where the ECG electrodes go (Fig. 3.25.1)
   - how and where to attach the wires
   - how to set the paper speed
   - how to interpret the ECG and possibly
   - recognise some common technical faults in a recorded ECG
     - baseline wander (Fig. 3.25.2)

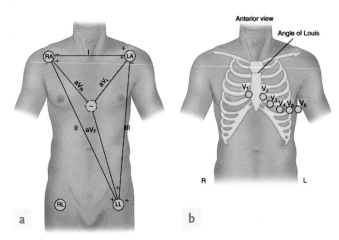

Figure 3.25.1 ECG electrode placement: **(a)** Standard limb leads. Leads are located on the extremities: right arm (RA), left arm (LA), and left leg (LL). The right leg electrode serves as a ground. Leads I, II, and III are bipolar, with each using a positive electrode and a negative electrode. Leads aVR, aVL, and aVF are augmented unipolar leads that use the calculated centre of the heart as their negative electrode **(b)** Precordial leads. V1 to V6 are the six standard precordial leads and are placed as follows: V1, fourth intercostal space, right sternal border; V2, fourth intercostal space, left sternal border; V3, equidistant between V2 and V4; V4, fifth intercostal space, left midclavicular line; V5, anterior axillary line, same horizontal level as V4; V6, midaxillary line, same horizontal level as V4 (Stacy KM, Urden LD and Lough ME. *Critical Care Nursing: Diagnosis and Management* 9th edn. Elsevier Inc., 2021.)

- movement artifact, for example from a Parkinsonian tremor (Fig. 3.25.3)
- incorrect paper speed (Fig. 3.25.4)
- incorrect limb lead placement (Fig. 3.25.5)
- incorrect chest lead placement (Fig. 3.25.6)

Examiners' likely questions

Here they may show you some examples of technically unsatisfactory ECGs as listed above.

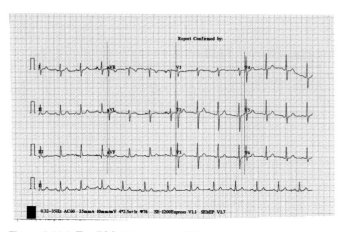

Figure 3.25.2 The ECG looks uneven. This is usually the result of movement, sometimes just breathing. It is more likely if the electrodes are not firmly attached (Figure reproduced courtesy of The Canberra Hospital.)

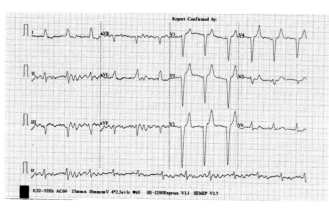

Figure 3.25.3 Movement of the patient during the recording – voluntary or involuntary, e.g. tremor — causes parts of the tracing to look shaky (Figure reproduced courtesy of The Canberra Hospital.)

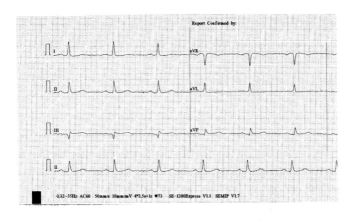

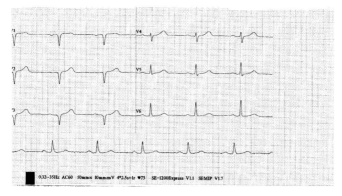

Figure 3.25.4 The normal paper speed is 25 mm/s but most ECG machines can be set at 50 mm/s. This is used occasionally to make the ECG intervals easier to measure but must be recognised or everything looks slow and long (Figure reproduced courtesy of The Canberra Hospital.)

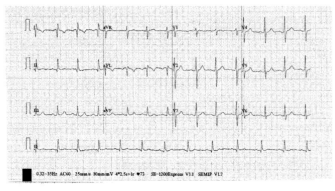

Figure 3.25.5 If the leads are placed on the wrong limbs, e.g. left and right arm leads reversed, the ECG axis looks abnormal and typically lead aVR has upright complexes instead of downward ones (Figure reproduced courtesy of The Canberra Hospital.)

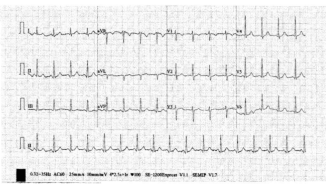

Figure 3.25.6 If the chest leads are put on in the wrong order (often V2 and V3 are reversed) the progression of R waves looks abnormal. For example, V2 has a taller R wave than V3 (Figure reproduced courtesy of The Canberra Hospital.)

- Baseline wander — make sure the electrodes are making good contact with the skin; shave hairy skin
- Tremor — put the arm leads on the shoulders
- Prosthetic leg — place electrode on the thigh if there is one, otherwise on lower abdomen.

Marking criteria table

Criteria	Satisfactory	Unsatisfactory
Introduces self, explains task, obtains consent, washes hands	1	0
Explains procedure to patient	1	0
Discusses skin preparation	1	0
Knows roughly where the electrodes are placed	1	0
Has some understanding of difference between limb and chest leads	1	0
Knows to label the tracing	1	0
Knows about calibration and paper speed	1	0
Recognises common technical problems	2	0–1

Pass mark: 6

Take a history — chronic cough

Background

Cough is a common presenting problem. The likely causes are often clear once a good history has been taken. This patient will often be an actor schooled in the answers she should give and may even be able to cough during the interview.

Introduction

This woman has a problem with cough. Take a history from her.

Rationale

Much information about the possible causes of a cough will come from the history. Students should be able to present a rational differential diagnosis after taking this history.

Method

Introduce yourself, then ask:

- May I ask you some questions? I gather you have had problems with a cough.
- How long have you had it? (acute versus chronic) Is the cough getting worse? Is it seasonal or with known triggers?
- Do you cough up any phlegm? How much? A teaspoon full, a cup full? (Large volumes usually mean bronchiectasis.)
- Is the phlegm discoloured? What colour is it (e.g. white, yellow)? Is it mixed with blood? (haemoptysis)
- Is the cough worse when you lie down and does it keep you awake? (suggests cardiac failure with paroxysmal nocturnal dyspnoea)

- Do you get wheezy or breathless? (asthma, especially if better with a bronchodilator; chronic obstructive pulmonary disease — COPD)
- How far can you walk before becoming too breathless to go on? How many flights of steps can you climb? (e.g. a dry cough with dyspnoea in COPD, interstitial lung disease)
- Have you had any problems with chest pain that makes it painful to take big breaths? (pleurisy)
- What do you do if the cough and breathlessness become worse or if you develop a fever? (Does the patient have an action plan, e.g. for asthma?)
- Do you have a postnasal drip (explain it to them), or rhinitis (upper airways cough)?
- Are you a smoker? Or in the past? How many a day for how many years? (Smoking and haemoptysis would suggest a lung cancer may be present.)
- Take a brief occupational history. (Hypersensitivity pneumonitis can occur from many different exposures (e.g farmer's lung). High risk occupations for asbestos include construction workers, boiler makers and shipyard workers.)
- What lung problems have been diagnosed in the past? When? How was this diagnosed?
- What treatment are you having at the moment? Do you take blood pressure medications? (Try to find out if they are on an angiotensin converting enzyme (ACE) inhibitor.)
- Do you have burning in the chest that rises up towards the throat (heartburn) or acid coming back into your mouth or a hoarse voice? (gastro-oesophageal reflux),
- Were you born overseas? (relevant for tuberculosis)
- Did you recently travel or have you recently had swelling in your legs? (venous thromboembolism)
- Do you have heart problems? Have you noticed any ankle swelling? (right heart failure)
- How has the cough interfered with your daily life and activities?

Present your findings

- Synthesise and present your findings. Mention especially the character and duration of the cough. Describe the sputum.

- Consider a differential diagnosis. Examples include:
  - long-term very productive cough — bronchiectasis
  - recent productive cough — chest infection, exacerbation of chronic obstructive pulmonary disease (COPD)
  - dry cough — interstitial lung disease, angiotensin converting enzyme (ACE) inhibitor drugs
  - cough at night — heart failure, gastro-oesophageal reflux disease
  - change in character of cough — infection, carcinoma of the lung
  - haemoptysis — tuberculosis, carcinoma of the lung

Examiners' likely questions

- What is the most likely diagnosis, based on your history?
  - This depends on whether it is an acute cough (<3 weeks, e.g. pneumonia, acute exacerbation of COPD) or a chronic cough (e.g. COPD, asthma, bronchiectasis, carcinoma of the lung, cardiac failure or a medication side effect).
- What physical findings would you expect to find on examination?
  - Say you would ask the patient to cough — loose or dry cough
  - You would like to see a sputum sample — bloody, purulent etc.
  - Coarse crackles and wheezes — bronchiectasis
  - Wheeze only (reversible) — asthma
  - Fine end-inspiratory basal crackles — interstitial lung disease.
  - Signs of consolidation — pneumonia (unlikely)
  - Normal examination — many patients with dry cough.
- What action plan does the patient have for asthma? Is it satisfactory?

Marking criteria table

Criteria	Satisfactory	Unsatisfactory
Introduces self, explains task, obtains consent	1	0
Asks sensible questions about the cough; character, duration etc.	3	0–2
Asks about associated features	2	0–1
Asks relevant questions about the patient's history, e.g. smoking, previous lung disease	2	0–1
Asks about current treatment (including ACE inhibitors)	1	0
Asks how much the cough has affected the patient's life	1	0
Gives a sensible differential diagnosis based on the history	2	0–1
Suggests likely examination findings for each of these diagnoses	2	0–1

Pass mark: 8

Take a history — breathlessness

Background

Breathlessness or dyspnoea is a very common presenting symptom. Dyspnoea is a subjective sensation of an increase in the work of breathing. Apart from pathological conditions, lack of fitness, advancing age and anxiety are all common causes.

Introduction

This man is short of breath. Take a history from him about this.

Rationale

Dyspnoea is a common symptom with many possible causes. A careful history may make the diagnosis or at least direct the examination and investigations. Methodical questioning is required.

Method

1. Introduce yourself, explain what you will be doing and obtain consent.
2. Ask him the following:
   - How long have you had shortness of breath? Does it come on very quickly? (e.g. asthma, pulmonary embolus, pneumothorax, or pulmonary oedema)
   - When are you short of breath? (on exertion; lying flat — orthopnoea or paroxysmal nocturnal dyspnoea)?
   - Do you find you are short of breath only when you try to do things? or Do you need to sleep propped up in

bed or in a chair because you are breathless at night? (orthopnoea)

- Do you wake up at night breathless and have to get up and walk around? (paroxysmal nocturnal dyspnoea)
- Is the feeling one of having difficulty getting a satisfying breath? (anxiety)
- How bad is the breathlessness? (New York Heart Association Grades I–IV; IV is dyspnoea at rest) Does it stop you walking upstairs or up hills?
- Did it come on very suddenly? Is it associated with chest pain? (suggests pulmonary embolus (PE) — ask about risk factors, previous PE, immobilisation, recent surgery)
- Is the shortness of breath getting worse? (more worrying)
- When you feel breathless, are you wheezy in the chest? (suggests asthma or chronic obstructive pulmonary disase (COPD))
- Is there a feeling of tightness or heaviness in the chest associated with it? (suggests angina)
- Do you have a cough?
- Do you cough up any sputum? Is it discoloured? How much do you cough up — would it be half a cup full or more? (suggests bronchiectasis)
- Have you had any chest pain that is worse when you breathe? (pleuritic pain; suggests pleurisy, chest infection or pulmonary embolus)
- Have you had a fever or problems with chest infections in the past? (pneumonia, exacerbation of COPD)
- Are you a smoker? If so, for how long? How many? Work out the number of packet years of smoking (20/day for a year = 1 packet year)
- Have you had heart problems in the past? Have you had a heart attack? Was there said to have been much damage to your heart? (suggests heart failure)
- Have you been found to have a murmur or valve problem? (suggests heart failure secondary to valvular disease or may be a symptom of aortic or mitral stenosis)
- Have you been told your heart is enlarged or you have a 'cardiomyopathy'? If so, ask about alcohol consumption

— a risk factor for cardiomyopathy or a family history of cardiomyopathy.
- Have you been told you have anaemia or a low blood count?
- How has your shortness of breath affected you?
- Have you been able to work? What sort of work do you do? Is it a physical job? Have there been financial problems as a result? Can you do ordinary things around the house?
- Do you know the results of any tests of your heart or lungs?
- Have you been started on any treatment? Ask about fluid tablets and inhalers.

Present your findings

- Summarise the nature and severity of the patient's symptoms. Try to present a differential diagnosis and indicate what you think is the likely problem.
- Explain what has led you to this conclusion, for example 'Mr Smith has been a very heavy smoker for many years and his breathlessness is associated with wheeze. He has never had orthopnoea or a diagnosis of heart disease. I think his breathlessness is most likely the result of chronic obstructive pulmonary disease.'

Examiners' likely questions

- What is your differential diagnosis for this man?
  - The examiners will want you to use the patient's answers to give a sensible differential diagnosis.
- Is this likely to be a cardiac or respiratory problem? Why?
  - Outline the features in the history that point to a particular cause.
- How badly has it affected his life?
  - Talk about the activities the patient can no longer do in relation to work, activities of daily living (ADLs).
- What are likely to be the most useful investigations in the first instance?
  - They do not want you to suggest random investigations but to direct these at the likely problem.

- They will also want you to comment on the way the patient and the family are coping with this acute or chronic problem.

Marking criteria table

Criteria	Satisfactory	Unsatisfactory
Introduces self, explains task, obtains consent	1	0
Asks about and quantifies severity and rapidity of onset	2	0–1
Asks about associated features	2	0–1
Is methodical in asking relevant questions in response to patient's answers	1	0
Finds out relevant aspects of past history and risk factors	2	0–1
Has a sensible approach to investigations based on the history	1	0
Gives a plausible differential diagnosis	1	0
Demonstrates an understanding of the effect of the patient's symptoms on ability to work or live normally	2	0–1

Pass mark: 7

Examination of a patient with breathlessness

Background

The history may suggest the likely system involved, but a focused examination of both heart and lungs is normally required.

Introduction

The examiners are likely to direct you to a particular system (usually the heart or lungs).

- This woman has been breathless for some months. Please examine her respiratory system.

  Otherwise a more general examination — heart and lungs — is required if time permits unless the general inspection suggests the appropriate system, for example pursed lips breathing and an overinflated chest indicating chronic obstructive pulmonary disease (COPD).

Rationale

Dyspnoea is a very common symptom with many possible causes — cardiac, respiratory, haematological (anaemia) and more general (e.g. psychogenic). A careful examination will help in establishing a sensible differential diagnosis and prevent unnecessary investigations. The examiners will expect you to have a sensible approach to the differential diagnosis and appropriate examination.

If the patient is breathless at rest the general inspection may give a clue to the cause and severity:

- use of the accessory muscles of respiration (severe)
- cyanosis (severe)

- sighing respiration (anxiety)
- rapid deep respiration (ketoacidosis)
- lack of respiratory effort, drowsiness (CO_2 narcosis); late sign audible wheeze (bronchoconstriction)
- over-expanded chest (COPD)
- obesity (obesity hypoventilation syndrome and obstructive sleep apnoea)
- anaemia.

Method

1. Examine her respiratory system based on the stem, including her chest back and front, assessing especially for:
   - cough (look at the sputum)
   - clubbing (suppurative lung disease or interstitial lung disease)
   - Hoover sign (COPD)
   - fever (chest infection, pneumonia)
   - wheeze
   - bronchial breathing (consolidation)
   - absent breath sounds (pneumothorax, pleural effusion and severe asthma)
   - stridor (tracheal obstruction)
   - diaphragmatic excursion on percussion (looking for diaphragmatic paralysis)
2. If there is time, examine the cardiovascular system, looking in addition for:
   - arrhythmia, such as atrial fibrillation with a rapid ventricular response rate
   - signs of cardiac failure (S3, displaced apex beat, basal crackles, elevated jugular venous pressure (JVP), positive hepatojugular reflux test)
   - aortic stenosis or regurgitation (or both)
   - mitral stenosis
   - Kussmaul sign — elevation of JVP during inspiration (pericardial tamponade — associated with severe dyspnoea, hypotension and tachycardia)

Present your findings

Describe the abnormal findings. Is the patient breathless at rest? Try to decide if the problem is cardiac, respiratory or something else.

Examiners' likely questions

- Is the cause of the patient's breathlessness obvious?
    - COPD, asthma, heart failure, asthma, valvular heart disease are possible obvious abnormalities.
- What questions might you ask the patient?
    - Have you had heart or lung problems in the past? What sort of problems? Are you breathless when you lie flat? (orthopnoea) Do you wake up breathless during the night? (paroxysmal nocturnal dyspnoea)
    - Have you been a smoker?
- What investigations might be useful?
    - Try to decide if the problem is respiratory or cardiac. A chest X-ray would be a useful test for either problem. Be prepared to discuss the possible findings.
    - If the problem seems cardiac, an electrocardiogram (ECG) might show atrial fibrillation or evidence of previous myocardial infarction.
    - An ECG will be helpful for measuring left ventricular function and assessing valvular disease.
    - Full blood count (FBC) for anaemia or evidence of acute infection (raised white cell count)
    - Consider asking for a blood gas and for a lactate measurement in an acute flair of asthma or COPD

Marking criteria table

Criteria	Satisfactory	Unsatisfactory
Introduces self, explains task, obtains consent, washes hands before and after	1	0
Makes a careful general inspection	2	0–1
Notes breathlessness, apparent increased work of breathing	2	0–1
Looks for peripheral signs of heart and lung disease	3	0–2
Performs an efficient respiratory examination	2	0–1
Performs an efficient cardiac examination	2	0–1
Describes important positive and negative findings	3	0–2
A sensible differential diagnosis	2	0–1
Gives a list of appropriate investigations	3	0–2

Pass mark: 14

Examine a patient with haemoptysis

Background

The patient may well be an actor, but the same signs must be looked for and explained to the examiners as for a real patient.

Introduction

This man has haemoptysis and weight loss. Please examine him.

Rationale

The possibilities include carcinoma of the lung and, much less likely in an OSCE, tuberculosis. General signs such as wasting and dyspnoea are as important as more specific ones such as tracheal deviation.

Method

1. Wash your hands. Introduce yourself, explain the task and obtain consent.
2. Stand back and look for obvious evidence of weight loss or cachexia.
3. Ask the patient to cough.
4. Ask if there is a sputum mug for you to inspect.
5. Carefully inspect the nails of his hands for clubbing and look for wrist swelling. (hypertrophic pulmonary osteoarthropathy)
6. Look for wasting of the small muscles of the hands. (Pancoast tumour)
7. Feel for cervical and other lymph node groups.

8. Palpate for tracheal deviation. Upper lobe tumours are associated with tracheal deviation — to the affected side if there is upper lobe collapse or fibrosis (Fig. 3.29.1).
9. Examine his chest systematically back and front. The examination may be normal.
10. Particularly look for unilateral signs that might indicate a lung cancer (e.g. evidence of mediastinal shift, local area of dullness, signs of an effusion, fixed inspiratory wheeze).
11. Palpate for tender ribs (from metastatic deposits).
12. Look also for previous thoracotomy scars and pleural drainage tube scars (Fig. 3.29.2).
13. If there are signs in the lung apex, look at the pupils for Horner syndrome on one (the same) side (unilateral constricted pupil, partial ptosis).

Present your findings

Describe the important positive and negative findings as outlined above. Suggest a differential diagnosis.

Examiners' likely questions

- What findings are consistent with your differential diagnosis?
- What investigations might be helpful?
    - Sputum cytology
    - Temperature chart
    - Chest X-ray
    - Bronchoscopy and washings
    - CT scan.
  Be able to say what information each of these might provide.
- What questions would you ask the patient?
    - Have you lost weight?
    - Have you been a smoker?
    - Have you been in contact with someone with tuberculosis?
    - Have you been in contact with asbestos? (increased risk of mesothelioma and non-small cell lung cancer)
- What are the extra-pulmonary manifestations of lung cancer?
    - This depends on the cancer type.

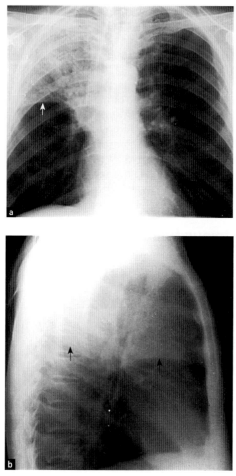

Figure 3.29.1 PA **(a)** and lateral **(b)** Right upper lobe consolidation. The right upper lobe is opacified and is limited inferiorly by the horizontal fissure (arrows). There must be some collapse as well, as the fissure shows some elevation. These changes could be due to a bacterial lobar pneumonia per se, but a central bronchostenotic lesion should be considered. If the pneumonia persists, a bronchoscopy is indicated to search for a central carcinoma (Talley NJ, O'Connor S. *Talley and O'Connor's Clinical Examination*. Elsevier Australia, 2017.)

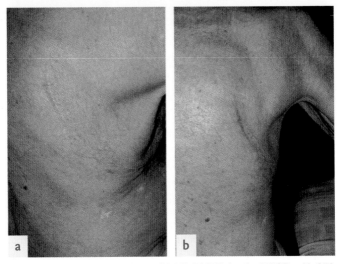

Figure 3.29.2 Thoracotomy scar (Hall T. *PACES for the MRCP: with 250 clinical cases*, 3rd edn. Elsevier, 2013.)

Marking criteria table

Criteria	Satisfactory	Unsatisfactory
Introduces self, explains task, obtains consent, washes hands before and after	1	0
Makes a general inspection, especially for wasting	1	0
Observes contact precautions if required	1	0
Asks patient to cough	1	0
Asks to see sputum mug	1	0
Looks for clubbing and hypertrophic pulmonary osteoarthropathy	2	0–1
Examines the chest for scars, drains etc.	2	0–1
Performs a competent chest examination	3	0–2
Has a sensible differential diagnosis	1	0
Has some sensible suggestions for investigations	2	0–1

Pass mark: 9

Take an occupational lung history

Background

Asking a patient about his or her occupation should be routine. It may be very important in deciding whether he or she can go back to work. Many occupations, such as commercial driving, require licensing, and some illnesses affect patients' ability to work legally.

Occupational lung disease is the result of work or hobbies and taking a careful history will help with the diagnosis.

Introduction

This man has been breathless. Take an occupational history from him.

Rationale

Occupational chest physicians consider themselves to be detectives. They are adept at uncovering details of a patient's past or present occupation that may be associated with lung disease. Students will be expected to have a basic knowledge of this important area.

Method

Ask him:

1. What is your job?
2. What does this involve, in detail?
3. How long have you been doing this work?
4. What ventilation arrangements or masks are provided at work? Do you use them all the time?

5. Are you more breathless as the working week goes on and better at weekends? (occupational asthma)
6. Are you or other workers or customers permitted to smoke at work?
7. Does your work involve exposure to dusts, solvents or animals? (if this is not already clear) (e.g. stone masons, who often work cutting kitchen benches or on repairing sandstone buildings and monuments, are at risk of silicosis).
8. Have you ever worked with asbestos? This might include:
   – mining
   – exposure to lagging on pipes (often in the navy)
   – demolition work
   – home renovations — asbestos insulation or cutting up of sheets of asbestos.
9. Has someone in the family worked with asbestos? (Contaminated clothing can lead to exposure of other family members.)
10. If you have worked as a miner, has there been regular screening of your lungs with X-rays and lung function assessment?
11. What previous work have you done? What did that involve?
12. Do you have any hobbies or pets? (Hobbies might involve exposure to dusts and solvents. Bird keepers are at risk of psittacosis.)

Present your findings

Outline the possible risk associated with the patient's work or hobbies (Table 3.30.1).

Examiners' likely questions

- Do you think this patient has had significant occupational exposure to dusts?
- Was adequate protection provided at work, and was it used?
- Have any respiratory investigations been performed? What investigations would you recommend?
  - Chest X-ray, chest CT
  - Pulmonary function tests (spirometry)

TABLE 3.30.1 Occupational exposure risks

Material implicated in lung disease	Consider with the following exposures or occupations
Silica	Stone masons, who often work cutting kitchen benches or on repairing sandstone buildings and monuments
Asbestos	Mining exposure to lagging on pipes (often in the navy) demolition work Home renovations — asbestos insulation or cutting up of sheets of asbestos
Allergens	Occupational asthma
Bird keepers	Psittacosis, hypersensitivity pneumonitis (also seen with many plant and animal exposures)

Marking criteria table

Criteria	Satisfactory	Unsatisfactory
Introduces self, explains task, obtains consent	1	0
Asks what work the patient does now and has done in the past	2	0–1
Goes on to detailed questions about the work and what it involves	1	0
Asks about protective measures provided at work	1	0
Asks about hobbies and weekend jobs that might involve dust exposure	1	0
Asks about smoking (currently and previously)	1	0
Asks about pets	1	0
Asks about previous investigations including X-rays — how often, how recently	2	0–1

Pass mark: 5

Smoking cessation

Background

Smoking is a major public health problem globally. In Australia, there are 19 000 smoking-related deaths per year. It increases risk of cancer (e.g. lung, oesophageal, oral, laryngeal, testicular) and causes poor wound healing, gingivitis, pregnancy complications, chronic pulmonary disease and ischaemic heart disease.

Patients may come asking for help with smoking cessation, especially after an illness. It should also be a routine part of patient assessment to ask, at every opportunity, about smoking and to offer help with cessation.

Introduction

You are the intern working on the respiratory team at a tertiary hospital. You are asked to review Mr Andrews, a 72-year-old male who is currently admitted under your team for an exacerbation of chronic obstructive pulmonary disease (COPD). You are informed that he is still smoking and asked to please provide brief intervention, counselling him regarding smoking cessation.

Rationale

As health professionals, we have many opportunities to intervene and encourage smoking cessation. It is crucial we are prepared for these conversations as they arise. See Box 3.31.1.

Box 3.31.1
Five A's of smoking cessation

Ask — are you a smoker? (Check if they've EVER been a smoker (they may have quit that day!)
Assess — take smoking history (including second-hand smoke), assess stage of change
Advice — provide advice
Assist — offer intervention
Arrange follow-up

Stages of change

There are five stages smokers may progress through and you need to assess in the station where the patient is now (also see page 221):

1. Pre-contemplation (NOT ready to quit)
2. Contemplation (considering a quit attempt)
3. Preparation (actively planning a quit attempt)
4. Action (actively involved in a quit attempt right now)
5. Maintenance (success in stopping smoking)

Useful strategies in approaching cessation

It is important to consider the patients as individuals to find appropriate and effective strategies for them. Let this be a two-way conversation; ask them what has worked for them in the past and what they perceive to be the biggest challenges they will have to overcome.

When craving a cigarette, patients may find it helpful to:

- delay
- deep breath
- drink water
- do something else.

What to expect

Withdrawing from cigarettes can result in a range of symptoms, as listed below. Patients can expect these symptoms to resolve after 10 days.

- Restlessness
- Cravings
- Hunger

- Irritability
- Impaired concentration
- Headache
- Insomnia
- Depression

Method

You obtain the following history.

Mr Andrews is a 72-year-old man currently admitted to hospital under the respiratory team for management of a COPD exacerbation. He presented feeling breathless and with a productive cough. Since admission, his symptoms have improved significantly, and he is hoping to be discharged home. He has no plans to stop smoking on discharge.

He has been a smoker for 45 years, smoking 20–30 cigarettes per day. He has tried to stop twice before, both times without any additional support, pharmacological or otherwise. The first time (5 years ago), he remained off cigarettes for 1 year after his first grandchild was born, but went back to smoking during a stressful period at work. The second time (last year), he remained off cigarettes for 3 months and started again when out drinking with friends who were smoking.

He drinks four alcoholic drinks (beer) on most days, and 10 on the weekend days when he is at the pub with friends. He occasionally smokes marijuana, about once a month, when offered by friends. He does not use any other drugs.

He lives with his wife and dog. He has three grandchildren, who live in the same suburb. They are his biggest motivation to quit. He would also like to be able to be more active and able to keep up with his wife and dog when he goes for a walk. He has supportive friends but finds it difficult to keep away from alcohol and cigarettes in their company.

If prompted, he would like to find out more about different strategies to help him quit, as well as different services available. He is not interested in pharmacological help.

Present your findings

- Outline the history you have obtained.
- Define the readiness to quit. Contemplation is the stage in this case.

- Give a realistic outline of what is possible to help the patient to become a non-smoker.

Examiners' likely questions

- Where do you think the patient currently falls in the stages of change?
- What medical information would you give to the patient with regard to the benefits of becoming a non-smoker?
  - Stopping smoking results in substantial health benefits, including a reduced risk of coronary artery disease, cancers, lung disease (COPD), and hip fracture (osteoporosis).
- How would you counsel this patient on nicotine withdrawal?
  - This depends on the stage. Providing resources and support, setting a quit date, counselling on controlling cravings and considering pharmacologic approaches (e.g. nicotine replacement) are all relevant.

Marking criteria table

Criteria	Satisfactory	Unsatisfactory
Asks about tobacco use	1	0
Quantifies current use	1	0
Quantifies duration of smoking	1	0
Assesses motivation to quit	1	0
Asks about previous attempts to quit	1	0
Asks about reasons to quit	1	0
Asks about obstacles to quitting	1	0
Assists the smoker in quitting	1	0
Offers brief advice on benefits of quitting	1	0
Offers available services	1	0
Correctly assesses stage of change	1	0
Answers patient's questions appropriately	1	0
Arranges follow-up	1	0

Pass mark: 10

Take a history — jaundice

Background

Jaundice may result from obstruction of the biliary tree (chole-static), acute or chronic liver disease (hepatocellular), or rarely haemolysis of red blood cells. The most common underlying disease is cirrhosis of the liver, often due to excessive alcohol consumption, although other possible causes need to be considered while taking the history.

Introduction

This man has noticed that his sclerae have turned yellow (Fig. 3.32.1). Please take a history from him.

Rationale

In many cases the cause of jaundice can be established from the history. If not, the information obtained from the history should at least direct investigations.

Method

This is likely to be jaundice (which should be obvious on inspection). Ask him the following:

1. Have you noticed a change in the colour of your skin and the whites of your eyes?
2. How long has it been present? Is it getting better or worse? Has it happened before?
3. Are you itchy? (An indication this may be obstructive — cholestatic — jaundice.)
4. Has the colour of your urine or stools changed? (dark urine and pale stools in obstructive jaundice)

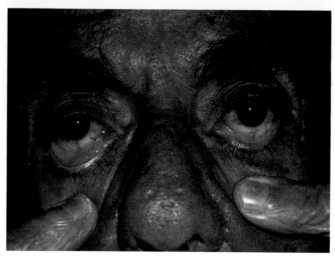

Figure 3.32.1 Jaundice (Talley NJ, O'Connor S. *Talley and O'Connor's Examination Medicine.* Elsevier Australia, 2020.)

5. Have you lost weight? (e.g. painless jaundice with malignancy involving the liver or pancreas)

6. Do you have any abdominal pain? Whereabouts? (Ask about the symptoms of biliary pain from stone obstruction or cholangitis complicating any cause of sluggish bile flow.)

7. Does your abdomen swell up? (ascites) Do you develop leg swelling? (oedema)

8. Have you ever vomited blood or passed black stools? (haematemesis and melaena — from bleeding oesophageal varices)

9. Have you ever had hepatitis? Have you travelled overseas? (infection, hepatitis)

10. Have you had fatigue, nausea, anorexia, myalgias, bruising? (common symptoms of liver disease)

11. Are you a diabetic? (haemochromatosis)

12. Do you now drink, or have you in the past drunk, large amounts of alcohol? (80 g a day for more than 10 years is

usually required to cause cirrhosis in men; women are at risk with less exposure.)

13. Do you suffer any memory loss or confusion? (hepatic encephalopathy) Have you been told to restrict your protein intake because of this?

14. Have you had a liver biopsy? Do you know what is wrong with your liver? Has excess alcohol or viral infection been mentioned as a cause? (probe for alcohol abuse and current alcohol consumption)

15. Do you have any history of blood transfusions, drug use, tattoos or body piercing? (e.g. hepatitis C or B) Has anti-viral treatment been commenced?

16. Have oesophageal varices been banded? Have there been regular ultrasounds to check for hepatocellular carcinoma? (an important complication of cirrhosis)

17. Take the medication history (drug-induced hepatitis).

18. Ask whether there is a family history of liver problems.

19. Ask if this disease (especially if it is chronic) has affected employment and the family.

20. Has liver transplant ever been mentioned as a possible treatment?

Present your findings

- If the aetiology of the jaundice is clear (e.g. excessive alcohol use), begin by outlining this.
- Talk then about whether this is a chronic or acute presentation.
- Outline the patient's current treatment regime, drugs, alcohol restriction etc.
- Explain how the disease has affected the patient's employment, life and family.

Examiner's' likely questions

- Has the patient a good understanding of his illness?
  - Explain what he seems to know about the cause and severity of the condition.
- How would you explain the severity of the problem and the likely prognosis to him and his family?
  - In cirrhosis, severity can be evaluated by the Childs–Pugh classification (which is scored A, B or C based on

the absence or presence of encephalopathy, ascites, and abnormal liver function as measured by the bilirubin, albumin and international normalised ratio (INR)). Ask the examiners for this information if not given to you. C has the worst prognosis (life expectancy 1–3 years).

- If the patient has advanced cirrhosis with evidence of chronic liver failure, the implications are very serious. You need to be able to outline in layman's terms the likely course of the disease and the treatment that may be required, such as preventing and treating variceal bleeding, treatment for ascites including abdominal paracentesis (drainage), diagnosing and treatment for spontaneous bacterial peritonitis, and diagnosis and treatment of hepatic encephalopathy and hepatorenal syndrome.

- How might you talk to him about ways of helping him to stop drinking alcohol?
    - Begin by outlining your assessment of the patient's awareness of the problem and the implications of his continuing to drink alcohol. Discuss any attempts he has made previously to stop drinking and how effective they were. Have a general approach to this problem and of how strategies such as joining groups like Alcoholics Anonymous may help. Discuss the role of the family and their current understanding of the problem.

Marking criteria table

Criteria	Satisfactory	Unsatisfactory
Introduces self, explains task, obtains consent	1	0
Asks about the duration of the changes	1	0
Asks about associated changes — weight, urine etc.	2	0–1
Asks about complications — melaena, ascites etc.	2	0–1
Asks about hepatitis and alcohol consumption	2	0–1
Asks about treatment	1	0
Asks about severity of effect on patient's life and family	2	0–1
Presents findings coherently	1	0
Comments on effect of illness and patient's insight	2	0–1

Pass mark: 10

Background

Patients with acute liver failure are always to be too sick to be involved in the exam, but chronic patients are often available as, of course, are actors.

Introduction

This man has been diagnosed as having liver failure. Please examine his abdomen.

Rationale

The examination of these patients can help with the assessment of severity and establish the presence of portal hypertension. There are often findings that help distinguish acute from chronic liver failure.

Method

1. Wash your hands.
2. Ask the patient's permission to examine his abdomen and ask him to lie flat with his abdomen exposed from the lower ribs to the symphysis pubis.
3. While the patient is undressing, stand back to look for obvious signs of chronic liver disease.
4. Ask whether any part of his abdomen is tender and to let you know if any part of the examination is uncomfortable.
5. Examine the abdomen systematically (inspect, palpate, percuss, auscultate). Assess particularly for ascites and hepatosplenomegaly (Fig. 3.33.1). Note any distended abdominal veins (Fig. 3.33.2).

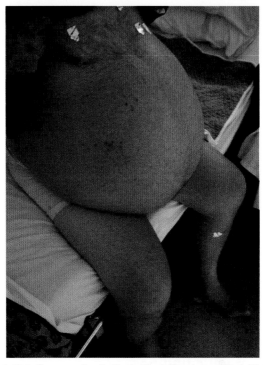

Figure 3.33.1 Gross ascites (patient sitting) (Courtesy of Dr A Watson, Infectious Diseases Department, The Canberra Hospital.)

6. Ask whether you may examine other regions. Note any jaundice or scleral pallor (anaemia).
7. Look for spider naevi and gynaecomastia on the chest wall (signs of chronic liver disease).
8. Look for finger clubbing, leukonychia and palmar erythema (signs of chronic liver disease) .
9. Test for a liver flap and fetor hepaticus.
10. Note any clues to the underlying aetiology. Obesity may indicate fatty liver disease. An enlarged parotid and Dupuytren contractures in the hands or feet may indicate excessive alcohol use.

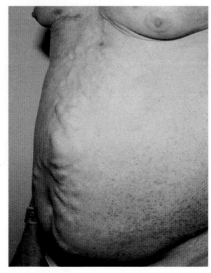

Figure 3.33.2 Distended abdominal veins in a patient with portal hypertension (Mir MA. *Atlas of Clinical Diagnosis*, 2nd edn. Edinburgh: Saunders, 2003.)

Present your findings

- Outline the important positive and negative findings. Mention particularly whether there is jaundice, ascites or hepatomegaly. Say if you think there is evidence of portal hypertension:
  - ascites
  - splenomegaly
  - distended abdominal veins.
- When the examiners begin their questions, keep in mind the causes of cirrhosis (Box 3.33.1).

Examiners' likely questions

- What are the possible causes of this man's cirrhosis and ascites?
  - See Box 3.33.1.
- How severe is it?

Box 3.33.1
Causes of cirrhosis

Alcohol
Post-viral (hepatitis C, B, delta)
Non-alcoholic steatohepatitis (NASH)
Drugs (e.g. methyldopa, chlorpromazine, isoniazid, nitrofurantoin, propylthiouracil, methotrexate, amiodarone)
Autoimmune chronic hepatitis
Haemochromatosis
Wilson disease
Primary sclerosing cholangitis
Primary biliary cirrhosis
Secondary biliary cirrhosis
Alpha$_1$-antitrypsin deficiency
Cystic fibrosis
Budd-Chiari syndrome
Cardiac failure, chronic constrictive pericarditis
Cryptogenic (idiopathic)

- Gross ascites and signs of hepatic encephalopathy suggest end-stage (advanced) severe disease.
- What future problems may occur?
  - See Box 3.33.2.

Box 3.33.2
Complications of cirrhosis

Hepatic encephalopathy
Portal hypertension and bleeding
Portal vein thrombosis
Ascites
Spontaneous bacterial peritonitis
Hepatic encephalopathy
Hepatorenal syndrome
Hyponatraemia
Portopulmonary hypertension
Hepatopulmonary syndrome
Hepatocellular carcinoma (may be underlying hepatitis B or C)

Marking criteria table

Criteria	Satisfactory	Unsatisfactory
Introduces self, explains task, obtains consent, washes hands before and after	1	0
Undresses and positions patient correctly	1	0
Makes a general inspection	1	0
Looks for peripheral signs of chronic liver disease	3	0–2
Asks patient about abdominal tenderness before beginning the examination	1	0
Examines abdomen systematically	2	0–1
Assesses for hepatic decompensation	1	0
Presents important positive and negative findings	2	0–1

Pass mark: 6

Alcohol cessation

Background

An actor schooled in the history needed will be the likely 'patient'. The questioning must still be sympathetic and matter-of-fact.

Introduction

There are a number of possible histories that you may be given with the introduction, including:

- This patient binges alcohol only every few weeks and does not see this as a problem.
- The patient is a university student presenting to his or her GP seeking a medical certificate after big night out.
- A patient complaining of insomnia who drinks alcohol at night to help him or her get to sleep.

  Please counsel your patient about alcohol reduction or cessation.

Rationale

Students will be expected to be familiar with the current safe alcohol guidelines, set out in Box 3.34.1.

The definition of a standard drink also is important to understand as you communicate with patients. The National Health and Medical Research Council (NHMRC) guidelines (2020) state a standard drink contains 10 grams of pure alcohol (Table 3.34.1).

Box 3.34.1
Safe alcohol guidelines

To reduce alcohol-related risk over a lifetime, current guidelines generally recommend:

- Not to exceed 10 standard drinks per week (previous guidance also recommended no more than 2 standard drinks per day and at least 1–2 alcohol free days)
- On any given day, consumption should not exceed four standard drinks
- There is no safe level of alcohol consumption for someone under 18
- No alcohol in pregnancy and breastfeeding is safest (do NOT drink if pregnant)
- Alcohol provides no clear health benefits and health risks are dose dependent (less is best).

TABLE 3.34.1 Standard drink equivalents

Alcoholic drink	Alcohol content (% alc/vol)	Volume equivalent to standard drink (mL)
Light beer	2.7	425
Mid strength beer	3.5	375
Full strength beer	4.9	285
Regular cider	4.9	285
Sparkling wine	13	100
Wine	13	100
Fortified wine e.g. sherry, port	20	60
Spirits e.g. vodka, gin, rum, whisky	40	30

https://www.nhmrc.gov.au/health-advice/alcohol

Method

1. Take a history focusing on alcohol intake.
   - Establish what the patient's drinking pattern is.
     - In a typical day, weekend?
     - Binge drinking? How often?
     - Any alcohol-free days?
     - Associated poly drug use?

- Convert to standard drinks. Remember to clarify strength of beer etc.
2. Look for any alcohol-related problems.
   - Medical history — any conditions related to or worsened by the alcohol consumed?
   - Mental health — anxiety, depression, insomnia, confusion, memory loss?
   - Domestic problems — relationship disruption, children with concerns and problems?
   - Employment — job stability or loss, sick days?
   - Legal — driving, drink-driving offences, assault?
   - Social — change in friends, recreational activities?
   - Finances?
3. Assess dependence (CAGE criteria are a reasonable option).
   - **C**ut down — have you ever attempted to cut down or been recommended to cut down?
   - **A**nnoyed — do people criticise the amount you drink?
   - **G**uilt — do you ever feel guilty over how much you drink or how it affects your life?
   - **E**ye opener — do you ever need to drink first thing in the morning to steady your nerves or to get rid of a hangover?
4. Education:
   - Explain the concept of a standard drink.
   - Explore the patient's beliefs about the health risks.
   - Correct or reinforce the patient's understanding and educate about other effects of alcohol. (Be prepared with information; however, a long list is also likely to put off the patient. Use what is relevant to the individual situation.)
     - Short-term consequences of alcohol consumption: accidents such as motor vehicle or pedestrian accidents, falls, fires, sports injury, drowning, violence, reduced cognitive function (especially reduced attention and increased reaction times)
     - Long-term health effects from significant alcohol consumption: cancer of the upper gastrointestinal tract, pancreatitis, hepatitis and cirrhosis, permanent cognitive deterioration, stroke, alcoholic

    cardiomyopathy, dependence and associated behaviours, peripheral neuropathy, erectile dysfunction, detrimental effects on finances and relationships

- Relate the patient's presenting symptoms or problem to drinking
- Describe the National Health and Medical Research Council drinking guidelines, as most people are surprised at how little alcohol is actually considered safe

5. Behavioural strategies
   - Delve into the issues preventing change
   - Discuss strategies to help reduce consumption:
     - Set limits
     - Avoid high-risk situations
     - Plan ahead
     - Pace drinks — sips, low-strength beer, alternate between alcoholic drinks and water
     - Coping mechanisms for everyday situations to avoid the need to drink
     - Enlist support people
     - Alcohol intake diary — cravings, abstinence, social situations and pressure
   - Reach a broad agreement for change and negotiate treatment goals. Patient-created solutions (even if suggested by you) are far more likely to be adhered to rather than a plan just dictated for the patient to follow.

6. Summarise and arrange follow up.
   - Summarise and check patient's understanding, concluding with a major plan
   - Arrange follow-up with the patient's general practitioner in 1–2 weeks
   - Patient may need referral to a drug and alcohol team
   - Patient may need referral for counselling and psychological support.

Present your findings

Summarise your discussion about the patient, the presenting complaint and how this was related to alcohol intake, whether you think this was a successful consultation and the plan created for alcohol reduction or cessation.

Examiners' likely questions

- How motivated is the patient? How ready is he or she for change? Will this affect adherence to recommendations for reduced alcohol intake?

  Be ready to discuss the recognised stages leading to control or relapse:

  - Pre-contemplation — the person has no intention to change, often because the behaviour is not seen as a problem. These patients will often place more emphasis on the negatives associated with trying to give up drinking than the health benefits they may receive from reducing or abstaining from alcohol
  - Contemplation — these people intend to start the healthy change in the future (<6 months); they are aware that they have a problem
  - Preparation (determination) — the person is intent on taking action soon (<30 days)
  - Action — the person has changed behaviour and intends to continue with the new, healthier, behaviour. This may be achieved by substitution of one behaviour for another or by modifying the old behaviour
  - Maintenance — patients have successfully changed their behaviour and have continued with their progress for at least 6 months. They have to monitor and prevent relapse
  - Termination — the person has no desire to return to the old behaviour and has no fear of relapse. Not many reach this stage; lifelong maintenance is most common.
  - Relapse — falling into old patterns of unhealthy behaviour. This restarts the pathway.

Marking criteria table

Criteria	Satisfactory	Unsatisfactory
Introduces self, explains task, obtains consent	1	0
Asks for more details about presenting problem, e.g. how often, how severe?	2	0–1
Quantifies alcohol consumption and duration of current pattern	1	0
Asks about problems possibly related to alcohol — work, family, health etc.	3	0–2
CAGE questions	3	0–2
Explains standard drink	1	0
Assesses patient's insight into problem	1	0
Outlines health risks	2	0–1
Outlines NHMRC guidelines	1	0
Discusses behavioural strategies	3	0–2
Makes a follow-up plan	1	0
Outlines the problem in relation to presenting situation	1	0
Discusses problem, insight and management with examiners	3	0–2

Pass mark: 17

Assessment of a patient with abdominal pain, diarrhoea and bloating

Background

Irritable bowel syndrome (IBS) is a common condition (prevalence 10%, 1.5:1 women:men). Patients present with chronic abdominal pain associated with bowel disturbance and often bloating.

Introduction

This 23-year-old woman has had a diagnosis of irritable bowel syndrome. Take a history from her.

Rationale

This condition is diagnosed from the history. Students need to know the main diagnostic features.

Method

1. Ask the patient: Have you been told the diagnosis? How long have you had symptoms? (Pain and disturbed defecation need to have been present for at least 6 months.)
2. Ask about the symptoms that have led to the diagnosis, their onset and duration. They include (by definition):
   - abdominal pain
   - pain relieved by (or worsened by) defecation
   - diarrhoea (describe stool frequency and stool form), or constipation, or a mixed pattern (see Fig. 3.35.1)

Type 1	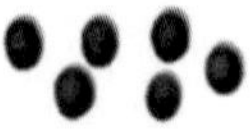	Separate hard lumps, like nuts
Type 2		Sausage-shaped but lumpy
Type 3		Like a sausage but with cracks on the surface
Type 4	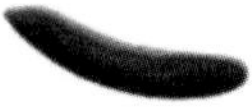	Like a sausage or snake, smooth and soft
Type 5	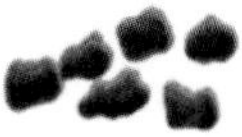	Soft blobs with clear-cut edges
Type 6	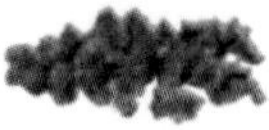	Fluffy pieces with ragged edges, a mushy stool
Type 7	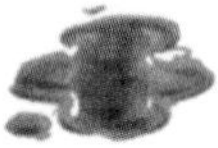	Watery, no solid pieces.

Figure 3.35.1 The Bristol Stool Form Scale shows seven categories of stool. Types 1 and 2 indicate slow colonic transit (constipation), while types 6 and 7 indicate fast colonic transit (diarrhoea) (© 2000 Rome Foundation, Inc. All Rights Reserved.)

- bloating. Some patients have visible abdominal distention (look like they're pregnant)
- other gastrointestinal symptoms commonly associated: heartburn, postprandial fullness and nausea.

3. Ask about the alarm symptoms that might suggest another diagnosis, such as colon cancer or inflammatory bowel disease or coeliac disease:
   - onset at age >50
   - anaemia
   - weight loss

- rectal bleeding
- family history of inflammatory bowel disease
- nocturnal symptoms
- family history of coeliac disease.

4. Ask about risk factors:
   - history of infection causing gastroenteritis — most accepted risk factor, but uncommon
   - family history of IBS
   - food intolerances
   - history of physical or sexual abuse
   - symptoms and history of anxiety and depression
   - sleep disturbances.

5. Ask about any tests. Consider the differential diagnosis:
   - coeliac disease — may be indistinguishable from IBS so serology testing (e.g. tissue transglutaminase) on a gluten-containing diet is routine
   - microscopic colitis — if diarrhoea in an older patient (diagnosis requires colon biopsy)
   - Inflammatory bowel disease (may present with IBS-like symptoms, causing confusion — routinely check a full blood count and C-reactive protein for evidence of anaemia and inflammation)
   - colon cancer (if older age of onset or there is a strong family history of colon cancer)
   - thyroid disease causing diarrhoea (hyperthyroidism) or constipation (hypothyroidism) is usally obvious on clinical examination so testing is not routine
   - colonoscopy is reserved for older patients with alarm features.

6. Find out what treatment and treatment strategies (including alternative therapies) have been tried.
   - A diet high in insoluble fibre (psyllium, ispaghula) is somewhat effective for constipation but soluble fibre diets (corn and wheat bran) are no better than placebo.
   - A low fermentable carbohydrate diet improves symptoms (pain, bloating, bowel disturbance) in over 50%.
   - Osmotic laxatives help with increasing bowel frequency in constipation but not with abdominal discomfort.
   - Loperamide can improve stool consistency and reduce frequency in diarrhoea but not pain or other symptoms.

- A low-dose tricyclic antidepressant can improve pain and other symptoms. They can be more helpful for IBS-diarrhoea because of their anticholinergic effects.

7. Ask how this chronic condition has affected the patient's life, work and family.

8. Ask if has it led to problems with depression.

9. Ask how she sees the future.

10. Attempt to confirm the likely diagnosis from the history (typical long-standing chronic symptoms, no alarm features, no history of organic disease).

T&O'C hint box

Remember the Rome IV definition of IBS. Two of the following:

1. Abdominal pain related to defecation (better or worse)
2. Abdominal pain associated with a change in stool frequency
3. Abdominal pain associated with a change in stool form (appearance: see the Bristol stool form scale Fig. 3.35.1)
   - Occurs over a period of at least 3 months and has been present for over 6 months.

Present your findings

- Indicate particularly if the presentation is typical (see T&O'C hint box) and there are no alarm features.
- Describe the effect the condition has had on the patient and her life.
- Mention and discuss previous investigations and comment on whether you feel they were appropriate.

Examiners' likely questions

- Are further investigations indicated?
  - These should generally be avoided if the presentation is typical.
  - Food allergy testing is not indicated.
- Is there a differential diagnosis?
  - Coeliac disease and inflammatory bowel disease should always be considered.

Marking criteria table

Criteria	Satisfactory	Unsatisfactory
Introduces self, explains task, obtains consent	1	0
Asks patient to describe her symptoms	2	0–1
Prompts with questions about typical symptoms that are not mentioned	1	0
Asks about the duration of the illness	1	0
Asks what investigations have been performed	1	0
Asks specifically about alarm features ('red flags')	1	0
Asks what treatment has been tried	1	0
Asks how badly her life and work have been affected	1	0
Presents a good summary of the history	1	0
Answers questions about the diagnosis	1	0

Pass mark: 7

Background

There are many presenting symptoms that would indicate a need for a rectal examination. It is part of the physical examination for colorectal disease (e.g. constipation, faecal incontinence, bleeding), and for diseases of the prostate (benign prostatic hyperplasia causing obstructive urinary symptoms; prostate cancer).

Introduction

This 60-year-old man reports the passage of bright red blood per rectum and a feeling of being unable to empty his bowels completely (tenesmus). Please conduct a rectal examination.

Rationale

The 'patient' will usually be a plastic model. Tenesmus and bleeding strongly suggest rectal pathology, and colon cancer needs to be excluded. Sensitive examinations require an explanation, consent and, where possible, a chaperone — though it is not needed for a plastic model, you should be able to talk about when a chaperone would be indicated.

Method

1. Introduce yourself.
2. Confirm the patient details (name, date of birth). (You don't want to perform a rectal exam on someone who doesn't need (or want) it.)
3. Explain why you want to perform the examination. (In this case, to look for evidence of abnormalities in the rectum.)

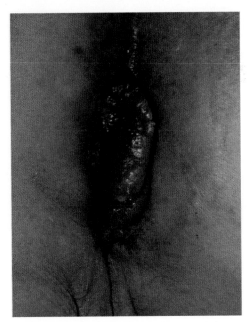

Figure 3.36.1 Haemorrhoids: Crohn 'piles'. This appearance is typical of Crohn 'piles'. They are pale and oedematous in contrast to ordinary haemorrhoids (Arulampalam THA, Biers SM, Quick CRG. *Essential Surgery: Problems, diagnosis and management*, 6th edn. Elsevier, 2020.)

4. Explain exactly what you are going to do (see steps below.) at the beginning and as you proceed. The examination is ordinarily uncomfortable but not painful.
5. Ask the patient for permission to proceed.
6. Make the area private (or ask to do so).
7. Ask the patient to remove his pants and underpants and lie in the left lateral position with his bottom over the edge and knees up (with you on the right side of the bed or couch).
8. Wash your hands. Don a pair of gloves then look for any obvious pathology (Figs 3.36.1, 3.36.2). and lubricate the right index finger.

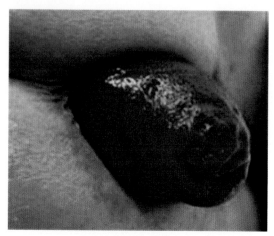

Figure 3.36.2 Rectal prolapse (Zitelli BJ, Nowalk AJ, McIntire SC. *Zitelli and Davis' Atlas of Pediatric Physical Diagnosis*, 7th edn. Elsevier Inc., 2018.)

9. Warn the patient about the cold jelly. Place your lubricated index finger over the anal area, ask the patient to strain (to relax the anal sphincter) and gently insert (Fig. 3.36.3). Ask about pain as you do this.
10. Palpate the rectum. Note if any masses are felt (or not). Note if any stool is in the rectum.
11. Note anal sphincter tone at rest then on squeezing. Ask the patient to bear down and note if the anal sphincter relaxes (as is normal to permit defecation; if it tightens this suggests pelvic outlet obstruction, which can be a cause of chronic constipation).
12. Assess the prostate gland (anterior: normally a smooth surface, feels firm and rubbery, midline groove present, no nodules, <3.5 cm). If there is enlargement with a hard, irregular nodule, be ready to describe your findings and suspect prostate cancer.
13. Take out your finger and inspect for blood or mucus, and the colour of any stool.
14. Dispose of the gloves and wash your hands.
15. Attend to the patient's comfort and address any questions he may have. Wash your hands again.

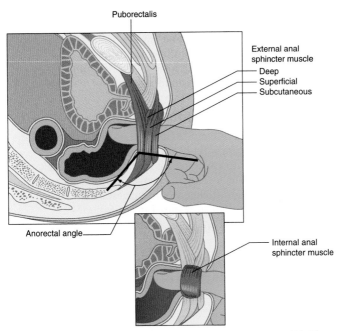

Figure 3.36.3 The rectal examination: regional anatomy (Talley NJ. How to do and interpret a rectal examination in gastroenterology. *American Journal of Gastroenterology* 2008; 108:802–803.)

Be ready to offer your summary of the findings and differential diagnosis, plus next steps in management.

T&O'C hint box

- Do not rush to examine — first spend time explaining, reassuring, and obtaining consent (yes, even to the plastic model).
- Each step in the rectal examination provides information on potential underlying pathology — anal pain (e.g. fissure), mass in the rectum (cancer, polyp), sphincter tone (e.g. reduced in faecal incontinence, paradoxical contraction on straining in a subgroup with constipation), prostate enlargement (e.g. cancer mass), and blood or mucus (e.g. inflammatory bowel disease).

Present your findings

- Describe relevant normal and any abnormal findings step by step (as you performed the examination).
- Provide a provisional diagnosis and a short differential diagnosis if there are any abnormalities.

Examiners' likely questions

- How would you differentiate benign prostatic hypertrophy from prostate cancer on rectal examination?
    - Smooth enlargement which may be asymmetrical and loss of the sulcus suggests benign prostatic hyperplasia (BPH). A hard nodule would suggest cancer.
- What would be your next initial investigation?
    - Depends on the introduction and findings!

Marking criteria table

Criteria	Satisfactory	Unsatisfactory
Introduces and confirms details	1	0
Explains why perform the examination and what it involves	2	0–1
Obtains consent	1	1
Sets up the patient correctly	1	1
Washes hands, dons gloves	1	1
Uses proper technique	2	0–1
Asks about pain on/during insertion	1	1
Checks anal sphincter tone	1	1
Examines prostate	2	0–1
Suggests differential diagnosis	2	0–1

Pass mark: 9

Assessment of a patient with inflammatory bowel disease

Background

Both ulcerative colitis and Crohn disease are common conditions in hospitals and outpatient clinics. They present both diagnostic and treatment problems. Ulcerative colitis (UC) typically presents in young adults with relapsing bloody diarrhoea, malaise, and fever and weight loss. Crohn disease can present like UC or can have a variable presentation, including an insidious onset of pain, diarrhoea, weight loss, malabsorption, intestinal obstruction or symptoms suggestive of appendicitis. The patient will usually know the diagnosis, but you may have to decide which type of inflammatory bowel disease (IBD) is present.

Introduction

Please take a comprehensive history from this woman, who has inflammatory bowel disease.

Rationale

These chronic relapsing diseases may affect people throughout their adult lives. Students should be able to obtain an outline of the course of the disease, its complications, treatments and effect on the patient's life. This is a long OSCE and you might be asked to question the patient only about certain aspects of the condition, such as the time course and current treatment or extra-colonic complications.

Method

1. Find out about symptoms at presentation and, if relevant, the current reason for admission.
2. Ask about local complications and extracolonic manifestations of the disease (Box 3.37.1).
3. Ask about any history of gastroenteritis and testing for infections (e.g. stool cultures) as infectious colitis may have a similar presentation.
4. Ask about any history of diverticular disease and diverticulitis.

Box 3.37.1
Complications of inflammatory bowel disease

Ulcerative colitis

Local
- Toxic megacolon (diameter of colon >6 cm on plain abdominal X-ray)
- Perforation
- Massive haemorrhage
- Strictures
- Carcinoma of the colon — often multicentric and related to disease extent and duration

Extracolonic

Liver disease
- Fatty liver
- Primary sclerosing cholangitis (large duct or small duct (pericholangitis))
- Cirrhosis
- Carcinoma of the bile duct
- Amyloidosis

Blood disorders
- Anaemia (owing to chronic disease, iron deficiency, ileal involvement, haemolysis from sulfasalazine or microangiopathy)
- Thromboembolism (as a result of antithrombin III deficiency, stasis, dehydration)

Arthropathy
- Peripheral (large joints)
- Ankylosing spondylitis

Skin and mucous membranes
- Erythema nodosum (coincides with active disease) (Fig. 3.37.1)
- Pyoderma gangrenosum (Fig. 3.37.2)
- Ulcers (Fig. 3.37.3)

Box 3.37.1
Complications of inflammatory bowel disease   *continued*

Ocular
- Uveitis, conjunctivitis, episcleritis

Crohn disease

Local
- Anorectal disease (including anal fissures or fistulas, pararectal abscess or rectovaginal fistula)
- Obstruction (usually terminal ileum)
- Fistula
- Toxic megacolon and perforation (rare)
- Carcinoma of the small and large bowel

Extracolonic
Similar to ulcerative colitis, except for the following:
- Liver disease — primary sclerosing cholangitis is less common
- Gallstones are more common (owing to decreased bile salt pool)
- Renal disease, including urate and calcium oxalate stones, pyelonephritis (owing to fistulas), hydronephrosis (ureteric obstruction), amyloidosis
- Malabsorption as a result of small bowel involvement
- Osteomalacia

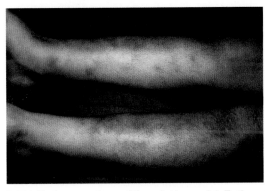

Figure 3.37.1 Erythema nodosum (Mana J, Marcoval J. Erythema nodosum. *Clinics in Dermatology*. 2007;25(3):288–294. Elsevier, with permission.)

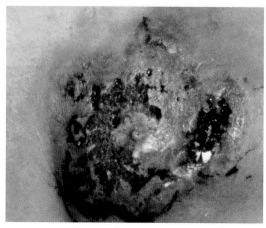

Figure 3.37.2 Pyoderma gangrenosum (Wierzbicka-Hainaut E et al. Pyoderma gangrenosum récidivant lors des grossesses. Recurring pyoderma gangrenosum in pregnancy. *Annales de dermatologie et de vénéréologie.* 2010; 137(3):225–229, Fig. 1.)

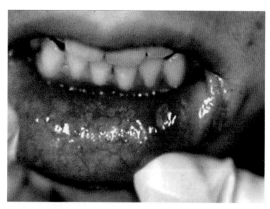

Figure 3.37.3 Aphthous ulcers (Akintoye SO, Greenberg MS. Oral soft tissue lesions: recurrent aphthous stomatitis. *Dental Clinics of North America.* 2005; 49(1):31–47, Fig. 2.)

5. Ask about all current and past medications. (NSAIDs can cause a similar picture; check point inhibitors for cancer are a cause of colitis.)
6. Determine the investigations at the time of presentation and subsequently.
7. Ask about the number of hospital admissions and how much these have interfered with normal life, work and schooling.
8. Ask whether regular follow-up colonoscopy has been performed in patients with longstanding colitis.
9. Find out about treatment, including medications such as sulfasalazine, 5-aminosalicylic acid preparations (mesalazine, olsalazine), local or systemic steroids, budesonide, metronidazole, immunosuppressants (e.g. azathioprine), other antibiotics (consider pseudomembranous colitis), biological agents such as infliximab or adalimumab (tumour necrosis factor antibody), and a detailed surgical history.
10. Inquire about family history of inflammatory bowel disease or bowel carcinoma.
11. Ask about smoking. (A greater proportion than average of Crohn disease patients are smokers and smoking can improve ulcerative colitis.)
12. Inquire about the patient's domestic arrangements and employment.

DIFFERENTIAL DIAGNOSIS

It is important to exclude other causes of colitis (Box 3.37.2).

Present your findings

- Begin by saying whether you think the diagnosis is Crohn disease or ulcerative colitis (and why), and whether the patient is unwell at the moment or in remission.
- Describe the time course of the illness and the number of hospital and intensive care admissions.
- State what treatments have been tried, drugs and surgical.
- Explain how the illness has affected the patient's life, family and work.
- State how the future seems to the patient.

Box 3.37.2
Causes of colitis

Inflammatory bowel disease
Infections, including pseudomembranous colitis
Radiation
Ischaemic colitis
Diverticulitis
Diversion colitis (colonic loops excluded from the faecal stream)
Medications (e.g. check point inhibitors, mycophenolate)
Microscopic or collagenous colitis

Examiners' likely questions

- What complications or extracolonic manifestations of the disease have there been?
  - See Box 3.37.1.
- Do you think the disease is under good control at the moment?
  - This depends on the current symptoms (clinical remission or not) and findings at colonoscopy (endoscopic and histologic remission or not).
- Is the patient's view of the prognosis realistic?
  - The disease course varies. Issues to consider include risk of resection surgery (10-year risk for Crohn disease is nearly 50%; UC risk of colectomy about 30%), colon cancer risk (increased with longer disease duration and more extensive colitis — screen with colonoscopy and biopsies), and mortality (overall only slightly increased versus the general population). Crohn disease is currently incurable; ulcerative colitis can be 'cured' by colectomy and ileoanal pouch but complications of surgery remain a limitation (e.g. pouchitis).

Marking criteria table

Criteria	Satisfactory	Unsatisfactory
Introduces self, explains task, obtains consent	1	0
Allows the patient to describe the course of the illness	1	0
Asks for more detail about specific areas, such as surgical treatment	1	0
Asks for a summary of previous and present drug treatment	1	0
Asks about side effects of treatment	1	0
Asks about extracolonic manifestations	1	0
Asks how the illness has affected the patient's life, family and work	2	0–1
Asks about the current state of the illness	1	0
Summarises the course and effect of the illness	1	0
Reflects on the patient's insight and thoughts about the future	1	0

Pass mark: 9

Examination of a hernia in the groin

Background

The anatomy of this part of the body is complicated. Surgeons are very keen that students have an understanding of it.

Introduction

This 56-year-old man has a hernia in the groin. Please examine him.

Rationale

Inguinal and femoral hernias, which are common conditions, are not always straightforward and are a test for discriminating good students from not quite so good students.

Method

1. Wash your hands, and this time don gloves.
2. Explain to the patient what you want to do and ask his permission.
3. Position the patient. A thorough examination for a hernia should be commenced with the patient standing, if possible. The patient should be asked to stand with full exposure from the thigh to the upper abdomen (Fig. 3.38.1).
4. Point sign: ask the patient to point to where the lump has been seen or felt.
5. Inspect, paying careful attention to scars from previous surgery, which may be difficult to see. Look for obvious lumps and swellings on both sides.

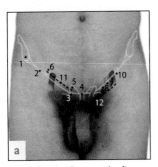

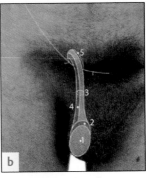

Inguinal region: bones and soft tissues
1 Anterior superior iliac spine
2 Inguinal ligament
3 Pubic tubercle
4 Symphysis pubis
5 Superficial inguinal ring
6 Deep inguinal ring
7 Femoral artery
8 Femoral vein
9 Femoral canal
10 Femoral nerve
11 Inguinal hernia incision
12 Femoral hernia incision

Testis and spermatic cord
1 Testis
2 Superior pole of epididymis
3 Spermatic cord
4 Vas deferens
5 Superficial inguinal ring

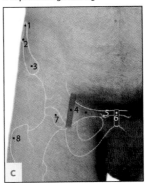

Pelvis and anterior thigh: palpable structures
1 Iliac crest
2 Tubercle of ilium
3 Anterior superior iliac spine
4 Femoral artery
5 Pubic tubercle
6 Symphysis pubis
7 Head of femur
8 Greater trochanter

Figure 3.38.1 Surface anatomy of the groin and key structures (Talley NJ, O'Connor S. *Talley & O'Connor's Clinical Examination Essentials: An introduction to clinical skills (and how to pass your clinical exams)*. Elsevier Australia, 2020.)

6. Check for cough impulse. Before palpation, ask the patient to turn his or her head away from you and cough. Fix your eyes in the region of the pubic tubercle and note the presence of a visible cough impulse. Ask the patient to cough again while you inspect the opposite side.

7. To palpate, place your fingers over the region of the pubic tubercle. Once again, ask the patient to cough, and seek a palpable expansile impulse. If a hernia is present, attempts at reduction should not be performed while the patient is erect, as it is more difficult and painful than when the patient is placed supine.

8. Ask the patient to lie supine on the examination couch. Perform the procedure of inspection and palpation in the same manner as above. The exact position of any hernia is usually easier to define with the patient lying supine. Assess if the hernia spontaneously reduces upon lying supine; if not, attempt gently to reduce it. A non-reducible hernia poses a higher risk of strangulation.

9. Identify the hernia type. If a lump is present, it must be determined whether this is a hernia and, if so, what sort of hernia. Identify the pubic tubercle. Remember, one cannot get above a hernia, but one can get above a hydrocele in the inguinal canal. Try to determine whether the hernia is inguinal (see Fig. 3.38.2a) or femoral, based on the position in relation to the pubic tubercle and inguinal ligament (see below).

10. Remember, femoral hernias are more dangerous. They are usually smaller and firmer than inguinal hernias and commonly do not exhibit a cough impulse. Because they are frequently irreducible they are commonly mistaken for an enlarged inguinal lymph node. A cough impulse is rare from a femoral hernia and needs to be distinguished from the thrill produced by a saphena varix when a patient coughs.

11. Ask to examine the testes and scrotum (usually not permitted). A large inguinal hernia may descend through the external ring immediately above the pubic tubercle into the scrotum. Gentle invagination of the scrotum with the tip of the gloved finger in the external ring may be performed to confirm an indirect hernia in men (Fig. 3.38.2b).

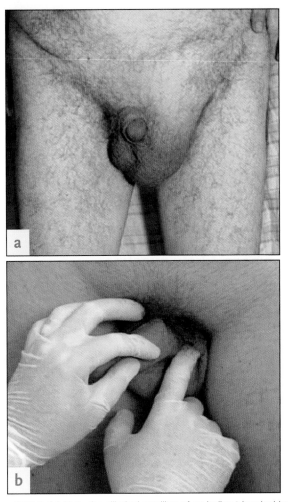

Figure 3.38.2 (a) Note the elliptical swelling of an indirect inguinal hernia descending into the scrotum on the right side. Also note the globular swelling of a direct inguinal hernia on the left side **(b)** To examine the inguinal canal in a male, invaginate the scrotum as shown. Always wear gloves (Swartz M. *Textbook of Physical Diagnosis.* Elsevier, 2014, Figure 15.31.)

12. A maldescended testis can be confused with an inguinal hernia, so always confirm (or ask to confirm) that there is a testis in each scrotum. A large inguinal hernia may present as a lump in the scrotum. It is important to ascertain whether one can get above the lump. If you can get above the lump, the lump is of primary intrascrotal pathology and is not a hernia.

Present your findings

- Describe the position and size of the hernia.
- What do you think the patient risk factors are? (Obesity and chronic cough are possible risk factors)
- Say whether you think it is an inguinal or femoral hernia, and why.
- Is it reducible or not, is it tender?

Examiners' likely question

- What is the differential diagnosis?
  - Consider a scrotal mass, saphena varix or enlarged lymph node, but see T&O'C hint box. Explain why it is not any of these.

T&O'C hint box

The examiners have told you it is a hernia. It is unlikely to be anything else.

Marking criteria table

Criteria	Satisfactory	Unsatisfactory
Introduces self, explains task, obtains consent, washes hands, puts on gloves	1	0
Positions patient	1	0
Asks patient to perform point sign	1	0
Inspects for scars and visible lumps	1	0
Tests for cough impulse	1	0
Palpates	1	0
Repositions patient, asks to examine scrotum	1	0
Provides an opinion on the likely hernia type and justifies it	1	0
Gives a sensible differential diagnosis	1	0

Pass mark: 5

Examination of polycystic kidney disease

Background

This an autosomal dominant condition and an important cause of hypertension and chronic kidney disease. The disease is associated with cerebral haemorrhage and cysts in other organs (liver).

Introduction

Please examine this man's abdomen. He has a family history of chronic kidney disease and hypertension.

> **T&O'C hint box**
>
> This introduction strongly suggests polycystic kidney disease.

Rationale

Polycystic kidneys can cause marked abdominal signs but are often (needlessly) confused with hepatosplenomegaly. See Fig. 3.39.1. This examination is a good test of a student's technique.

Method

1. As always, wash your hands.
2. Ask the patient's permission to examine his abdomen and ask him to lie flat with his abdomen exposed from the lower ribs to the symphysis pubis.

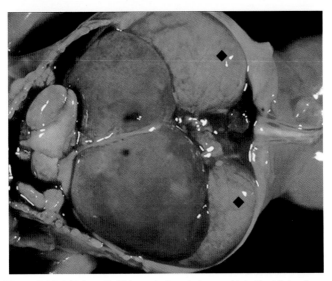

Figure 3.39.1 Polycystic kidneys in the abdomen. Note the bilaterally massively enlarged kidneys (♦) that nearly fill the abdomen below the liver, consistent with ARPKD in this fetus at 23 weeks' gestation that died from pulmonary hypoplasia as a result of oligohydramnios (Klatt EC. *Robbins and Cotran Atlas of Pathology.* Elsevier Inc., 2014.)

3. Look from the side for abdominal distension by squatting down beside the patient. Look from above for scars, especially the left or right lower quadrant scar of a renal transplant. See Fig. 3.39.2.

4. Ask about areas of tenderness and promise to be even more gentle than usual in examining those parts of the abdomen.

5. Examine the abdomen, paying particular attention to palpation of both kidneys.

6. Attempt to outline the size of the kidneys and detect the characteristic cystic shape.

7. Ballot the kidneys (with a two-handed technique) and demonstrate that you can get above them (i.e. that there is renal enlargement, not hepatosplenomegaly).

8. Feel for a possible transplanted kidney under any lower quadrant scars (will be superficial and easily felt).

9. Assess the liver and spleen (may also be polycystic). The liver edge may feel 'bumpy'.

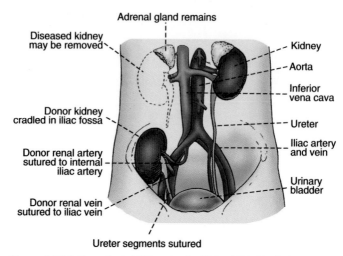

Adrenal gland remains

Diseased kidney may be removed

Kidney

Aorta

Inferior vena cava

Donor kidney cradled in iliac fossa

Ureter

Iliac artery and vein

Donor renal artery sutured to internal iliac artery

Urinary bladder

Donor renal vein sutured to iliac vein

Ureter segments sutured

Figure 3.39.2 Transplanted kidney in situ (Shiland BJ. *Medical Terminology & Anatomy for Coding.* Elsevier Inc., 2020.)

10. Take the blood pressure, but *not* in the arm where you have noticed an arteriovenous fistula for haemodialysis (Fig. 3.39.3).

PRESENT YOUR FINDINGS

- Describe the size and texture of the kidneys.
- Comment on the presence of a suspected transplanted kidney, if relevant.
- Comment on the liver size and texture (polycystic?).
- Comment on the presence of a haemodialysis fistula in the forearm.
- Give the blood pressure reading.

EXAMINERS' LIKELY QUESTIONS

- Is there a differential diagnosis?
  - If the kidneys are the cause of the abdominal masses, stick to your guns. Note there could be confusion with splenomegaly.

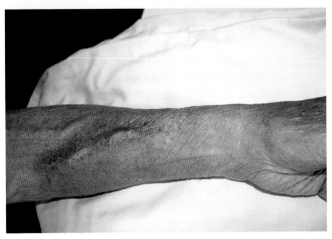

Figure 3.39.3 Arteriovenous fistula in the arm for haemodialysis (Talley NJ, O'Connor S. *Talley and O'Connor's Clinical Examination*. Elsevier Australia, 2017)

- Are you concerned about the blood pressure?
  - Good blood pressure control is important in these patients because they are prone to hypertension and to cerebral aneurysms.
- What other manifestations of this condition do you know?
  - Amaze the examiners by memorising Box 3.39.1.

Box 3.39.1
Additional manifestations of polycystic kidneys

Liver cysts
Pancreatic cysts
Splenic cysts
Thyroid cysts
Seminal vesicle cysts
Intracranial cerebral aneurysms
Hypertension
Diverticular disease
Hernias

Marking criteria table

Criteria	Satisfactory	Unsatisfactory
Introduces self, explains task, obtains consent, washes hands before and after	1	0
Positions patient correctly and asks about tenderness	2	0–1
Inspects abdomen	1	0
Palpates systematically	1	0
Assesses for enlarged kidney	2	0–1
Examines for hepatosplenomegaly	1	0
Asks to take blood pressure	1	0
Presents positive and negative findings	2	0–1

Pass mark: 6

Examination of a patient with lymphoma

Background

A knowledge of the major lymph node groups and their names will be required here. Palpable but small lymph nodes are often found in normal people, especially in the inguinal region. Students need to have an idea what is normal and what is not. In addition, search carefully for splenomegaly.

Introduction

This woman has a lymphoma. Please examine her abdomen.

Rationale

This specific introduction means students are expected to know what to look for when examining someone with lymphoma — at least enlarged lymph nodes and splenomegaly. See Fig. 3.40.1.

Method

1. Wash your hands.
2. Ask the patient's permission to examine her abdomen and ask her to lie flat with her abdomen exposed from the lower ribs to the symphysis pubis.
3. While the patient is undressing, look for wasting, abdominal distension and surgical scars.
4. Ask about tenderness or discomfort.
5. Examine her abdomen (inspect, palpate, percuss and auscultate).
6. Pay particular attention to the size of the liver and spleen. Both will typically be enlarged.

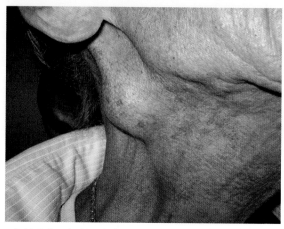

Figure 3.40.1 Cervical lymphadenopathy (Bird DL., Robinson DS. *Modern Dental Assisting*. Elsevier Inc., 2020.)

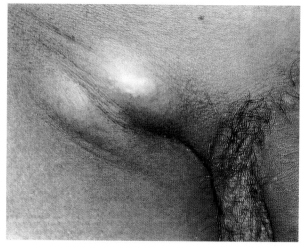

Figure 3.40.2 Inguinal lymphadenopathy (Rao SD, Rao KD. *Essentials of Surgery for Dental Students*. Elsevier Inc., 2016.)

7. Palpate for enlarged abdominal lymph nodes.
8. Examine all the other lymph node groups, starting with the inguinal nodes (Fig. 3.40.2).

9. Ask whether you have time to examine the chest (usually you won't have time). There may be a pleural effusion. Look for radiotherapy tattoo marks on the abdomen or chest.
10. Look for signs of infection, especially the rash of herpes zoster.
11. Look at the sclerae for signs of anaemia (pale).
12. Ask to see the temperature chart (fever a systemic ('B') sign, with night sweats and weight loss).

Present your findings

- Comment on the patient's general appearance; that is, well or ill.
- Describe any palpable lymph nodes — the groups involved, their size and consistency. In lymphoma, nodes are firm, rubbery and non-tender.
- Comment on the presence or absence of splenomegaly and hepatomegaly.
- Note associated findings.

Examiners' likely questions

- Can you stage the disease?
  - The correct answer is 'yes'. See Table 3.40.1.

TABLE 3.40.1 Staging lymphoma (Lugano classification)	
Stage	Description
Stage I	Disease confined to a single lymph node region or a single extralymphatic site (Ie)
Stage II	Disease confined to two or more lymph node regions on the same side of the diaphragm, plus or minus splenic involvement
Stage III	Disease confined to lymph node regions on both sides of the diaphragm (III1 = upper abdomen; III2 = lower abdomen), with or without localised involvement of the spleen (IIIs), other extralymphatic organ or site, e.g. liver (IIIe), or both
Stage IV	Diffuse disease of one or more extralymphatic organs (with or without lymph node disease)

- What questions might you ask the patient?
  - Have you had fevers or weight loss >10% in 6 months or night sweats? (No symptoms = stage A, symptoms = stage B.)

Marking criteria table

Criteria	Satisfactory	Unsatisfactory
Introduces self, explains task, obtains consent, washes hands	1	0
Performs a general inspection e.g. for tattoo radiation marks, herpes zoster	2	0–1
Positions patient correctly, asks about tenderness	1	0
Examines abdomen correctly, including liver and spleen	3	0–2
Examines inguinal nodes	1	0
Asks to examine the other lymph node groups (knows how to so if told to go ahead)	2	0–1
Can stage the disease	1	0

Pass mark: 7

Take a history from a patient with rheumatoid arthritis

Background

Students need to be able to assess patients with this relatively common chronic disease. It can be very severe and cause intense disruption to patients' lives. The treatment (e.g. use of steroids) can be complicated and associated with significant side effects. This OSCE tests students' clinical knowledge of rheumatoid arthritis and their approach to chronic disease in general.

Introduction

This 42-year-old woman has rheumatoid arthritis. Please assess her illness and its effect on her social situation.

Rationale

This case is an example of a chronic and possibly disabling disease (Fig. 3.41.1). Similar cases would include (for example) chronic obstructive pulmonary disease, heart failure or scleroderma.

Method

1. Introduce yourself and explain the purpose of the interview.
2. Ask:
   - How long have you had arthritis?
   - How was the diagnosis made?
   - Which joints were affected first?
   - How was the diagnosis made?

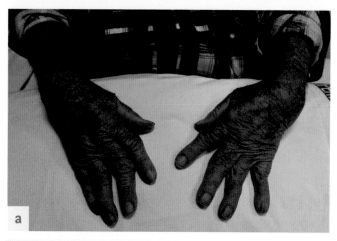

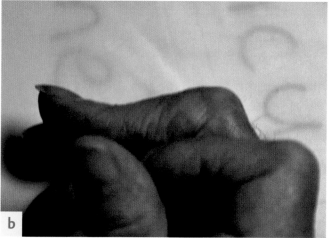

Figure 3.41.1 **(a)** Rheumatoid hands showing swan neck deformity and DIP. **(b)** Boutonnière deformity of the PIP and DIP joints (Talley NJ, O'Connor S. *Talley and O'Connor's Clinical examination.* Elsevier Australia, 2018.)

- How long was it before the diagnosis was made? (There can be delays in diagnosis, especially if the presentation was atypical. The patient may know what blood tests were done.)
- Which joints are affected?
- Are they swollen and tender?
- For how long are your joints stiff in the morning? (The duration of morning stiffness is an indication of the activity of the disease.)
- Has the disease affected any other parts of your body than the joints? (e.g. lung involvement)
- Can you bathe yourself, go to the toilet, dress yourself, cut food, and eat? (activities of daily living — ADLs)
- How do you manage shopping, cooking, cleaning, transport and driving, managing medications and finances? (instrumental activities of daily living — IADLs)
- What medications do you take? (The patient's previous and current medication regimes are very important. You may need to prompt with questions about the use of steroids, nonsteroidal anti-inflammatory drugs (NSAIDs) and immunosuppressants and biological agents.)
- Have (give the trade name) NSAIDs caused problems with stomach ulcers, kidney damage or high blood pressure? Find out whether steroids (prednisone) have been used. At what doses and for how long they have been needed? Ask about tests (bone mineral density scans) and treatment (vitamin D analogues, bisphosphonates) for osteoporosis.
- Have azathioprine or biological agents (use trade names) been used? Have these been helpful? Have there been any problems with their use (infections)? Have they had to be stopped because of this?
- Do you know the results of any of the tests or investigations?
- Are you rheumatoid factor positive?
- Have you needed operations on any of your joints? What was done, for example joint replacement or tendon release?

- Have there been any other complications of the disease — with your lungs (infection, fibrosis) or heart (pericarditis) or kidneys (failure) or spleen (enlarged with or without anaemia), or legs (numbness from peripheral neuropathy, weakness)?
- Do you work?
- What sort of work do you do — physical or sedentary?
- Have you needed much time off work?
- Has your employer been helpful?
- Have you had financial worries as a result of your illness?
- Who lives at home with you? What support do you get?

Present your findings

- Summarise the course of the illness.
- Outline how the patient copes — at home and at work and with activities of daily living.

Examiners' likely questions

- Do you think the disease is active at the moment?
  - Describe her joint symptoms and the duration of morning stiffness. She may know the results of tests such as inflammatory markers.
- How has she coped with this chronic illness from the point of view of her independence, finances and her family?
  - Summarise her answers to your questions about these important matters.
- Have there been problems with her treatment? What?
  - Discuss drug side effects, for example from steroids (Cushing syndrome), including risk of and treatment to prevent osteoporosis.

- Is she aware of her prognosis and of future potential side effects?
  - Discuss your impression of the patient's understanding of the severity of her disease and the implications of treatment.
- Has she had any other complications of the disease?

Marking criteria table

Criteria	Satisfactory	Unsatisfactory
Introduces self, explains task, obtains consent, appears sympathetic	1	0
Asks questions that help establish the severity and course of the illness	3	0–2
Finds out about treatment, including non-drug treatment	1	0
Asks about treatment side effects	1	0
Performs detailed analysis of patient's domestic and financial situation, taken in a sympathetic fashion	2	0–1
Makes an overall assessment of the effect of the illness and the patient's insight into her disease and its prognosis	2	0–1

Pass mark: 6. The examiners would also pay close attention to the interaction between student and patient, looking for an appropriate mixture of sympathy and professionalism.

Examine the hands

Background

Modern treatment of inflammatory arthritis has reduced patients' problems with joint deformity, but acute arthritis, severe osteoarthritis and patients with preexisting deformity are plentiful.

Introduction

- This 67-year-old woman has arthritis. Please examine her hands.
- This man has had pain in his hands. Please examine him. (The use of the word *pain* makes it likely the examination is a rheumatological one rather than a neurological one.)
- This patient has had difficulty using her hands. Please examine her. (This stem is more ambiguous and the decision about which examination to perform will depend on what changes are seen during inspection of the hands.)

Rationale

Chronic arthritis can cause many structural and functional changes in the hands. Students need to know how to perform this examination smoothly. (The examiners should not think this is the first time you have seen arthritic hands.)

Method

1. When you are asked to examine the hands, consider the possibilities of arthropathy, acromegaly, a peripheral nerve lesion, a myopathy or a neuropathy. The stem will usually help.

2. Remember the principles of joint examination:
   - Look (inspection)
   - Feel (palpation)
   - Move (function)
   - Presence of extraarticular manifestations of arthritis.

T&O'C hint box

The diagnosis of arthritis is usually made during the inspection. Note the nature of the joint abnormalities and the pattern of joint involvement. Time spent on inspection is not wasted.

If there is obvious joint disease, examine as follows.

3. Look at the patient for cushingoid features (steroid treatment is more likely if the problem is rheumatoid arthritis or systemic lupus erythematosus — SLE).

4. Look around the room for walking sticks, wheelie walkers or other aids to mobility.

5. Make the patient comfortable, then expose as much of the hands and forearms as possible.

6. Ask the patient to show you her elbows. Look for ease of movement of the elbows and shoulders and for rheumatoid nodules or a psoriatic rash on the elbows or extensor tendons.

7. Now place the patient's hands on a pillow, palms down.

8. Take some time to look at the hands, as the diagnosis is often made by inspection. Is there a symmetrical deforming polyarthropathy involving the wrists and hands? Are the distal interphalangeal (DIP) joints spared (as you would expect in rheumatoid arthritis)?

9. Look at the skin for erythema, ecchymosis or skin atrophy (this may indicate steroid use), scars (tendon release or transfer) and rashes.

10. Then look for swelling and its distribution, wrist deformity, and muscle wasting involving the forearms and interosseous muscles.

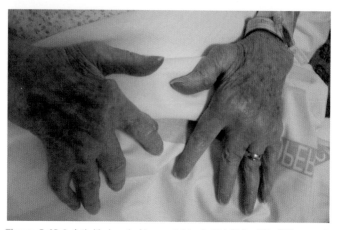

Figure 3.42.1 Arthritic hands (rheumatoid arthritis) (Talley NJ, O'Connor S. *Talley and O'Connor's Examination Medicine.* Elsevier Australia, 2020.)

11. Go on to the metacarpophalangeal (MCP) joints. Note, if present, any skin abnormalities, swelling and deformity (Fig. 3.42.1), particularly ulnar deviation and volar subluxation, 'swan necking' and boutonnière deformity of the fingers, and Z deformity of the thumb, seen in advanced rheumatoid arthritis.
Sausage-shaped phalanges and telescoping of the fingers with predominant interphalangeal joint disease usually means psoriatic arthropathy (Fig. 3.42.2) or Reiter disease (reactive arthritis) (see Fig. 3.42.3). Small joint ankylosis is common. Look for telangiectasia.

12. Next look at the nails and describe any psoriatic nail changes (present in the great majority of patients with psoriatic arthritis), namely pitting, onycholysis, hyperkeratosis, ridging and discoloration. Note the signs of vasculitis (splinter haemorrhages or black to brown 1–2 mm skin infarcts, usually in a periungual location) and mention this to the examiners.

13. Now ask the patient to open and close the hands. This will reveal tendon ruptures and fixed flexion deformities.

14. Turn the wrists over and look at the palms for scars (Fig. 3.42.4), palmar erythema and muscle wasting.

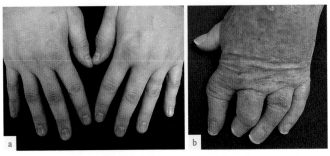

Figure 3.42.2 **(a)** and **(b)** Swollen joints in psoriatic arthritis over the second and third metacarpophalangeal joints of the hands (Garg A, Gladman D. Recognizing psoriatic arthritis in the dermatology clinic. Capsule Summary. *Journal of the American Academy of Dermatology* 2010; 63(5):733–48, Figs 3 and 5. American Academy of Dermatology Inc., with permission.)

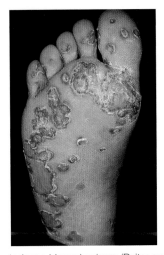

Figure 3.42.3 Keratoderma blenorrhagicum (Reiter syndrome). The palms and soles are commonly involved. There are keratoic papules, plaques and pustules that coalesce to form circular borders like those seen on the penis (Habif TP. *Clinical Dermatology*, 5th edn. Fig. 8.13. Mosby, Elsevier, 2009, with permission.)

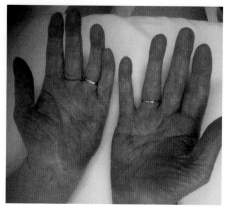

Figure 3.42.4 Scars from previous tendon surgery and palmar erythema (Talley NJ, O'Connor S. *Talley and O'Connor's Examination Medicine.* Elsevier Australia, 2020.)

T&O'C hint box

If the DIP joints are spared, the diagnosis is likely to be rheumatoid arthritis or SLE. If the DIP joints are involved, consider osteoarthritis, gouty arthritis or psoriatic arthritis.

15. Next, describe the proximal interphalangeal (PIP) and DIP joints. Symmetrical wrist, MCP and proximal joint swellings suggest rheumatoid arthritis. Swelling (hard, bony) in the PIP joints and DIP joints is suggestive of osteoarthritis.

T&O'C hint box

The DIP joints may look to be in the wrong position because of arthritis and deformity of the PIP and MCP joints, even when they are not involved.

T&O'C hint box

Be gentle while examining — do not hurt the patient. During the examination, look up periodically at the patient's face for signs that the examination is uncomfortable.

16. Palpate each joint, starting with the wrists.
17. Feel for synovitis (boggy swelling) and effusions. As you feel, remember that the joint line is the place where these changes occur.
18. Note the range of passive movement of the joint.
19. Feel for any joint crepitus.
20. Palpate the ulnar styloid for tenderness.
21. When examining the MCP joints, also feel for subluxation.
22. Test for palmar tendon crepitus (tenosynovitis).

Now test for function.

23. Test grip strength, key grip and opposition strength (thumb and little finger).
24. Ask the patient to perform a practical procedure, such as undoing a button or writing something.

A formal neurological examination of the hand is not required in assessing arthropathy. However, a ganglion or tenosynovitis may cause carpal tunnel syndrome.

25. Ask the patient to flex both wrists together for 30 seconds — paraesthesiae will often be precipitated in the affected hand if carpal tunnel syndrome is present (Phalen wrist flexion test). Tap over the carpal tunnel while the wrist is held in extension for Tinel sign (paraesthesiae in the distribution of the median nerve). These tests have similar but limited specificity and sensitivity.
26. If there is time, check sensation in the median and ulnar nerve distributions.
27. Look for extraarticular manifestations and the extent of the disease.

At this point, if there is time, you need to decide whether to ask to examine other joints or look for other abnormalities.

28. If other joints seem obviously abnormal or are on display (e.g. shoes are off), ask to look at them.
29. If you have found evidence of psoriasis, look at common sites for psoriatic rashes — scalp (just at the hairline), umbilicus and elbows.

By now you will be out of time. If the patient is seated in a chair with a number of layers of clothing covering the chest, it is unlikely the examiners will want you to examine the heart or lungs. However, if you feel strongly that you want to do this (and

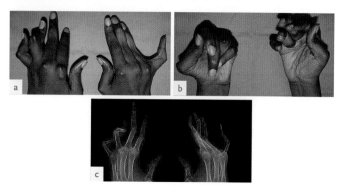

Figure 3.42.5 A 40-year-old patient with bilateral rheumatoid hand deformities. **(a)** Boutonnière deformities of the left small, left ring, and right small fingers with simultaneous swan neck deformities of the left long, right long, and right ring fingers **(b)** Note the inability to make a fist on the right hand (predominantly swan neck deformity) compared with the left hand (predominantly boutonnière deformity) **(c)** Radiograph (Sebastin SJ, Chung KC. Reconstruction of digital deformities in rheumatoid arthritis. *Hand Clinics* 2011; 27(1):87–104, Fig. 1, with permission.)

you have time), it is better to ask to put the patient onto the bed and remove the shirt rather than to try to examine the chest through layers of clothing.

Present your findings

You should now have an idea of the pattern and severity of the deformity, as well as the extent of loss of function and the activity of the disease. Always consider the differential diagnosis of a deforming polyarthropathy.

- Rheumatoid arthritis (see Figs 3.42.5, 3.42.6, 3.42.13 and 3.42.14)
- Seronegative arthropathies — particularly psoriatic arthritis (see Figs 3.42.7, 3.42.8, 3.42.15 and 3.42.16)
- Polyarticular gout (look for tophi) (Figs 3.42.9a, b and 3.42.17) or pseudogout (see Fig. 3.42.10)

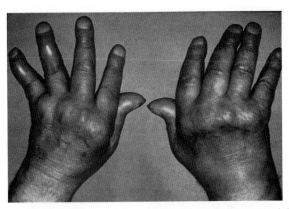

Figure 3.42.6 The hands of a patient with severe inflammatory arthritis, showing symmetrical deformity (Dacre JE, Worrall JG. Rheumatology part 1 of 2: the rheumatological history. *Medicine* 2010; 38(3):129–132, Fig. 1, with permission.)

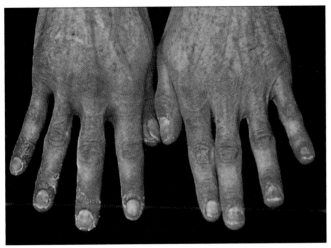

Figure 3.42.7 Psoriatic arthritis of the hands (Talley NJ, O'Connor S. *Talley and O'Connor's Examination Medicine*. Elsevier Australia; 2020)

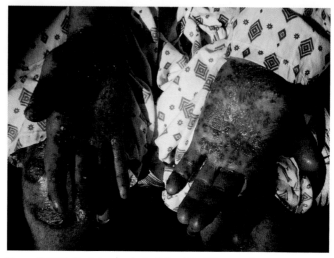

Figure 3.42.8 Pustular psoriasis (Talley NJ, O'Connor S. *Talley and O'Connor's Examination Medicine*. Elsevier Australia, 2020.)

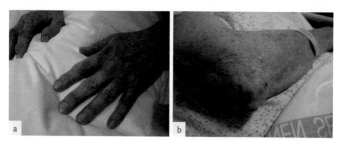

Figure 3.42.9 **(a)** and **(b)** Tophaceous gout (Talley NJ, O'Connor S. *Talley and O'Connor's Examination Medicine*. Elsevier Australia, 2020.)

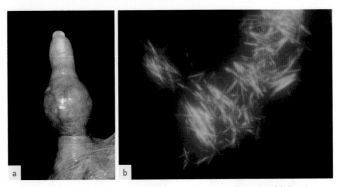

Figure 3.42.10 **(a)** Pseudogout. The swollen interphalangeal joint **(b)** Calcium pyrophosphate crystals (Alexandroff A, Kirkham N, Nayak N. Reprinted with permission from Elsevier (*The Lancet*, 2008; 371(9618):1114).)

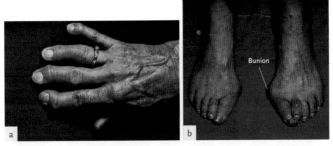

Figure 3.42.11 **(a)** and **(b)** Primary generalised osteoarthritis (Talley N, O'Connor S. *Clinical Examination*, 7th edn. Fig. 24.5a and b. Elsevier Australia, 2013, with permission.)

- Primary generalised osteoarthritis (where DIP and PIP joint involvement is common) (see Figs 3.42.11, 3.42.12 and 3.42.18).

Examiners' likely questions

- Can you describe the pattern of this patient's arthritis?
  - Which joints are involved — large or small, peripheral or spine? Is it symmetrical?

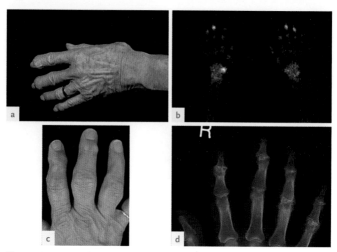

Figure 3.42.12 (a)–(d) Osteoarthritis of the hands (Vincent TL, Watt FE. Rheumatology, part 1 of 2: osteoarthritis practice points. *Medicine* 2009; 38(3):151–156, Fig. 2, with permission.)

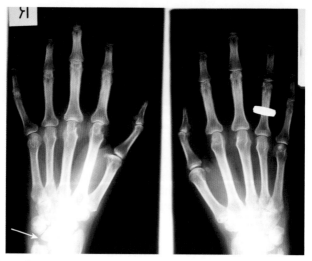

Figure 3.42.13 X-rays of the hands of a patient with early rheumatoid arthritis. Note the erosions of the metacarpal heads, reduced cartilage in the joint spaces and erosion of the ulnar styloid (arrow) (Figure reproduced courtesy of The Canberra Hospital.)

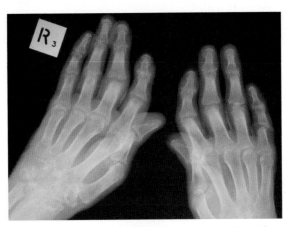

Figure 3.42.14 X-ray of the hands showing advanced destructive changes in a patient with rheumatoid arthritis. Note the ulnar deviation, Z deformity of the thumb, destruction of the PIP and MCP joints, and bone erosion (Figure reproduced courtesy of The Canberra Hospital.)

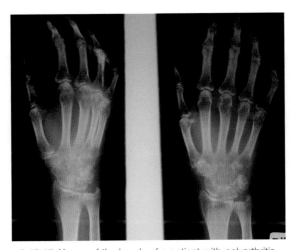

Figure 3.42.15 X-rays of the hands of a patient with polyarthritis secondary to connective tissue disease (CREST syndrome). Calcinosis, Raynaud (atrophy distal tissue pulp), Esophageal dysmotility, Sclerodactyly, Telangiectasia. There are destructive changes in all the joints (the DIP joints are not spared), and bony erosions are prominent (Figure reproduced courtesy of The Canberra Hospital.)

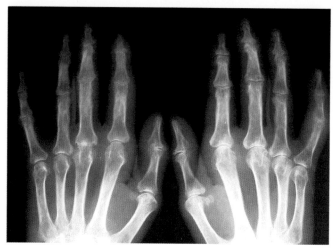

Figure 3.42.16 X-ray of the hands of a patient with psoriatic arthritis. Note bone erosion, loss of joint space and 'pencil in cup deformity' of the PIP joints (Figure reproduced courtesy of The Canberra Hospital.)

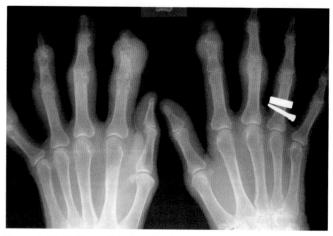

Figure 3.42.17 X-ray of the hands of a patient with severe gouty arthritis. Note the large soft-tissue masses and severe joint destruction (Figure reproduced courtesy of The Canberra Hospital.)

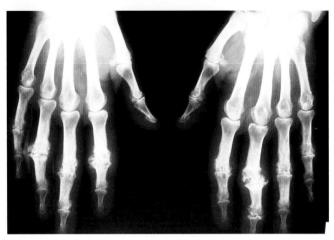

Figure 3.42.18 X-ray of the hands of a patient with severe osteoarthritis. Note Heberden nodes and DIP joint involvement (Figure reproduced courtesy of The Canberra Hospital.)

- – Is the arthropathy deforming?
- Do you think the disease is active?
  - – Are there signs of inflammation or of the boggy swelling of synovitis?
  - – Are the joints tender?
- Have you noticed any extraarticular features?
  - – Mention rheumatoid nodules, signs of psoriasis, skin changes etc.

QUESTIONS MORE LIKELY FOR SENIOR STUDENTS

- What is your differential diagnosis?
- Please comment on these X-rays.
  - – Look for the changes seen in Figs 3.42.13–3.42.18.
- What blood tests might be helpful?
  - – Mention rheumatoid factor (positive in 70% of rheumatoid patients, anticitrullinated peptide antibody (ACPA, 97% specific), tests for inflammation (C-reactive protein — CRP or erythrocyte sedimentation rate — ESR) and evidence of chronic disease (haemoglobin for anaemia). It is unlikely more detail than this would be expected of you.

T&O'C hint box

Severe osteoarthritis can cause hand deformity. Sometimes more than the DIP and PIP joints are involved, but these are usually the worst.

Destructive changes (especially shortening and telescoping of digits) and DIP disease suggests seronegative arthropathy — look carefully for the rash of psoriasis.

Marking criteria table

Criteria	Satisfactory	Unsatisfactory
Introduces self, explains task, obtains consent, washes hands before and after	1	0
Positions patient and hands	1	0
Inspects for and recognises pattern of joint involvement	2	0–1
Looks for skin changes and signs of vasculitis	2	0–1
Looks for rheumatoid nodules and gouty tophi	1	0
Tests hand function	2	0–1
Asks to examine other joints likely to be involved and other relevant systems	1	0
Answers examiners' questions correctly	3	0–2
Makes sense when interpreting X-rays	2	0–1

Pass mark: 10

Examine the knees

Background

The knee is a complicated joint and knee problems are common and varied. This examination tests students' understanding of knee anatomy and of common knee problems.

Introduction

- This man has had painful knees. Please examine him. (arthritis)
- This woman has noticed swelling in her knees. Please examine her. (arthritis or effusions)
- This woman has had difficulty walking. Please examine her knees. (arthritis or muscle weakness)

T&O'C hint box

If the introduction includes a statement about difficulty walking, it would be a good idea to begin by asking the patient to walk.

Rationale

Students must have a systematic approach to this examination (look, feel, move, function), which is often neglected and performed badly. Always ask the patient to walk at some point in the evaluation if he or she can — this is clearly what the knees are for!

Method

1. **Look** around the room for walking aids.

2. Perform a general inspection of the face, body and hands. Note the patient's general appearance, such as rheumatoid hands or cushingoid facies (from steroid use). A fit athletic patient may have a meniscal tear or patellar dislocation. A tall patient with marfanoid features may have arthritis or dislocations. An elderly overweight patient may have osteoarthritis (important to mention when reporting findings).

3. Expose both knees and thighs fully and carefully inspect from the front.
    * Look for quadriceps wasting
    * Inspect over both knees for any skin abnormalities (scars or rashes)
    * Note any swelling and deformity. Synovial swelling is seen medial to the patella and in the suprapatellar area
    * Fixed flexion deformity must be assessed: inspect the knee from the side (a space beneath the knee will be visible when the patient is asked to extend fully).

4. **Feel** the quadriceps for wasting.

5. Ask the patient if there is any pain or tenderness and next palpate for warmth and synovitis over the knee joint and for joint line tenderness.
    * Examine for an effusion on both sides — the patella tap (ballottement) is used to confirm a large effusion. The fluid from the suprapatellar bursa is pushed by the hand into the joint space by squeezing the lower part of the quadriceps and then pushing the patella downwards with the fingers. The patella will be ballotable if fluid is present under it. In patients with a smaller effusion, pressing over the lateral knee compartment may produce a noticeable medial bulge as a result of fluid displacement.
    * Test flexion and extension passively and note the range of movement and the presence or absence of crepitus.
    * Examine again for fixed flexion deformity by gently extending the knee.

6. Test the ligaments next (**move**). The lateral and medial collateral ligaments are tested by having the knee slightly flexed, holding the leg with the right hand and arm, steadying the thigh with the left hand and moving the leg

laterally and medially. Movements of more than 5–10° are abnormal. The cruciate ligaments are tested by steadying the foot with your elbow and moving the leg anteriorly and posteriorly with the other hand. Again, laxity of more than 5–10° is abnormal.

7. Apply McMurray's test for assessing meniscal integrity. Holding the lower leg and foot, flex and extend the knee while internally and externally rotating the tibia. Pain or clicking is very suggestive of a meniscal tear.

8. Ask the patient to stand up and look for varus (bow-leg) and valgus (knock-knee) deformity.

9. Examine from behind for a Baker cyst. It is felt in the popliteal fossa and is more obvious when the knee is extended.

10. **Test function**. Ask the patient to walk.

11. Ask to complete your assessment by going on to examine other joints that may be involved, as directed by your general inspection and findings. (You usually won't be allowed.)

Present your findings

- Say if the disease is active (e.g a tender hot joint, or an effusion), symmetrical, and whether there is impaired function.
- Mention the most likely diagnosis and the differential diagnosis.

Examiners' likely questions

- Do you think the problem here involves the knee joints themselves or other structures?
  - This question is a hint that the problem is not the joint but perhaps the bursa or muscles.
- What is the differential diagnosis for this patient's knee joint problems?
  - Consider osteoarthritis — if there are no signs of inflammation or an inflammatory arthritis.

FOR FINAL YEAR STUDENTS

- What tests might help?

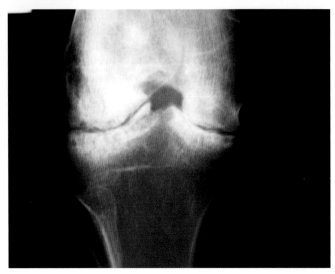

Figure 3.43.1 X-ray of the knee joint of a patient with arthritis secondary to haemophilia. Note loss of joint space. The juxtaarticular aspects of the tibia and femur appear sclerotic, but the bones are generally osteoporotic (Figure reproduced courtesy of The Canberra Hospital.)

- You've examined the patient; you need the history before ordering tests. Particularly ask about the onset, any history of trauma, knee pain, stiffness, locking, swelling, instability, and sexual activity (gonococcal oligoarthritis) and previous surgery.
- Ask for sensible blood tests, for example for inflammatory markers, and serology for rheumatoid arthritis. You may consider aspiration of the joint for septic arthritis or gout or pseudogout if there is an acutely swollen hot red single joint.
- Ask to look at X-rays (Figs 3.43.1 and 3.43.2) and make comments about findings, such as loss of joint space, soft tissue swelling or erosions, but do not make anything up. If you can't see anything wrong, comment on what you would ordinarily look for.
- What other joints might be involved?
  - If osteoarthritis seems likely, mention interphalangeal joints, hips and metatarsophalangeal joints.

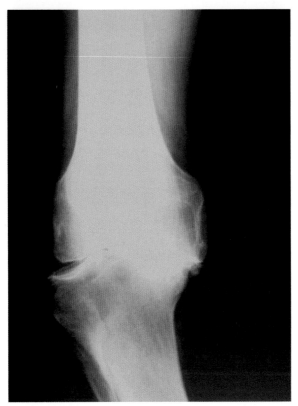

Figure 3.43.2 X-ray of the knee of a patient with rheumatoid arthritis. Here there is more severe joint space loss (Figure reproduced courtesy of The Canberra Hospital.)

T&O'C hint box

The knees and other hinge joints are commonly affected in patients with arthritis secondary to haemophilia. The pattern of joint involvement and juxtaarticular bony sclerosis on X-ray helps to distinguish this from rheumatoid arthritis involving the knees (see Figs 3.43.1 and 3.43.2).

Marking criteria table

Criteria	Satisfactory	Unsatisfactory
Introduces self, explains task, obtains consent, washes hands	1	0
Undresses patient adequately	1	0
Asks patient to walk next if walking is mentioned in the introduction	1	0
Inspects knees and notes swelling, scars or deformity	1	0
Asks about tenderness before beginning to examine	1	0
Feels for warmth and swelling	1	0
Tests flexion and extension, notes range of movement	1	0
Tests for ligamentous laxity	1	0
Tests for meniscal problems	1	0
Looks for a Baker cyst	1	0
Presents findings — positive and negative	2	0–1
Interprets X-rays satisfactorily	2	0–1

Pass mark: 9 for final year students, 7 for others

Examine the feet

Background

Again, remember that feet are used for walking, so at some point ask if you may get the patient to walk.

Introduction

- This woman has painful feet. Please examine her. (arthritis)
- This man has difficulty walking. Please examine his feet. (arthritis or neurological abnormality)

The stem is unlikely to be ambiguous in this way unless the problem is very clear on inspection. Look carefully before deciding which examination to do.

Rationale

This examination is even more neglected than the knee assessment. It is not difficult but requires some practice.

Method

1. **Look**. As usual, glance around the room for walking aids and at the patient for signs of systemic disease, rashes and other clues.
    - Start by inspecting the ankles. Look at the skin of the feet and toes (for scars, ulcers and rashes), and look for swelling, deformity and muscle wasting.
    - Examine the midfoot and forefoot similarly. Deformities affecting the forefoot include hallux valgus and clawing and crowding of the toes (in rheumatoid arthritis). If pes cavus is present, consider a hereditary motor and sensory neuropathy (Fig 3.44.1).

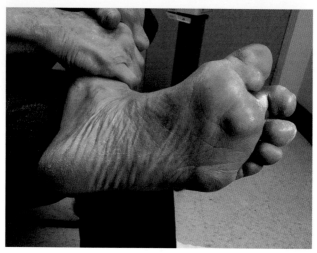

Figure 3.44.1 Pressure ulcers are most likely to occur at areas of deformity on or over the plantar region of the metatarsophalangeal joints. This patient has large rheumatoid nodules on the plantar foot, creating shoe wear issues and increased risk for pressure sores (Koretzky GA, Gabriel SE, O'Dell JR et al. *Firestein & Kelley's Textbook of Rheumatology*, 11th edn. Elsevier Inc., 2021.)

- Note any psoriatic nail changes (e.g. pitting, ridging, onycholysis, hyperkeratosis, discolouration).
- Look at the transverse and longitudinal arches (lost in neuropathies including due to diabetes mellitus).
- Look for callus over the metatarsal heads, which occurs in subluxation.
- Note any obvious gross deformities that suggest Charcot joints.

2. **Feel**. Palpate, starting with the ankle, feeling for synovitis, stress fractures, plantar fasciitis (medial calcaneal tubercle tenderness) and effusion.

- Passive movement of the talar joints (dorsiflexion and plantarflexion) and subtalar joints (inversion and eversion) must be assessed.
  The best way to examine the subtalar and midtarsal joints is to fix the os calcaneus and ankle joint with the left hand while inverting and everting the midfoot with the right. Tenderness on movement is more

important than range of movement. The midfoot (midtarsal joint) allows rotation of the forefoot on a fixed hindfoot.

- Squeeze the metatarsophalangeal joints for tenderness.
- Examining the individual toes is useful in seronegative spondyloarthropathies. (A sausage-like swelling of the toe is characteristic in psoriatic arthritis.)
- Feel the Achilles tendon for nodules and palpate the inferior aspect of the heel for tenderness. (plantar fasciitis) Consider a neurological examination — test pinprick sensation and proprioception (important for senior students).

3. If difficulty walking was part of the stem, ask the patient to walk.
4. Ask to go on to examine other joints as appropriate.

Present your findings

- Say if the disease is active (e.g a tender hot joint, or an effusion), symmetrical, and whether there is impaired function.
- Mention the most likely diagnosis and the differential diagnosis.

Examiners' likely questions

- Which joints seem most involved?
- Do think this is arthritis, or a different problem?
  - Pes cavus and muscle wasting suggest a myopathic process.
- Did you find evidence of systemic disease?
  - Often a hint that the patient has rheumatoid or psoriatic arthritis

QUESTIONS FOR SENIOR STUDENTS

- What tests might be useful?
  - X-rays of the feet are the most likely investigations that will be available (see Figs 3.44.2–3.44.6). Patients with rheumatoid arthritis can have involvement of the cervical spine, hips and shoulders, and X-rays of these may also be available.
  - Serological tests may be relevant.

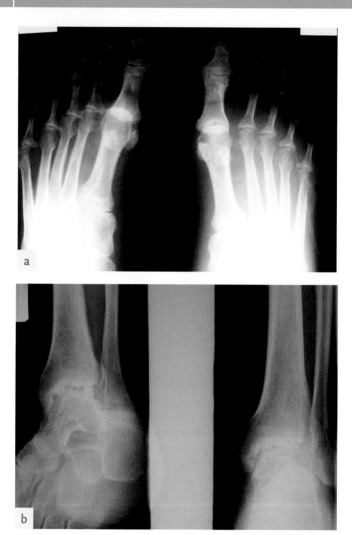

Figure 3.44.2 (a) X-ray of the feet of a patient with early rheumatoid arthritis. Note the joint erosions and deformity of some of the metatarsophalangeal (MTP) and proximal interphalangeal (PIP) joints (Figure reproduced courtesy of The Canberra Hospital.) **(b)** X-ray of the ankles of a patient with rheumatoid arthritis. There is generalised loss of joint spaces, and early destructive changes are present (Figure reproduced courtesy of The Canberra Hospital.)

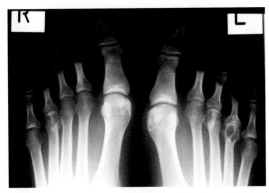

Figure 3.44.3 X-ray of the feet of a patient with early psoriatic arthritis. Note the large erosions and absence of osteoporosis. There is already some joint deformity, and a spiculated bony growth is visible (Figure reproduced courtesy of The Canberra Hospital.)

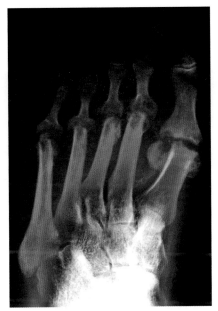

Figure 3.44.4 X-ray of the feet of a patient with severe psoriatic arthritis: arthritis mutilans (Figure reproduced courtesy of The Canberra Hospital.)

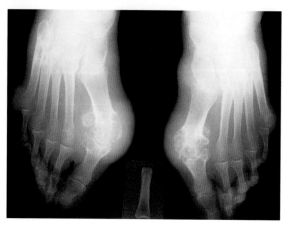

Figure 3.44.5 X-ray of the feet of a patient with severe gouty arthritis. Note the relative preservation of the joint spaces with erosions and overhanging edges. The area of the junction of the forefoot and midfoot has numerous erosions, which is a common finding (Figure reproduced courtesy of The Canberra Hospital.)

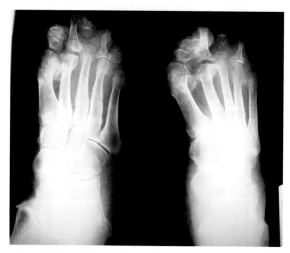

Figure 3.44.6 X-ray of the feet of a patient with diabetic arthropathy. Note the gross joint destruction (Charcot joints) (Figure reproduced courtesy of The Canberra Hospital.)

Marking criteria table

Criteria	Satisfactory	Unsatisfactory
Introduces self, explains task, obtains consent, washes hands	1	0
Makes usual general inspection for walking aids, special shoes and signs of frailty or other disease	2	1
Removes patient's shoes and socks	2	0–1
Looks at feet and ankles; checks for scars, deformity (especially the severe deformity of a Charcot joint), swelling etc.	3	0–2
Looks at transverse and longitudinal arches	1	0
Feels for swelling and heat	1	0
Tests for movement and tenderness (gently)	2	0–1
Squeezes metatarsophalangeal joints	1	0
Gives a summary and interpretation	2	0–1
Satisfactory-X-ray interpretation	2	0–1

Pass mark: 12 for senior students, 10 for others

Examine the back (ankylosing spondylitis)

Background

Back pain is very common; the aetiology may be inflammatory or a result of injury or not at all obvious. The presence of neurological symptoms and signs as a result of spinal cord or cauda equina involvement indicates the problem is urgent.

Introduction

- This man has had back pain for many years. Please examine him.
- This man has ankylosing spondylitis. Please examine him and assess the severity of his disease. (Fig. 3.45.1).

Rationale

Only limited examination of the back is possible. Most signs of arthritis are to be found in patients with ankylosing spondylitis, and they are rather over-represented in exams compared with other chronic back problems.

Method

1. **Look**. The initial inspection confirms that this is a case of ankylosing spondylitis (see Table 3.45.1). Ask the patient to undress to his underpants and stand up.
   - Look for deformity, inspecting from both the back and the side, particularly for loss of kyphosis and lumbar lordosis.

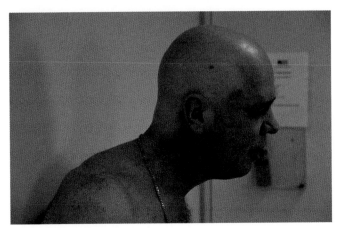

Figure 3.45.1 Ankylosing spondylitis. Note the occiput-to-wall distance (Talley NJ, O'Connor S. *Talley and O'Connor's Examination Medicine*. Elsevier Australia; 2020)

TABLE 3.45.1 The seronegative spondyloarthropathies	
Spondyloarthropathy	HLA-B27 (%)
Ankylosing spondylitis	95
Psoriatic spondylitis	50
Reactive arthritis, including Reiter syndrome	80
Enteropathic arthritis	75

2. **Feel**. Palpate each vertebral body for tenderness and palpate for muscle spasm.
3. **Test function.** Measure the finger–floor distance. (Inability to touch the toes suggests early lumbar disease.)
   - Next look at extension, lateral flexion and rotation of the back. Get him to run each hand down the corresponding thigh to test lateral flexion.
   - Ask whether you may perform a modified Schober test. This involves identifying the level of the posterior iliac spine on the vertebral body (approximately at L5). Place a mark 5 cm below this point and another 10 cm above this point. Ask the patient to touch his toes. There should normally be an increase of 5 cm or more in the

distance between the marks. In ankylosing spondylitis there will be little separation of the marks, since all the

movement is taking place at the hips.

- Next test the occiput-to-wall distance. Ask the patient to place his heels and back against the wall and to touch the wall with the back of his head without raising his chin above the carrying level. (Inability to touch the wall suggests cervical involvement.) Measure the distance from

occiput to wall.

- Before asking the patient to lie down, test for active sacroiliac disease by springing the anterior superior iliac spines. Pain felt in the region of the sacroiliac joints suggests activity. A simple (and unreliable) test for sacroiliac disease is to push with the heel of the hand on the sacrum and note the presence of tenderness in either sacroiliac joint on springing. (*Note:* Usually there is bilateral disease in ankylosing spondylitis.)
- Ask the patient to lie down. Examine the heels for Achilles tendinitis and plantar fasciitis, which are characteristic of the spondyloarthropathies.
- Ask to evaluate the other large joints, particularly the knees, hips and shoulders.

EXTRA-ARTICULAR MANIFESTATIONS (ANKYLOSING SPONDYLITIS)

1. You need to know these manifestations although usually you won't have time to examine for them unless the OSCE stem points you in a specific direction to start with.

- Examine the chest for decreased lung expansion (chest expansion of less than 3 cm at the nipple line suggests early costovertebral involvement) and for signs of apical fibrosis.
- Examine the heart for aortic regurgitation or mitral valve prolapse.
- Inspect the eyes for uveitis (red painful eye).
- Examine the gastrointestinal system. Ask for results of a rectal examination (for evidence of inflammatory bowel disease). Rarely there may be signs of amyloid deposition (e.g. hepatosplenomegaly, abnormal urine analysis results).
- Remember also to check for signs of psoriasis and Reiter syndrome, which may cause spondylitis and unilateral sacroiliitis (so may be confused with ankylosing spondylitis).
- Rarely, patients with ankylosing spondylitis have signs of a cauda equina compression (bilateral leg weakness, perineal (saddle) sensory loss (S2–4), urinary catheter).

Present your findings

If the stem has mentioned activity of the disease or limitation of function, make special mention of these.

Examiners' likely questions

- Do you think this disease is active?
  - This is unlikely, but joint tenderness is suggestive.
- What extraarticular manifestations of ankylosing spondylitis did you look for?
  - List the main ones as above.
- How severe is the arthritis?
  - Discuss limitation of spinal movements and occiput-to-wall distance. Report you would examine for nerve root impingement including signs of cauda equina.

SENIOR STUDENTS

- What tests do you want?
  - Ask for X-rays. X-ray changes are described in Box 3.45.1 and illustrated in Figs 3.45.2–3.45.4.

Box 3.45.1
X-ray changes in ankylosing spondylitis

Sacroiliac joints
Cortical outline lost (early)
Juxtaarticular osteosclerosis
Erosions
Joint ankylosis

Lumbar spine
Loss of lumbar lordosis
Squaring of vertebrae
Syndesmophytes (thoracolumbar region)
Bamboo spine (bony bridging of vertebrae) and osteoporosis
Apophyseal joint fusion

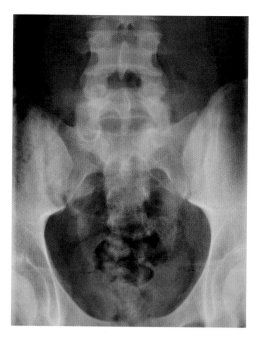

Figure 3.45.2 X-ray of the pelvis of a patient with Reiter syndrome. Note the loss of joint space in the two sacroiliac joints and lumbar spine ankylosis (Figure reproduced courtesy of The Canberra Hospital.)

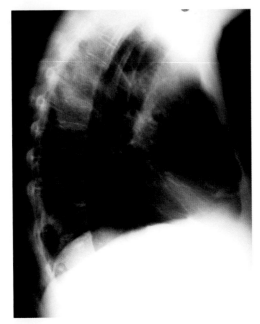

Figure 3.45.3 Lateral chest X-ray of a patient with ankylosing spondylitis. Note the loss of joint space and squaring of the vertebrae (Figure reproduced courtesy of The Canberra Hospital.)

- Know the right words to use to describe the X-ray findings — syndesmophytes, loss of joint space, squaring of vertebrae, ankylosis of joints etc. Do not, however, use these words if these things are not actually present on the X-rays.
- Ask for appropriate serology and inflammatory markers.

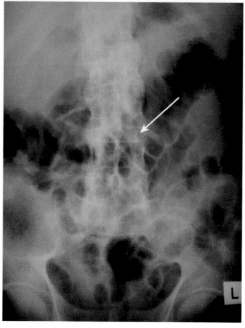

Figure 3.45.4 X-ray of the pelvis of a patient with ankylosing spondylitis. Note the lateral bridging syndesmophytes (arrow) (Figure reproduced courtesy of The Canberra Hospital.)

Marking criteria table

Criteria	Satisfactory	Unsatisfactory
Introduces self, explains task, obtains consent, washes hands	1	0
Undresses patient sufficiently	1	0
Inspects	1	0
Asks about tenderness	1	0
Feels for spinal tenderness	1	0
Tests movement of spine and function	3	0–2
Asks to go on to examine other specific relevant areas	3	0–2
Decides about severity and disease activity	2	0–1
Asks for and satisfactorily interprets X-rays	2	0–1

Pass mark: 11 for senior students, 9 for others

Take a history from a patient with osteoarthritis

Background

Osteoarthritis involves synovial joints. Weight-bearing joints (the hip and the knee) and the proximal interphalangeal (PIP) and distal interphalangeal (DIP) joints of the hands and the first meta-tarsophalangeal (MTP) joint of the foot are most often affected. There is usually loss of articular cartilage, meniscal damage, laxity of surrounding ligaments, formation of osteophytes and changes to sub-chondral bone.

Risk factors include obesity (for the knee especially), a family history and joint injury, which can be repetitive or acute.

Introduction

This man has been troubled by arthritis for some years. Please take a history from him.

(Do not be put off by the arrival of an athletic and mobile-looking youth — he is likely to be an actor, well-schooled in what symptoms to describe.)

Rationale

This common problem affects many people, many of whom are keen to talk about this chronic condition and are available for OSCEs. Osteoarthritis affects 80% of the population over age 55 and 95% of people over 65 years. It is associated with obesity and diabetes mellitus, and may be one of the reasons a patient cannot exercise and lose weight. It should be possible from the history and examination to distinguish this from an inflammatory arthritis, although many patients may have both.

Method

THE HISTORY

1. Introduce yourself and explain what you would like to do. Ask:
   - How long has the arthritis been a problem?
   - What joints have been involved? (Distal interphalangeal, shoulders, hips, knees and proximal metacarpophalangeal joints are often affected in osteoarthritis.)
   - Has there been swelling or inflammation (redness and warmth) of the joints? (if not after an injury, suggests an inflammatory arthritis rather than osteoarthritis)
   - Has there been joint instability? Have you noticed any deformity? Locking?
   - Is there any loss of function (e.g. use the hands, walk, climb stairs)?
   - Are the joints stiff in the morning? (Patients with osteoarthritis do not have much morning stiffness; more than 30 minutes of morning stiffness suggests an inflammatory arthritis not osteoarthritis.)
   - Is there a family history of arthritis and is the type known?
   - Have there been injuries to the joints, for example, from playing sport?
   - Have you been able to lose weight?
   - What limitations are there as far as mobility and exercise?
   - Do you need a walking stick or frame?
   - How do you manage around the house? (activities of daily living — ADLs — etc.)
   - Are you able to drive or work?
   - What drugs are you currently using and what have you used in the past for your arthritis?
   - Have there been side effects? (especially from non-steroidal anti-inflammatory drugs — NSAIDs)
   - Have complementary medicines been tried, such as glucosamine?
   - What other treatment has been tried? (joint injections, exercise and physiotherapy, weight loss, alternative treatments, surgery including joint replacement)
   - Have these treatments helped?

Present your findings

- What joints are involved?
- How badly are the patient's life, work etc. affected?
- Is weight a problem? What strategies have been tried to help with weight loss?
- What other treatments have been tried?
- How successful have they been?
- Have there been complications of treatment?

Examiners' likely questions

- Tell us more about how much the patient's daily life is affected. Can he or she drive? Do the shopping etc.?
  - Discuss work, sport, finances, ADLs.
- What else might be done?
  - Discuss weight loss, including the possibility of bariatric surgery, joint replacement (including possible risks of surgery), physiotherapy and further drug treatment, such as large regular doses of paracetamol or more risky NSAIDs.

Marking criteria table		
Criteria	Satisfactory	Unsatisfactory
Introduces self, explains task, obtains consent	1	0
Takes a comprehensive history of the course of the arthritis	2	0–1
Asks about extent of joint involvement	2	0–1
Asks about morning stiffness	1	0
Asks about previous joint injuries	1	0
Asks about non-drug treatment	1	0
Asks about current and previous drug treatment	1	0
Asks about drug side effects	1	0
Asks about weight and attempts at weight loss	1	0
Asks about surgery, including joint replacement	1	0
Asks about the effect on the patient's life, work and family	2	0–1

Pass mark: 10

Examine a patient diagnosed as having osteoarthritis

Background

Remember what the hands and knees are for. Tests of function — use of the hands, and walking — are essential. If the actor is a circus performer he may complain of difficulty walking on his hands, but for most people you want to check fine movement such as pincer grasp (picking up a 10 cent coin) and unbuttoning.

Introduction

This man has osteoarthritis and has had particular problems with his hands and knees. Please examine him.

Rationale

This is a test of your ability to examine the joints of the hands and the knees.

Method

1. Introduce yourself, wash hands, explain what you plan to do, and obtain consent.
2. Ask the patient to undress to his underpants.
3. Note the patient's weight and general mobility, for example difficulty undressing.
4. Examine the joints the patient has had problems with (see Boxes 3.47.1–3.47.3) — here, the hands and knees (as described in the stations covering hands and knees, but focus here on osteoarthritis signs).

Box 3.47.1
Examination findings — osteoarthritis of the hands

Interphalangeal joints affected
Heberden and Bouchard nodes
Joints enlarged, due to osteophyte formation (Fig. 3.47.1)
Onset in middle age
Women more often affected
Usually good eventual function of hand

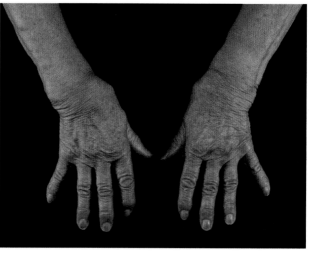

Figure 3.47.1 Severe osteoarthritis of the hands (Firestein GS, Budd RC, Gabriel SE, McInnes IB, O'Dell JR. *Firestein & Kelley's Textbook of Rheumatology*. Elsevier Inc., 2020.)

Box 3.47.2
Examination findings — osteoarthritis of the knees

Jerky, antalgic gait, favouring worse side
Varus or sometimes valgus deformity
Weakness and wasting of quadriceps
Joint-line or periarticular tenderness
Flexion and extension reduced
Joint crepitus
Bony swelling around the joint line

> ### Box 3.47.3
> ### Examination findings — osteoarthritis of the hips
>
> Antalgic gait
> Gluteal and quadriceps wasting
> Restriction and pain on internal rotation of the hip when it is flexed. This is the earliest and most sensitive finding
> Later all movements are restricted and there may be fixed flexion and external rotation deformity
> Tenderness of the anterior part of the groin lateral to the femoral pulse
> Ipsilateral leg shortening may occur when the femoral head has migrated and there is severe joint space loss

5. Assess for scars from previous surgery, passive and active movement, joint pain on movement, deformity, loss of range of movement, any effusions, and ligamentous laxity.
6. Test joint function. Test hand function, for example by getting the patient to do up buttons or remove the lid from a jar (if you happen to have one).

   Ask the patient to walk, without walking aids at first if this is possible, and then with. Does the gait appear painful? Ask the patient to turn around and walk back. How slow and limited does this movement seem? You may then want to ask to examine the hips.
7. Look at the effectiveness of walking aids by comparing walking with and without them, if that is possible.

Present your findings

If the stem has mentioned activity of the disease or limitation of function, make special mention of these.

Examiners' likely questions

If you have described the findings and, in particular, how badly the patient is affected, the examiners may turn to management.

- What non-pharmacological measures might be helpful?
  - Unleash the following suggestions on the examiners.
  - Exercise
    - Stretching and mobility exercises can help maintain joint range of motion

- Aquatic exercise may be possible for patients with severe restriction
- Exercise bicycle so that exercise is not weight bearing
- Supervised or group exercise works better for reduction of pain than independent exercise at home
- Use of mobility aids
  - A stick used in the opposite hand
  - Knee braces and foot orthoses
- Loss of weight. This is the most important modifiable risk factor for osteoarthritis. A 10% loss of weight achieved by diet and exercise has been shown to reduce symptoms by 50%.
- Surgery. Joint replacement can be very helpful when other treatment has failed. Arthroscopic procedures have not been shown to be effective for knee arthritis beyond what medical treatment can achieve.
  - All right then, what about drug treatment?
  Again, you are ready for this.
- **Non-steroidal anti-inflammatory drugs (NSAIDs)** are the usual first-line treatment. They are probably somewhat more effective than paracetamol but at the expense of their well-known gastrointestinal and cardiovascular side effects. The COX-2 inhibitors cause less dyspepsia (12%). Using a proton pump inhibitor with a NSAID reduces dyspepsia risk by 66%. There is no good information about the best duration of treatment.
- **Paracetamol** (up to 4 g/day) has been a common choice for osteoarthritis because of concerns about the side effects of NSAIDs. There is not much evidence, however, that it is more effective than placebo, especially for knee pain, and there have been concerns about an increase in cardiovascular events with prolonged use of large doses. It is no longer recommended as first-line treatment.

- **Topical NSAIDs** have been shown to be useful for knee and hand arthritis and seem safer than oral NSAIDs.
- **Intraarticular injections of steroids** give 1–2 weeks of relief and improve mobility. They are useful for acute exacerbations. Frequent use can cause cartilage and joint damage and involve some risk of infection.
- **Opioids** should generally be avoided. Their use is associated with more adverse events than NSAIDs. These include cardiovascular events, fractures and an increased mortality.
- **Duloxetine** is a centrally acting serotonin and norepinephrine uptake inhibitor. It has been shown to be superior to placebo and can be used in combination with NSAIDs.
- **Complementary medicines:** the most commonly used of these drugs is glucosamine. It seems no more effective than placebo in controlled trials.
- **Fish oil** and **chondroitin** have similarly failed to show advantages over placebo for knee pain.

Marking criteria table

Criteria	Satisfactory	Unsatisfactory
Introduces self, explains task, obtains consent, washes hands before and after	1	0
Makes a general inspection, including using the opportunity of patient's walking in or undressing to look for limitation	2	0–1
Undresses patient appropriately	1	0
Satisfactorily examines most likely joints to be affected: hands, knees	3	0–2
Looks for muscle wasting	1	0
Assesses mobility, use of aids etc.	2	0–1
Summarises findings	3	0–2
Discusses management	2	0–1

Pass mark: 9

Take a history — systemic lupus erythematosus

Background

Remember that the diagnosis of systemic lupus erythematosus (SLE) requires at least four of the 11 published criteria, either currently or in the past (Box 3.48.1). Fewer than four criteria are often labelled 'possible lupus'. Non-specific positive autoimmune tests with some evidence of inflammation can be referred to as 'undifferentiated connective tissue disease'.

Introduction

This 40-year-old woman has had a diagnosis of SLE. Please take a history from her.

Rationale

This chronic multisystem disorder affects women more often than men (8:1). It usually begins in patients between 20 and 40 years of age. Most patients are well informed about their illness and can give a good history. By taking a good history, students should be able to establish:

- how the diagnosis was made
- the time course of the illness
- the effect of this chronic disease on the patient and her family.

Method

1. Introduce yourself and say you have been asked to talk to her about her diagnosis of systemic lupus erythematosus. Obtain permission.

Box 3.48.1
American Rheumatism Association criteria for SLE

Four or more manifestations of the following 11 must be present serially or simultaneously.

- Malar rash — sparing the nasolabial folds (Fig. 3.48.1)
- Discoid rash
- Photosensitivity rash
- Oral ulcers
- Arthritis — non-erosive, and affecting two or more peripheral joints
- Serositis — pleurisy or pericarditis, with audible rub, effusion or electrocardiogram (ECG) changes
- Renal disorder — persistent proteinuria >0.5 g/day or cellular casts
- Neurological disorder — seizures or psychosis not related to drugs or metabolic abnormalities
- Haematological disorder — haemolytic anaemia, leucopenia (<4000/μL), lymphopenia (<2000/μL), thrombocytopenia (<100 000/μL)
- Immunological disorder — anti-DNA antibodies in abnormal titre, or anti-Smith (anti-Sm) antibody, or positive antiphospholipid antibodies
- Antinuclear antibody (ANA) disorder — abnormal ANA titre >1 : 160

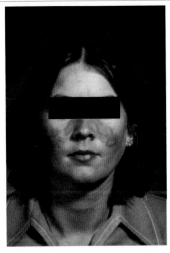

Figure 3.48.1 Butterfly rash of systemic lupus erythematosus (Talley NJ, O'Connor S. *Talley and O'Connor's Clinical Examination*. Elsevier Australia, 2017.)

> **Box 3.48.2**
> **Summary of systems review for SLE**
>
> Aphthous ulcers
> Serositis
> Raynaud phenomenon
> Alopecia
> Photosensitivity rashes
> Dry eyes and mouth
> Thrombosis
> Miscarriages
> Nephritis (haematuria, kidney failure)

2. Ask about symptoms. As for most chronic conditions, it is best to focus on drawing a mental image of the timeline of the disease. Begin with what symptoms are present now as patients find this easiest to remember (and allows you more control over the conversation when time is limited!) — start with open-ended questions then narrow down your questions (Box 3.48.2).

3. Then ask methodically about any organ system involvement. Symptoms may be elicited for some; otherwise you can ask if they have been told they had the disease or diagnosis.

   - Ask about general symptoms — malaise (nearly all patients), weight loss (60%), nausea and vomiting (50%), clotting (thrombosis) of veins or arteries (15%)
   - Ask about musculoskeletal symptoms (95%) — arthralgia, arthritis (typically symmetrical and non-erosive), myalgia and myositis
   - Ask about dermatological symptoms (85%) — skin rash, alopecia, oral or nasal ulcers
   - Ask about any history of recurrent fevers (77%)
   - Find out about neuropsychiatric symptoms (60%) — convulsions, abrupt involuntary movements (chorea should be obvious), memory loss, neuropathy, loss of vision (optic neuritis), stroke, headache, anxiety and depression
   - Ask about kidney symptoms (50%) — haematuria, oedema (just about any type of glomerulonephritis can be present)

Box 3.48.3
Drugs that may induce SLE

Procainamide (most patients are ANA-positive within 1 year; 15–20% develop SLE)
Hydralazine (most patients are ANA-positive within 1 year; 5–10% develop SLE)
Isoniazid
Methyldopa
Penicillamine
Chlorpromazine
Anticonvulsants, particularly phenytoin (not sodium valproate)

- Lung symptoms (45%) — ask about pleuritic chest pain (pleurisy)
- Heart symptoms (40%) — ask about palpitations, dyspnoea/orthopnea or ankle swelling (pericarditis, myocarditis, valvular lesions, premature coronary artery disease from increased atherosclerosis)
- Haematological symptoms (50%) — symptoms of anaemia, clots (thromboembolism), large lymph nodes
- Gastrointestinal symptoms (30%) — nausea, diarrhoea
- A history of thrombophlebitis, recurrent spontaneous abortion or fetal death in utero (suggests antiphospholipid syndrome)
- Dry eyes and dry mouth (sicca symptoms, secondary to Sjögren syndrome)
- Reduced activities of daily living and ability to work as a result of the effect of this chronic and relapsing disease on her life.

4. Ask about any drug history (e.g. procainamide, hydralazine — causes of an SLE-like syndrome) (Box 3.48.3).
5. Ask about any treatment given and any complications of treatment. Particularly obtain information on any long-term steroid use. Ask about steroid doses and duration of treatment. Has osteoporosis been diagnosed (bone mineral density scan or low impact fracture)? Has the patient developed diabetes mellitus?
6. Ask about problems during pregnancy and use of contraception. (Pregnancy is especially risky if the disease

is active. Progesterone or low dose oestrogen contraception is advisable.)

7. Does she know if her renal function is normal or if there is protein in the urine? Has the renal function been getting worse?

8. Ask about protection from sunlight. (This reduces the risk of photosensitivity rashes and flares of systemic disease.)

9. Inquire about the family history.

10. Inquire about the patient's understanding of the implications of this chronic and incurable disease and its prognosis.

Remember though that current treatment allows a 90% 10-year survival rate compared with 50% 30 years ago.

Present your findings

- Outline the presenting symptoms and the time course of the illness.
- Discuss the investigations the patient knows of that have led to the diagnosis.
- Give your understanding of how the patient's life has been affected.

Examiners, likely questions

- How definite is the diagnosis in this case, do you think?
  - Consult Box 3.48.1.
- Do you think the disease is active at the moment?
  - Discuss any current symptoms and say you would like to see the results of recent blood tests, for example for inflammatory markers.
- Have there been any complications from the use of steroids over many years?
  - Consider obesity, diabetes mellitus and osteoporosis.

SENIOR STUDENTS

- Can you tell us some of the serological tests used in making the diagnosis of SLE?
  - Refer to Table 3.49.1.

Marking criteria table

Criteria	Satisfactory	Unsatisfactory
Introduces self, explains task, obtains consent	1	0
Asks questions about how the diagnosis was made	1	0
Finds out about the time course	1	0
Asks in a methodical way about the major groups of symptoms	3	0–2
Finds out what effect this chronic illness has had on her, her family and her work	2	0–1
Asks about treatment, its effectiveness and side effects e.g. osteoporosis as a result of steroid use	3	0–2
Knows the basics of serological testing	1	0

Pass mark: 8

Systemic lupus erythematosus examination

Background

As outlined in Station 48, almost any part of the body may be affected by systemic lupus erythematosus (SLE). The examination needs to be very general unless directed to a particular area by the history (or the examiners).

Introduction

Please examine this 40-year-old woman, who was diagnosed with SLE at the age of 25.

Rationale

Depending on the current activity and severity of the disease, there may or may not be many signs. The examiners, however, will expect you to know the important signs that you should look for. Refer to Fig. 3.49.1 to refresh your memory.

The examination

Method

1. Introduce yourself and, of course, wash your hands.
2. Would you mind if I had a look at you for changes caused by this disease?
3. Inspect the patient for weight loss and cushingoid appearance (because of steroid treatment) and assess the patient's general mental state.

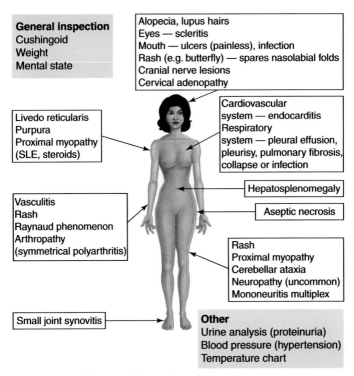

| **General inspection** Cushingoid Weight Mental state | Alopecia, lupus hairs Eyes — scleritis Mouth — ulcers (painless), infection Rash (e.g. butterfly) — spares nasolabial folds Cranial nerve lesions Cervical adenopathy |

Livedo reticularis
Purpura
Proximal myopathy
(SLE, steroids)

Cardiovascular system — endocarditis
Respiratory system — pleural effusion, pleurisy, pulmonary fibrosis, collapse or infection

Hepatosplenomegaly

Aseptic necrosis

Vasculitis
Rash
Raynaud phenomenon
Arthropathy
(symmetrical polyarthritis)

Rash
Proximal myopathy
Cerebellar ataxia
Neuropathy (uncommon)
Mononeuritis multiplex

Small joint synovitis

Other
Urine analysis (proteinuria)
Blood pressure (hypertension)
Temperature chart

Figure 3.49.1 Where to look for physical signs of systemic lupus erythematosus

4. Examine all the skin for a discoid lupus erythematosus (DLE) raised rash (Fig. 3.49.2), a photosensitivity rash and a classical malar rash (Fig. 3.49.3).
   Remember that DLE occurs in 20% of SLE patients. This disfiguring skin disease leads to permanent hair loss with telangiectasia, scaling, circular erythematous lesions and follicular plugging. There is often destruction of skin appendages. DLE can occur without other features of SLE.
5. Look at the hands for vasculitis, which can produce nail-fold infarcts and ischaemia or gangrene, and rash (e.g. photosensitivity, diffuse maculopapular rash).

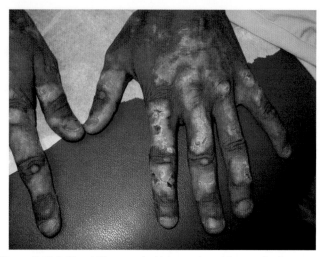

Figure 3.49.2 Discoid lupus rash. Note sparing of the proximal interphalangeal joints, a typical SLE feature (Dall'Era M. *Kelley's Textbook of Rheumatology*. Saunders Elsevier, 2013, with permission.)

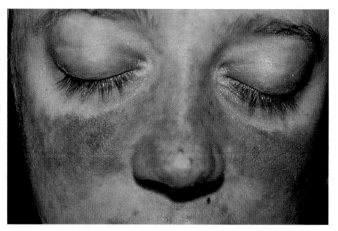

Figure 3.49.3 Malar rash in SLE (face) (Beck BJ. Mental disorders due to a general medical condition. *Comprehensive Clinical Psychiatry*. Ch 21:257–281. Online Archives of Rheumatology, 2008, with permission)

6. Look for Raynaud phenomenon and arthropathy (fusiform swelling of the proximal interphalangeal (PIP) joints or synovitis, possibly in a rheumatoid arthritis distribution — 10% develop swan neck deformity and ulnar deviation of the fingers).

7. Look at the forearms for livedo reticularis and purpura as a result of vasculitis or thrombocytopenia. Test for proximal myopathy caused by actual disease or secondary to steroid treatment.

8. Inspect the head. Look for alopecia. Lupus hairs are characteristic: they occur above the forehead and are short, broken hairs that grow back quickly after hair loss.

9. Look at the eyes for keratoconjunctivitis sicca and for pale conjunctivae owing to anaemia.

10. Look in the mouth for ulcers and infection. Note any facial rash (butterfly photosensitivity rash (30%), discoid lupus or diffuse maculopapular rashes). Feel the cervical and axillary nodes.

11. Examine the cardiovascular system, note signs of pericarditis (pericardial rub) and murmurs (Libman-Sacks endocarditis).

12. In the respiratory system, note signs of pleural effusion (absent breath sounds and stony dull percussion note), pleuritis (a pleural rub), and interstitial lung disease (fine basal crackles).

13. Examine the abdomen for splenomegaly (usually mild) and hepatomegaly. Feel for abdominal tenderness.

14. Examine for proximal weakness in the legs, cerebellar ataxia, hemiplegia and transverse myelitis. Assess mental status (cognitive changes, even psychosis).

15. Also examine for neuropathy (mainly sensory) and mononeuritis multiplex, as well as thrombophlebitis and leg ulceration.

16. Look at the urine analysis for evidence of renal disease (haematuria and proteinuria).

17. Take the blood pressure (it may be elevated in renal disease). Also look at the temperature chart for fever, indicating active disease or secondary infection.

Present your findings

Summarise the important positive and negative findings, beginning with the general inspection and then skin and joint changes. If there were no cardiac or respiratory abnormalities, just say that these examinations were normal. Comment on any signs that the disease is active, such as rashes, ulcers or joint swelling.

Examiners' likely questions

- What possible abnormalities were you looking for in your cardiac and respiratory examination?
  - Mention rubs and effusions from serositis (pleura and pericardium), inspiratory crackles from interstitial lung disease, arterial or venous thromboembolism from overlying antiphospholipid syndrome and the rare sterile endocarditis (Libman-Sacks endocarditis).
- Did the patient appear cushingoid?
  - The patient may have some but not all cushingoid features; a good answer would outline which ones are present and which are lacking.
- Tell us about some of the useful blood tests for lupus.
  - See Table 3.49.1, but also discuss tests for inflammation (e.g. C-reactive protein — CRP) and chronic disease

TABLE 3.49.1 Antibodies associated with SLE

Antibody	Comments
Anti-single-stranded DNA	Not specific (useless!)
Anti-double-stranded DNA	70% — high titres are specific
Anti-Smith (anti-Sm)	30% — specific for lupus
Anti-ribonuclear protein (anti-RNP)	30% in low titre — high titre in mixed connective tissue disease (MCTD)
Antihistone	drug-induced SLE, usually from hydralazine or procainamide; 95%
Antiphospholipid	50% — include anticardiolipin and lupus anticoagulant
Anti-erythrocyte	60% — occasionally causes anaemia
Antilymphocyte	70% — possible leucopenia

(e.g. normocytic anaemia) and of renal function — so important for prognosis (estimated glomerular filtration rate — eGFR).

Criteria	Satisfactory	Unsatisfactory
Introduces self, explains task, obtains consent, washes hands	1	0
Begins with a general inspection	1	0
Examines the hands and arms for skin and joint changes	2	0–1
Examines the head and neck for skin, hair changes and lymphadenopathy	2	0–1
Examines the chest for interstitial lung disease, effusions	1	0
Examines the abdomen for splenomegaly	1	0
Examines other joints for arthropathy	1	0
Examines the legs for peripheral neuropathy	1	0
Presents findings coherently	2	0–1

Pass mark: 7

Take a history — diabetes mellitus

Background

Juvenile diabetes (immune-mediated diabetes) is called type 1 and maturity-onset diabetes (non-immune-mediated diabetes) is called type 2. Most type 1 diabetes (type 1A) is associated with autoimmune destruction of islet cells, but a small proportion of these diabetics do not have these abnormalities (type 1B). Type 2 diabetes is increasingly found in obese adolescents and children. More than 90% of diabetics have type 2 disease.

- Remember the criteria for diagnosis of diabetes mellitus — a fasting (overnight) blood sugar level (BSL) of 7.0 mmol/L or higher on at least two separate occasions or, in the absence of fasting hyperglycaemia, a 2-hour postprandial glucose level of 11.1 mmol/L or higher.
- Fasting blood glucose levels of 6.1–7.0 mmol/L are considered to represent impaired fasting glucose levels. In a patient with symptoms of diabetes, a random BSL of >11.1 mmol/L is diagnostic.
- There is evidence that complications of diabetes may occur in some populations when the fasting glucose level is over 6.1 mmol/L.
- An HbA1c level of >48 mmol/mol (>6.5%) is consistent with a diagnosis of diabetes and is often used in place of a formal 75 g glucose tolerance test to make the diagnosis, except in pregnancy.

Introduction

This man has diabetes mellitus. Please take a history from him.

Rationale

This common condition (type 2 more common than type 1) has numerous complications involving most regions of the body. Treatment can be complicated. The examiners will be looking for an efficient approach that results in a comprehensive history. This is a very big OSCE and will likely be constructed as a more focused topic for the OSCEs, such as optimising current treatment or the various complications of the disease.

Method

Ask about the age at which diabetes was diagnosed and its manner of presentation, including thirst, polyuria and polydipsia, weight loss, infection, ketoacidosis, asymptomatic glycosuria.

Remember the rare causes of glucose intolerance (Box 3.50.1).

1. Ask about the treatment initiated at diagnosis and any major changes that have occurred over time (insulin is

---

Box 3.50.1
Causes of glucose intolerance

Diabetes mellitus
Counter-regulatory hormone excess (rare)
- Acromegaly
- Cushing syndrome
- Phaeochromocytoma
- Glucagonoma (associated with necrolytic erythema)
Pregnancy
Drugs
- Steroids or oral contraceptives
- Streptozotocin
- Thiazide diuretics (temporary and mild, secondary to hypokalaemia)
- Phenytoin, diazoxide (insulin secretion inhibited)
Pancreatic disease
- Chronic pancreatitis or carcinoma
- Haemochromatosis (decreased insulin production with or without increased insulin resistance)
Chronic liver disease (insulin resistance)

> **Box 3.50.2**
> **Recommended contribution to daily energy for type 1 and type 2 diabetes**
>
> Protein 10–20% kJ/day
> Saturated fat <10% kJ/day
> Polyunsaturated fat 10% kJ/day
> Carbohydrate (50–55%) and monounsaturated fats for the rest
> Artificial sweeteners as required
> Fibre 30g/day

required for survival in type 1 diabetes, which usually has an onset below age 30 years; in type 2 diabetes, control typically becomes more difficult with time).

2. Ask about the diet prescribed (Box 3.50.2). The previous strict dietary rules using exchanges and portions have largely been abandoned, but some patients may still use them (one exchange = 15g of carbohydrate = 60 calories = 250kJ (but the definition does vary). For example, for an average-sized male, three exchanges for each main meal and two exchanges for morning and afternoon tea and supper are required to provide an even carbohydrate distribution — 50% of the diet.
Ask whether the patient knows about the glycaemic index (GI) factor. What has happened to the patient's weight since the diagnosis was made? Newly diagnosed type 2 diabetics who lose weight and exercise may lose their glucose intolerance.

3. Ask whether oral hypoglycaemic drugs have been used or are being taken. Which ones? Have there been problems with any of them?

4. Ask about insulin treatment — how much, and when taken. The usual dose is 0.5 units/kg/day, with 40% of the dose comprising a long-acting insulin. Also ask where the insulin is injected and by whom, and find out the type of insulin syringe used (e.g. a pen injector).

5. Ask about the progress of the disease:
   - When did the patient last see a diabetic educator or endocrinologist and how often do these visits occur?
   - Assess adequacy of control — does the patient use a home blood glucose monitoring meter? If the patient is

blind, is the glucometer a talking version? Inquire how often the test is done, the usual results, at what time of day the test is performed (pre- or postprandial or both) and whether the dose is adjusted at other times (e.g. gastrointestinal upset). Ask about recent glycosylated haemoglobin (HbA1c) results.

-   Ask about symptoms of poor control:
    -   hyperglycaemia — polyuria, thirst, weight loss, intermittent blurring of vision, hospital admissions with ketoacidosis (type 1 diabetes only)
    -   hypoglycaemia/hypoglycaemia occurrence and awareness — ask about any previous episodes of hypoglycaemia and the precipitating factors. Ask the patient to describe the symptoms and how they are managed; ask specifically about morning headaches, morning lethargy and night sweats (symptoms suggestive of nocturnal hypoglycaemia), weight gain and seizures; ask about the time of day in relation to food, alcohol, exercise and insulin injection.

6. Ask about involvement of other systems:
    -   vascular system — ischaemic heart disease, intermittent claudication, cerebrovascular disease (macrovascular complications)
    -   nervous system — peripheral neuropathy, autonomic neuropathy (causing erectile dysfunction, fainting, nocturnal diarrhoea), amyotrophy
    -   eyes — regular visits to an ophthalmologist or retinal photography at the diabetes clinic, and treatment received (ask especially about laser treatment)
    -   renal system — dysuria, nocturia, oedema, hypertension; is the patient taking an angiotensin-converting enzyme (ACE) inhibitor or angiotensin receptor (AR) blocker for renal protection? has there been proteinuria?
    -   skin — boils, vaginitis and balanitis, *Candida*, necrobiosis lipoidica.

7. Ask about prevention and treatment of diabetic foot disease (special footwear, nail cutting, podiatry reviews and history of ulcers).

8. Ask about drug history — steroids, thiazides, oral contraceptives and beta-blockers are associated with

> **Box 3.50.3**
> **Risk factors for type 2 diabetes**
>
> Family history (first-degree relatives)
> Age over 45
> Overweight (body mass index (BMI) $>27\,kg/m^2$)
> Race (Australian Aboriginals are at risk with BMI $>22\,kg/m^2$;
>   Pacific Islander)
> Previous abnormal fasting glucose (6.1–7.0 mmol/L)
> Gestational diabetes
> Hypertension
> Polycystic ovaries

hyperglycaemia, while beta-blockers may blunt hypoglycaemia awareness. All of those medications are commonly used and not contraindicated in diabetes.

9. Ask about associated other diseases — history of pancreatitis, Cushing syndrome, acromegaly.
10. Inquire about social background — type of work, living conditions (living alone or with family), coping with giving insulin (associated blindness etc.), eating habits, financial situation, driving (type of licence held).
11. Ask about variations in weight and a regular exercise program. Have diet and exercise led to a fall in weight since the diabetes was diagnosed?
12. Ask about cardiovascular risk factors, including family history, serum cholesterol level, smoking and hypertension, and drug and non-drug attempts at control of these factors (except family history).
13. Inquire about family history of diabetes and obstetric history (e.g. gestational diabetes suggested by large babies and stillbirths), and other risk factors for type 2 diabetes (see Box 3.50.3).
14. Ask whether the patient has an action plan for hypoglycaemic symptoms and what this involves.
15. Try to assess the patient's understanding of the disease and its prognosis. See Box 3.50.4. How does he or she feel about his or her future?

Present your findings

- Begin by naming the type of diabetes.

> **Box 3.50.4**
> **Particular considerations for type 1 diabetes**
>
> Insulin is always required
> Absolute lack of insulin makes BSLs unstable
> BSL testing at least four times a day is optimal
> Much higher risk of severe hypoglycaemia (10-fold at least)
> Much higher risk of life-threatening ketoacidosis
> Severe disruption to normal life from >1000 BSL tests a year
> Complicated and constant adjustments of insulin doses
> Vascular and renal complications occur later but still at a young age
>   for most patients
> Vascular complications common once proteinuria occurs
> Lifelong aggressive control of cardiovascular risk factors is essential
> Associated autoimmune abnormalities are common — if clinically
>   indicated, test for thyroid and coeliac disease

- Outline the symptoms at diagnosis and the time since diagnosis.
- Describe the changes in treatment over time.
- What is the current treatment regime? Include discussion of blood sugar monitoring and results of HbA1c tests if the patient knows them.
- Have there been treatment complications — hypoglycaemic episodes, gain in weight, and fat atrophy at injection sites?
- Go through the various complications of the disease systematically and say which have occurred and which have not.
- Has there been regular screening for complications — eye examinations, tests of renal function, foot care etc.?
- Have cardiovascular risk factors been assessed and controlled? Remember, this is the most common cause of mortality.

Examiners' likely questions

- How well controlled is this patient's diabetes?
    - Discuss the HbA1c, patient's blood sugar measurements and management of complications.
- How good is this patient's understanding of the disease?
    - Talk about the way complications are managed and the patient's approach to blood sugar readings, hypoglycaemic episodes and weight.

- What do you think the prognosis is?
  - Talk about complications, especially cardiovascular and renal ones. Has renal dialysis been discussed? These factors affect the prognosis.

Marking criteria table

Criteria	Satisfactory	Unsatisfactory
Introduces self, explains task, thanks patient for help, obtains consent	1	0
Asks about the way the disease presented and was diagnosed	2	0–1
Establishes the time course of treatment, including non-drug measures	2	0–1
How does the patient manage BSL testing, hypos etc.?	2	0–1
Perfoms thorough questioning about complications and their management	3	0–2
Asks about effect of this chronic disease on the patient's life, work and family	2	0–1
Asks about mood and expectations for the future	1	0
Makes a coherent, usually chronological presentation of the findings	2	0–1
Answers the examiners' questions	2	0–1

Pass mark: 11

Examine a patient with type 1 diabetes

Background

Patients with type 1 diabetes are often very different from type 2 diabetics. They are not usually overweight, they are usually taking insulin and they are often well informed about their disease.

Introduction

- This woman has diabetes. Please examine her.
- This man has diabetes. Please examine his eyes (or even his legs).

Rationale

Students are expected to have a systematic approach to the detection of the many complications of diabetes. This big OSCE will often be broken into parts, such as eyes, legs, neurological examination.

Method

See Box 3.51.1.

1. Do the usual with your possibly germ-laden hands.
2. Expose the patient's legs. This is the only case in which there is an advantage in starting at the legs.
3. Look for pigmented scars, skin atrophy, ulceration and infection, and for necrobiosis lipoidica over the shins (a central yellow scarred area with a surrounding red margin, if active, owing to atrophy of subcutaneous collagen — it is rare) (Fig. 3.51.1).

Box 3.51.1
Diabetes mellitus examination

1. General inspection
Weight — obesity
Hydration
Endocrine facies
Pigmentation — haemochromatosis etc.

2. Legs
Inspect:
Skin — necrobiosis, hair loss, infection, pigmented scars, atrophy, ulceration, injection sites
Muscle wasting
Joint destruction — Charcot's joints
Palpate:
Temperature of feet (cold, blue owing to small or large vessel disease)
Peripheral pulses:
Femoral (auscultate)
Popliteal
Posterior tibial
Dorsalis pedis
Oedema:
Neurological assessment
Femoral nerve mononeuritis
Peripheral neuropathy

3. Arms
Inspect:
Injection sites
Skin lesions
Pulse

4. Eyes
Fundi — cataracts, rubeosis, retinal disease, III nerve palsy, etc.

5. Mouth and ears
Infection

6. Neck
Carotid arteries — palpate, auscultate

7. Chest
Signs of infection

8. Abdomen
Liver — fat infiltration; rarely haemochromatosis
Fat hypertrophyt — insulin injection sites

9. Other
Urine analysis — glycosuria, ketones, proteinuria
Blood pressure and pulset — lying and standing

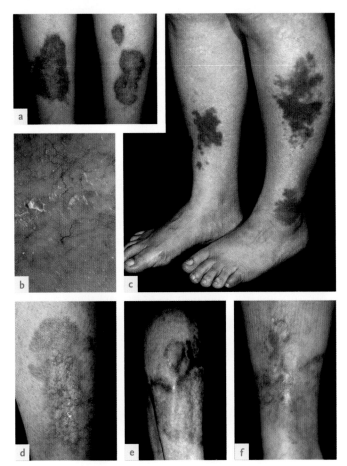

Figure 3.51.1 Necrobiosis lipoidica. **(a)** Erythematous violaceous plaques on the anterior surface of the lower legs **(b)** The central area atrophies and has a waxy surface with prominent telangiectasias **(c)** The mid lower legs are most often affected **(d)** The central area is waxy yellow with prominent telangiectasia **(e)** End-stage disease with severe atrophy and telangiectasia **(f)** Severe disease with dense fibrosis and ulceration (Dinulos GH. *Habif's Clinical Dermatology: A color guide to diagnosis and therapy*, 7th edn. Elsevier Inc., 2021.)

4. Look at the thigh for injection sites, fat atrophy (owing to the use of impure insulin) or fat hypertrophy (owing to repeated injections into the same site, which leads to scarring and hypertrophy) and quadriceps wasting, from femoral nerve mononeuritis — called (inaccurately) diabetic amyotrophy.

5. Inspect the feet and toes very carefully. Look for loss of hair, skin atrophy and blue, cool feet (small vessel vascular disease), ulcers and foot deformity.

6. Feel all the peripheral pulses and note capillary return.

7. Test proximal muscle power (hip flexion) and test the reflexes (knee jerk). (diabetic amyotrophy)

8. Assess for peripheral neuropathy, including dorsal column loss with impaired proprioception and vibration sense (diabetic pseudotabes), which are the first modalities to be impaired. Check for temperature and pin-prick (spinothalamic pathway) and light touch (medial lemniscal pathway).

9. Charcot joints (owing to proprioceptive loss) may be present (Fig. 3.51.2). (*Note:* neuropathic joint disease; sensory loss (e.g. from diabetes or leprosy) allows repeated

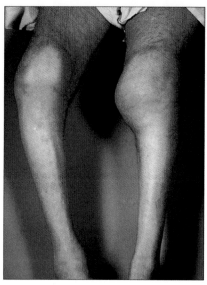

Figure 3.51.2 Charcot knee joints showing gross destructive changes (Gravallese EM, Hochberg MC, Smolen JS et al. *Rheumatology*, 7th edn. Elsevier Inc., 2019.)

joint trauma, producing bony overgrowth, synovial effusion and joint distortion and instability.)

10. Go to the upper limbs. Look at the nails for *Candida* infection.
11. Feel the upper arm injection sites.
12. Ask for the blood pressure or take the pulse and blood pressure lying and standing to detect autonomic neuropathy.
13. Now examine the eyes for visual acuity. Remember, episodes of poor control cause lens abnormalities acutely (Fig. 3.51.3). Next assess the pupils and light reflex. Remember, a diabetic third nerve palsy is usually pupil-sparing — infarction affects the inner more than the outer fibres, whereas compressive lesions affect the outer fibres first and so involve the pupil early.
14. Ask to look in the fundi (Fig 3.51.3). Know the changes expected — non-proliferative (dot and blot haemorrhages, microaneurysms, hard and soft exudates) and proliferative (scars, retinal detachment). While performing fundoscopy

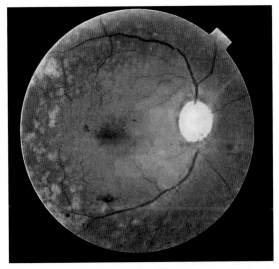

Figure 3.51.3 Diabetic retinopathy. Small hemorrhages (blots), micro-aneurysms (dots), and hard yellow exudates (Talley NJ, O'Connor S. *Talley and O'Connor's Examination Medicine*. Elsevier Australia, 2020.)

for diabetic retinopathy, also note the presence of cataracts and any new blood vessel formation over the iris (rubeosis).

15. Test the III, IV and VI cranial nerves and remember that other cranial nerves may be affected. Do so by examining the range of eye movements — see Fig. 2.11.6.

16. Look in the mouth for *Candida* and other infections. If there is time:

17. Examine for hepatomegaly as a result of fatty infiltration and then ask for the results of urine analysis with respect to glucose and protein.

18. There may be signs of chronic kidney disease with advanced diabetes.

19. Ask whether you may weigh the patient.

> **T&O'C hint box**
>
> The examination is directed at looking for the complications of diabetes and these may be hinted at by the introduction; for example, numbness in the legs usually means peripheral neuropathy.

Present your findings

- Try to address any problems suggested by the introduction.
- Describe the important positive and negative findings.
- Comment on the patient's weight.

> **T&O'C hint box**
>
> The sophisticated student will use the signs that have been elicited to make a diagnosis. For example 'I found evidence of a peripheral sensory neuropathy to the knees and a Charcot joint at the left ankle' rather than 'there was numbness when I tested pin-prick sensation in the legs and the left ankle looked swollen'.

- Ask for certain important routine investigations:
  - the patient's blood sugar recordings or HbA1c
  - Retinal photographs
  - Urinalysis for proteinuria
  - Creatinine and estimated glomerular filtration rate (eGFR)
  - Doppler ultrasound assessments of blood flow in the legs.

Examiners' likely questions

- What questions might you ask the patient?
  - How long have you had diabetes? (Complications are more likely over time.)
  - Do you know your last HbA1c result? (Well informed patients manage their diabetes better.)
  - What is your current treatment? (insulin or oral hypoglycaemic drugs)
  - Have you had problems with complications of the disease? (Prompt the patient with questions about kidneys, eyes, heart, nerves etc.)
- Can you give us an idea of the patient's prognosis?
  - This will depend on the time the disease has been present and what complications, especially vascular ones, have occurred.

If you are going very well there may be some questions about the value of improving the patient's blood sugar control and how this might be achieved.

Marking criteria table

Criteria	Satisfactory	Unsatisfactory
Introduces self, explains task, obtains consent, washes hands	1	0
Follows examiners' instructions; e.g. when told to examine legs, does so	1	0
Assesses systematically the area being examined	1	0
Looks for important diabetic complications likely to be present	2	0
Presents findings accurately	2	0–1
Asks for appropriate test results and can justify the request	2	0–1
Answers examiners' questions	2	0–1

Pass mark: 9

Take a history from a patient with suspected osteoporosis

Background

- The patient is often a postmenopausal woman or is taking corticosteroids for an acute or chronic inflammatory illness.
- Osteoporosis will commonly form part of another medical problem.
- Osteoporotic fractures can affect 30% of postmenopausal women over their lifetime. Many older women have undergone screening bone densitometry and may be aware that they have asymptomatic osteoporosis.
- Patients who have had a hip fracture or who have evidence of an endocrine disorder, malabsorption, liver disease, Crohn disease or bone marrow disease, or who are taking certain medications, should have the possibility of osteoporosis considered while they are being evaluated (see Box 3.52.1).
- Screening questions that help assess the risk of osteoporosis should form part of a general history taking.

Introduction

This woman has had a diagnosis of osteoporosis. Please take a history from her.

Rationale

Osteoporosis is the result of decreased bone mass with increased bone fragility. Students need to know how to identify women at

Box 3.52.1
Major secondary causes of osteoporosis

Drugs
Steroids (chronic, usually high dose use)
Chronic heparin therapy
Thyroxine over-replacement
Phenytoin

Gastrointestinal diseases
Malabsorption syndromes (e.g. coeliac disease, Crohn disease)

Malnutrition
Anorexia nervosa
Scurvy
Alcoholism

Connective tissue diseases
Ehlers-Danlos syndrome
Osteogenesis imperfecta
Rheumatoid arthritis

Endocrine diseases
Hyperthyroidism
Hyperparathyroidism
Cushing syndrome
Hyperprolactinaemia
Hypogonadism

risk of osteoporosis and particularly of fractures. These have a high morbidity and mortality in elderly women. You want to ask about the history of low-impact fractures, back pain and height loss, and the presence of risk factors for osteoporosis. The advanced student might be asked about investigations and therapy. A good student will also consider osteomalacia in the differential diagnosis and ask further relevant questions. (Osteomalacia is defective bone mineralisation, usually due to low vitamin D levels.)

Method

1. Ask about a history of fractures, particularly fractures of the wrist (risk increases from age 55), hip (risk increases from age 70), humerus and ribs, and vertebral compression

fractures (especially T12), which may have occurred with minimal stress (risk increases from age 55). Has the patient had any episodes of prolonged immobilisation?

2. Has there been sudden back pain which took weeks or months to subside? (Vertebral compression fractures often present like this and may recur.) Has the patient's height decreased?

   If the patient has had a hip fracture, ask about any secondary complications, including pulmonary thromboembolism and nosocomial infections.

3. Ask about symptoms of diffuse bone pain and proximal muscle weakness, which suggests osteomalacia (characterised by defective bone mineralisation in adults).

4. Ask if the patient is a smoker (and ask about the details). (Cigarette smoking reduces skeletal mass.)

   Determine the menstrual history and age of onset of menopause. Inquire about symptoms of thyroid excess or thyroid hormone replacement (thyroxine).

   Take a past history with a focus on relevant chronic diseases that can cause osteoporosis (Box 3.52.1).

5. Ask about bone pain and proximal weakness (osteomalacia, usually due to vitamin D deficiency; then you must exclude malabsorption).

6. Take a careful drug history. Medications that cause osteoporosis include steroids (dose and how long — normally occurs after 3 months of steroid treatment), alcohol, heparin, thyroxine over-replacement, and chronic anticonvulsants (by affecting vitamin D metabolism).

   Also ask about medications used to treat osteoporosis (e.g. calcium and vitamin D, or a bisphosphonate, which may be delivered orally or intravenously).

7. Inquire about a poor diet (a low-fat diet often limits calcium intake) or inadequate sunlight exposure if the patient is a nursing home resident, or has a history of renal disease or phenytoin use (all risk factors for osteomalacia) (Boxes 3.52.2 and 3.52.3).

8. Ask about the patient's exercise history, as physical activity throughout life preserves bone mass.

9. Determine any risk factors for falls: a greater risk of falls increases the risk of fracture at any level of osteoporosis.

Box 3.52.2
Sunlight requirements

Inadequate sunlight exposure can lead to osteomalacia.
 Sun exposure and maintenance of normal vitamin D levels in moderately fair-skinned people requires:
- 6–7 minutes of sun exposure to the arms, face and hands in the mid-morning or afternoon in summer
- 9–13 minutes of exposure in winter in northern Australia
- 11–15 minutes of exposure in winter in central Australia (Brisbane or Perth)
- 16 (Sydney) –30 minutes (Hobart) of exposure of as much skin as practical in winter in the middle of the day

Box 3.52.3
Causes of osteomalacia

Unavailability of vitamin D:
- vitamin D malabsorption (e.g. coeliac disease, pancreatic insufficiency, cirrhosis)
- abnormal vitamin D metabolism (e.g. chronic kidney disease, pseudohypoparathyroidism)
- decreased vitamin D bioavailability (e.g. inadequate sunlight, nephrotic syndrome, peritoneal dialysis)
 Phosphate unavailability caused by phosphate-binding antacids, hereditary hypophosphataemia, tumour-induced osteomalacia (e.g. fibrous dysplasia of bone)
 Normal anion gap metabolic acidosis (e.g. distal renal tubular acidosis (type 1) with hypokalaemia and hypercalciuria, often caused by autoimmune disease such as Sjögren syndrome or systemic lupus erythematosus (SLE))

10. Ask if there is a family history of osteoporosis (a risk factor for osteoporosis).
11. Determine the social effect of the disease (e.g. immobility, pain, fear of falling).
12. Have vitamin D levels been measured? Were they reduced?

13. Ask if a bone density (DEXA) scan has been performed. The patient may know the result and whether it means she qualifies for treatment for osteoporosis. A previous minimal trauma fracture or prolonged use of steroids is an indication for treatment of osteoporosis without the need for a DEXA scan.

Present your findings

- Describe any features of the history that suggest osteoporosis.
- Outline the relevant positive and negative risk factors.
- List the investigations the patient knows about.
- What treatment has been prescribed?

Examiners' likely questions

- How definite is the diagnosis of osteoporosis for this patient?
    - Describe any minimal trauma fractures and the results of a DEXA scan if the patient has had one.
- Is she at risk of more fractures?
    - Discuss the severity of the disease as far as you have been able to tell, and the risk of falls.
- How has the condition affected her life?
    - Is she in constant pain? Can she manage at home with or without help?

Marking criteria table

Criteria	Satisfactory	Unsatisfactory
Introduces self, explains task, obtains consent	1	0
Asks if patient knows she has osteoporosis	1	0
Asks how diagnosis was made and if she knows how severe it is	1	0
Asks about fractures and whether these have occurred with minimal trauma	1	0
Is the patient anxious about falls and the risk of fractures to the point of limiting her activities?	1	0
Asks if vitamin D has been measured	1	0
Asks about drug treatment that may increase risk and treatment for osteoporosis — especially steroids	2	0–1
Asks about other risk factors for osteoporosis	2	0–1
Has a DEXA scan been performed? What was the result?	1	0
Understands the difference between osteoporosis and osteomalacia	1	0

Pass mark: 7

53

Take a history from a patient with suspected acromegaly

Background

Although an uncommon condition, three to four new cases per million people a year, acromegaly is a chronic illness and patients are available for exams as a history-taking or examination OSCE.

Introduction

The examiners will usually give you the diagnosis but sometimes the introduction is more oblique.

- This man has had a diagnosis of acromegaly. Please ask him about his illness.
- This woman has noticed an increase in the size of her hands. Her rings no longer fit. Ask her about this and her health problems.

Rationale

This tests your knowledge of the features of acromegaly and the effect of this chronic condition on the patient's life.

Method

The patient will probably know the diagnosis.

1. Find out when the diagnosis was made and how long ago; in retrospect, the patient may have had symptoms for years. The average time taken to make the diagnosis is more than 10 years.
2. Ask why the diagnosis was suspected. The onset of abnormalities is usually very gradual. The common features of the condition are listed in Box 3.53.1.

Box 3.53.1
Symptoms and signs in acromegaly

Acral enlargement*
Cardiac failure
Carpal tunnel syndrome
Diabetes mellitus
Enlarged jaw and facial features* (see Fig. 3.53.1)
Erectile dysfunction and hypogonadism
Galactorrhoea
Goitre
Headache*
Hypertension
Hypopituitarism
Macroglossia
Muscle weakness
Osteoarthritis
Paraesthesiae
Peripheral neuropathy
Skin tags and colon polyps
Soft-tissue enlargement*
Sweating*
Symptoms of sleep apnoea
Visual disturbance (field defect): bitemporal hemianopia as with other
    pituitary tumours

*In >50% of patients

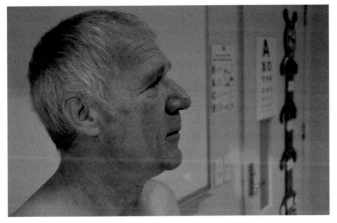

Figure 3.53.1 Acromegalic appearance (Talley NJ, O'Connor S. *Talley
and O'Connor's Examination Medicine*. Elsevier Australia, 2020.)

3. Ask what changes the patient has been aware of and whether these have improved with treatment. (Bony and acral changes are irreversible.)

4. Ask about the associations and complications of the condition. Any history of heart disease or myocardial infarction? Has the patient been screened for colon cancer and, if so, how and when? The mortality rate for untreated acromegaly is about twice that of the age-matched population, mostly as a result of an increased risk of cardiovascular disease. There is also an increase in the incidence of colonic polyps and carcinoma of the colon.

5. There is an association with obstructive sleep apnoea and questions should be asked about snoring, daytime sleepiness and other relevant symptoms. The reason for the association is the enlargement of the tongue and swelling of the upper airway.

6. Ask if the patient knows what investigations have been performed (see investigations below).

7. Ask about current and past treatment and how helpful this has been. (Pituitary surgery and radiotherapy have a number of possible complications.)

   Have hormone replacement treatments been necessary because of loss of pituitary gland function? What do these involve (steroids, thyroid hormone, sex hormones)?

8. As with any chronic illness, the effect of acromegaly on the patient's life may be severe. Ask about occupation and ability to work.

Present your findings

- Outline the course of the disease as it has occurred in this patient.
- Include information about how the diagnosis was made, what investigations the patient knows of and what treatment has been used.
- List any complications or side effects of treatment.
- Explain what effect the illness has had on the patient's life, work and family.

Examiners' likely questions

- How can the definitive diagnosis be made?
  - The preferred test is measurement of insulin-like growth factor 1 (IGF-1). Unlike growth hormone (GH), which is affected by exercise and diet, the level of IGF-1 does not fluctuate and the absolute level reliably reflects the average GH level. The result must be interpreted according to the patient's age — levels are highest at puberty and decline with age. There is also physiological elevation of the level in pregnancy.
  - The diagnosis is usually confirmed with a glucose tolerance test, where growth hormone suppression (normal to <0.3 mcg/L) is measured in response to a glucose load. Failure of suppression is characteristic of acromegaly, but the test is non-specific and may be abnormal in renal impairment, thyrotoxicosis and diabetes.
  - Imaging is performed once an elevated IGF-1 is confirmed. MRI scanning is the modality of choice as it provides excellent anatomical definition of the tumour (see Fig. 3.53.2). Seventy per cent of tumours are macroadenomas (>1 cm).
  - If the tumour is close to the optic chiasm, formal visual field assessment should be performed.
- How would you test pituitary function?
  - Basal tests of pituitary function
  - 9 a.m. cortisol
  - Testosterone or oestradiol
  - Luteinising hormone (LH) and follicle-stimulating hormone (FSH)
  - Prolactin
  - Thyroid-stimulating hormone (TSH) and free T4.
- What long-term screening is indicated?
  - Cardiovascular: echocardiography 5- to 10-yearly (heart failure, valve disease)
  - Gastrointestinal: colonoscopy for polyps — at diagnosis and as required for surveillance
  - Thyroid: thyroid examination and thyroid function tests (TFTs) regularly

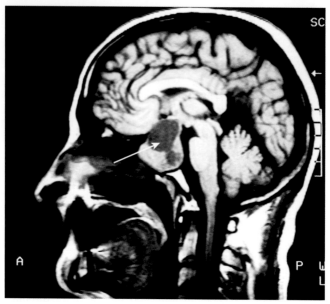

Figure 3.53.2 MRI of the brain, showing a large pituitary tumour (arrow) (Figure reproduced courtesy of The Canberra Hospital.)

- – Metabolic: check blood pressure, check lipids annually, fasting blood sugar level (BSL) annually
- – Musculoskeletal: ask about symptoms; carpal tunnel, arthropathy.
- ● How has the patient coped with this chronic illness?

NOTES ON INVESTIGATIONS

In 25% of acromegalic patients, the prolactin level is elevated and this can be associated with galactorrhoea. Other pituitary hormone levels may be low because of interference with normal pituitary function by the large mass of the tumour. Baseline pituitary function should be assessed with measurements of prolactin, cortisol, thyroxine, FSH, LH.

Marking criteria table

Criteria	Satisfactory	Unsatisfactory
Introduces self, explains task, obtains consent	1	0
Asks about the diagnosis, presenting symptoms and investigations	2	0–1
Goes through the list of common symptoms	3	0–2
Asks what treatment, drug and surgical, has been tried	3	0–2
Asks about the effect of the disease on life, work and family	2	0–1
Asks about follow-up and monitoring	1	0

Pass mark: 8

Acromegaly examination

Background

The changes of acromegaly are very gradual and often not noticed by the patient, his or her family or the usual doctor. Old photographs will often demonstrate what striking changes have occurred over time.

Introduction

- This man has noted some change in his facial appearance. Please examine him.
- This man has acromegaly. Please examine him for activity and features of the disease.

Rationale

This endocrine disease can affect many parts of the body and provides a suite of possible findings. The examiners will expect some comment on disease activity (Box 3.54.1).

Method

The order and direction of the examination obviously depend on the stem. However, if a 'change of appearance' of any part of the body is mentioned in the stem, it is likely you are expected to make a spot diagnosis. Look very carefully at the patient before deciding where to examine.

1. Make a general inspection, looking especially for the acromegalic facies.
2. Wash your hands. Have the patient stand or sit on the side of the bed. Look at the hands. Look for coarse features and spade-like shape (Fig. 3.54.1 a, c), as well as increased

Box 3.54.1
Evidence of activity in acromegaly

Skin tag number
Excessive sweating
Presence of glycosuria
Increasing visual field loss or development of cranial nerve palsies of
    III, IV, VI and V
Enlarging goitre
Hypertension
Symptoms of headache, or increasing ring size, shoe size or
    dentures

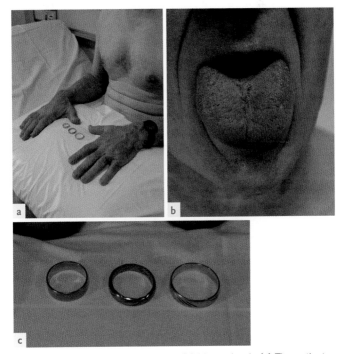

Figure 3.54.1 **(a)** Acromegalic hands **(b)** Macroglossia **(c)** The patient
has conveniently brought his rings with him (Talley NJ, O'Connor S.
Talley and O'Connor's Examination Medicine. Elsevier Australia, 2020.)

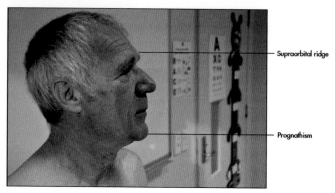

Supraorbital ridge

Prognathism

Figure 3.54.2 Acromegalic facies (Talley NJ, O'Connor S. *Talley and O'Connor's Examination Medicine*. Elsevier Australia, 2020.)

sweating and warmth. Osteoarthritis-like changes are frequent in the hands, shoulders, hips and knees.

Perform Phalen wrist flexion test for carpal tunnel syndrome (median nerve entrapment). Feel the ulnar nerve at the elbow for thickening.

3. Go to the arms and test for proximal myopathy. Also look in the axillae for skin tags (molluscum fibrosum), greasy skin and acanthosis nigricans (brown-to-black velvety elevation of the epidermis owing to multiple confluent papillomas).

4. Go on to the face (Fig. 3.54.2). Look for frontal bossing as a result of a large supraorbital ridge (which may also occur in rickets, Paget disease, hydrocephalus or achondroplasia). Note whether there is a large tongue (sometimes too big to fit into the mouth neatly — Fig. 3.54.1b). Enlargement of the lower jaw (called prognathism) and splaying of the teeth may be present. Notice any acne or hirsutism in women and test the voice, which may be deep, husky and resonant.

5. The eyes must be carefully examined. Visual fields should be checked — look particularly for bitemporal hemianopia, but many field defects are possible.

Ask if you may examine the fundi for optic atrophy, papilloedema and angioid streaks (red, brown or grey streaks three to five times the diameter of the retinal veins appearing to emanate from the optic disc and owing to degeneration of Bruch membrane with resultant fibrosis).

There may also be diabetic (growth hormone excess is diabetogenic) or hypertensive changes in the fundi.

6. Examine the thyroid gland for diffuse enlargement or a multinodular goitre.

7. Examine the cardiovascular system for signs of congestive cardiac failure, the abdomen for organomegaly — of liver, spleen and kidney — and for signs of hypogonadism (secondary to an enlarging pituitary adenoma).

8. Examine the lower limbs for osteoarthritis and pseudogout. Large osteophyte formation and ligamentous laxity are common features. Also look for foot drop (entrapment of common peroneal nerve) and heel pad thickening.

9. Assesses for evidence of hypothyroidism (including skin changes, e.g. cool, dry, cold hands; puffiness of the eyes; bradycardia; neck for a goitre).

10. Do not forget to ask for the results of a urine analysis to exclude glycosuria secondary to glucose intolerance and to take the blood pressure (hypertension is an association).

11. Decide whether the acromegaly is active (see Box 3.54.1). Ask whether any photographs taken of the patient over the years are available for inspection (typically, manifestations begin in middle age). See Box 3.54.2 for the diagnostic evaluation.

Present your findings

- List the features of acromegaly that are present and any important ones that are not.
- Try to decide if the disease is active (it probably won't be).
- If you are feeling confident (lucky), ask to see an MRI scan of the pituitary and for the results of IGF-1 testing.

Box 3.54.2
Diagnosis of acromegaly

Biochemical
Insulin-like growth factor (IGF-1) (somatomedin C) level in plasma
   (elevated in active acromegaly)
Glucose tolerance test (no suppression or a paradoxical rise in
   growth hormone level)

Anatomical (99% pituitary adenoma)
Skull X-ray (enlarged sella, double floor) — not routine
MRI scan (if normal, exclude extrapituitary acromegaly)

Examiners' likely questions

- Are the acral changes likely to improve?
  - No
- What screening for complications may be indicated?
  - See history taking (Station 53).
- Why might the patient need hormone replacement
  treatment?
  - There may have been damage to pituitary function by
    tumour or treatment (radiotherapy or surgery).

Marking criteria table

Criteria	Satisfactory	Unsatisfactory
Introduces self, explains task, obtains consent, washes hands before and after	1	0
Positions patient, starts with hands	1	0
Looks for arthritis and carpal tunnel syndrome	2	0–1
Offers to take blood pressure	1	0
Tests for proximal myopathy	1	0
Looks for skin tags	1	0
Looks for enlarged supraorbital ridge and macroglossia	2	0–1
Looks for prognathia	1	0
Asks to examine the fundi	1	0
Looks and feels for thyroid enlargement	1	0
Asks to look for organomegaly elsewhere	1	0
If prompted, asks for urine analysis	1	0

Pass mark: 9

Examine a patient with hypothyroidism

Background

Hypothyroidism is easily missed but is eminently treatable. Signs suggesting hypothyroidism include coarse cool dry skin, periorbital puffiness, hoarse voice, loss of the outer one-third of eyebrow hair and a slow pulse rate.

Introduction

This woman has been diagnosed with hypothyroidism. Please examine her.

Rationale

This OSCE tests the student's knowledge of the signs of hypothyroidism. Don't just focus on trying to find a goitre (many won't have one). It will soon be obvious to the examiners if you do not know what the signs are.

Method

If you are told the patient has *hypothyroidism*, proceed as follows.

1. Introduce yourself, explain what you will be doing and obtain consent. Wash your hands, then pick up the hands. Note peripheral cyanosis, swelling, and dry, cold skin. Look at the palmar creases for anaemia (see Box 3.55.1).

2. Feel the pulse for bradycardia and a small volume pulse.

3. Test for carpal tunnel syndrome. Ask the patient to flex both wrists for 30 seconds — paraesthesiae will often be precipitated in the affected hand if carpal tunnel syndrome is present (Phalen wrist flexion test).

> **Box 3.55.1**
> **Causes of anaemia in patients with hypothyroidism**
>
> 1. Chronic disease (direct or erythropoietin-mediated depressive effect on bone marrow)
> 2. Folate deficiency secondary to bacterial overgrowth
> 3. Pernicious anaemia associated with myxoedema
> 4. Iron deficiency in women owing to menorrhagia
> 5. Haemolysis secondary to hypercholesterolaemia-induced spur-cell anaemia

4. Test for delayed relaxation of the biceps jerk (advanced students — best shown testing the ankle jerk). Rarely you'll also find proximal weakness.
5. Proceed to the face. Note here any general swelling and periorbital oedema. Look for loss of the outer one-third of the eyebrows and periorbital xanthelasma. Touch the face. Note whether the skin is dry, fine and smooth. There may be signs of carotenaemia, alopecia or vitiligo.
6. Look at the tongue, which may be swollen, then ask the patient to tell you her name and address and note any hoarseness or slowness of speech.
7. Test for nerve deafness, which may be bilateral.
8. **Examine the neck for a goitre** (inspect while the patient sips some water, palpate from behind, percuss for retrosternal extension, auscultate if enlarged, Pemberton sign for a retrosternal goitre).
9. Go to the legs next. Look for swelling and check it's non-pitting. Examine the legs neurologically, starting with the ankle jerks, noting particularly any evidence of slow relaxation. This is best seen with the patient kneeling on a chair.

> **T&O'C hint box**
>
> Many cases of hypothyroidism are not associated with an enlarged thyroid gland but those with severe iodine deficiency, late Hashimoto's and treated thyrotoxicosis may have this finding.

10. If there is time, then examine for peripheral neuropathy, proximal myopathy and cerebellar signs that can all be manifestations of hypothyroidism but are uncommon.
11. Examine the chest if there is time (or ask to do so). A pleural effusion may be present. A pericardial effusion can also occur.

Present your findings

- Outline your findings after a general (but not derogatory) statement about the patient's appearance.
- Try to decide if the patient is hypothyroid, euthyroid or thyrotoxic.
- Decide if there is a goitre and any retrosternal extension of the gland.
- If there is time to talk about investigations, thyroid function tests (starting with thyroid-stimulating hormone — TSH) and a thyroid ultrasound (size and consistency of the gland) may be indicated.

Examiners' likely questions

- Do you think the disease is active?
  - This applies if you suspect thyrotoxicosis. Discuss the presence or absence of tachycardia, sweating, tremor, brisk reflexes and a bruit over the gland.
- Describe the patient's reflexes.
  - Brisk (thyrotoxicosis) or hung up (hypothyroidism) — a hung-up reflex is best demonstrated when the patient kneels on a chair.

Marking criteria table

Criteria	Satisfactory	Unsatisfactory
Introduces self, explains task, obtains consent, washes hands	1	0
General inspection	1	0
Examines hands and pulse	2	0–1
Assesses biceps jerk	1	0
Examines face	2	0–1
Assesses ankle jerks, if possible with patient kneeling; can describe a hung-up jerk	2	0–1
Looks for myxoedematous changes	1	0
Examines neck for goitre	1	0
Presents findings accurately	1	0
Offers a sensible discussion about investigations	1	0

Pass mark: 8

Weight gain (suspected Cushing syndrome) examination

Background

Remember the difference between Cushing disease and Cushing syndrome. Each is due to steroid excess: Cushing disease is due to pituitary overproduction of adrenocorticotropic hormone (ACTH); Cushing syndrome, which is much more common, is from excess steroid production of any cause including administration of steroids (often as treatment to induce immune suppression).

Introduction

- This woman has noted weight gain. Please examine her.
- This woman has had difficulty standing up from a chair and changes in her appearance. Please examine her.

Rationale

Steroids are prescribed for many inflammatory conditions and their side effects should be understood by students. Only rarely will a patient with Cushing disease be available for the exams.

Method

See Box 3.56.1.

1. This type of introduction may mean Cushing syndrome in the clinical examination (Fig. 3.56.1). It helps if the patient is undressed to her underwear. Ask her to stand.

Box 3.56.1
Cushing syndrome examination

Standing

1. General inspection
- Central obesity and thin limbs
- Skin bruising, atrophy
- Pigmentation (ACTH tumour — rare — or bilateral adrenalectomy)
- Poor wound healing

2. Arms
- Purple striae (proximally)
- Proximal myopathy

Sitting

3. Face
- Plethora, hirsutism, acne, telangiectasia
- Moon shape
- Eyes — visual fields (pituitary tumour), fundi (atrophy, papilloedema, signs of hypertension or diabetes)
- Mouth — thrush (with exogenous steroids)
- Neck — supraclavicular fat pads, acanthosis nigricans

4. Back
- Interscapular fat pad
- Kyphoscoliosis (osteoporosis)
- Tenderness of vertebrae (osteoporotic fractures)

5. Legs
- Squat (proximal myopathy)
- Striae (thighs)
- Bruising, oedema

6. Mental state
- Depression
- Psychosis
- Irritability

Lying flat

7. Abdomen
- Purple striae
- Adrenal masses, adrenalectomy scars
- Liver (tumour deposits)

8. Other
- Urine analysis (glycosuria, evidence of renal stone disease)
- Blood pressure (hypertension)
- Signs of ectopic tumour (e.g. lung small cell carcinoma or carcinoid) — rare
- Hirsutism

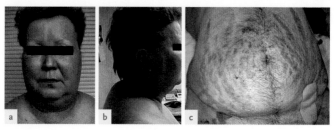

Figure 3.56.1 Cushing syndrome **(a)** Moonfaced **(b)** Buffalo hump **(c)** Abdominal striae (Townsend CM. *Sabiston Textbook of Surgery: The biological basis of modern surgical practice*, 18th edn. Fig. 39.11. Saunders, Elsevier, 2007, with permission.)

2. Look at the patient from the front, sides and behind. Note central obesity with peripheral sparing and look at the skin for bruising, atrophy and pigmentation of extensor areas. Is there an obvious underlying problem that may have led to steroid use, for example chronic rheumatoid arthritis, a transplanted kidney or sometimes chronic obstructive pulmonary disease (COPD)?

3. Test for proximal myopathy of the arms and also of the legs (initially by getting the patient to squat).

4. Examine the back for a buffalo hump and feel it. Look for kyphoscoliosis and tap the spine for bony tenderness as a result of osteoporotic vertebral crush fractures.

5. Ask the patient to sit on the side of the bed. Look at the face for plethora, hirsutism, acne, telangiectasia and a moon shape.

6. Test the eyes for visual field defects (which are uncommon) and ask to look in the fundi for papilloedema (caused by benign intracranial hypertension or a pituitary tumour) and optic atrophy, as well as hypertensive or diabetic changes.

7. Inspect the neck for supraclavicular fat pads and acanthosis nigricans.

8. Ask the patient to lie down. Examine the abdomen for adrenalectomy scars, pigmentation, striae and adrenal masses.

9. Say you would like to look at the genitalia (you probably won't be allowed). Virilisation in women or gynaecomastia in men suggests that adrenal carcinoma is more likely.
10. Next, look at the legs for oedema, bruising and poor wound healing.
11. Do not forget to ask for the results of urine analysis (glucose) and take the blood pressure (hypertension).
12. Diagnostic tests are summarised in Box 3.56.2.

Present your findings

- List the features of Cushing syndrome that you have found and any important negative findings.
- Say if any abnormalities are present that suggest a reason for steroid use.

Examiners' likely questions

- How severe are the changes?
  - Consider the weight of the patient and the severity of the skin changes.
- What questions might you ask the patient?
  - Have been taking prednisone or cortisone tablets? For how long? What doses have been used?
  - Why were they prescribed?
  - How are you and your family affected by the condition?
  - Have you had tests of your bone health? (osteoporosis)
- How can the diagnosis be made?
  - Refer to Box 3.56.2. Most cases, however, are due to steroid administration.

Box 3.56.2
Diagnosis of Cushing syndrome*

Screening tests
- Cortisol levels morning and evening (serum or salivary): loss of diurnal rhythm (evening cortisol level should be less than half the morning value) of little diagnostic value
- 24-hour urine collection for urinary free cortisol determination (an indirect assessment of cortisol production). Should be threefold increased (above normal)
- Overnight dexamethasone suppression test (1 mg dexamethasone at midnight causes suppression of cortisol in normal subjects at 9.00 a.m.). No suppression is found in Cushing syndrome, but this may also occur with alcoholism, induction of hepatic enzymes (e.g. phenytoin) or depression, in patients taking the contraceptive pill and in some obese patients
- Blood count (secondary polycythaemia, neutrophilia, leucocytosis, eosinopenia)
- Electrolyte levels (hypokalaemic alkalosis, particularly with ectopic ACTH-producing tumours)
- Blood sugar level (hyperglycaemia)

Definitive tests
- 2 mg dexamethasone suppression test (0.5 mg 6-hourly for 48 hours). No suppression of plasma cortisol or urinary free cortisol occurs in Cushing syndrome, but usually suppression does occur in normal subjects, obese patients and depressed patients
- 8 mg dexamethasone suppression test (2 mg 6-hourly for 48 hours). Suppression occurs in Cushing disease, but no suppression is usually found in adrenal adenoma or carcinoma or in the presence of ectopic ACTH production. False-positive results can occur in patients taking anticonvulsants (which accelerate dexamethasone metabolism)
- ACTH level — high in ectopic ACTH production, low with adrenal adenoma or carcinoma, high or normal in Cushing disease. Ectopic secretion of corticotropin-releasing hormone (CRH) by tumours is a very rare cause of Cushing syndrome
- Petrosal sinus ACTH sampling — a central-to-peripheral venous cortisol ratio of >2 : 1 is diagnostic of Cushing disease; lateralisation of ACTH production helps the neurosurgeon plan trans-sphenoidal exploration of the sella

*Cushing disease is specifically pituitary ACTH overproduction To diagnose Cushing syndrome, at least two definitive tests should be abnormal
Note: If Cushing disease is present, pituitary assessment is necessary. If adrenal disease is suspected, CT scanning is useful to assess the anatomy. Remember, ectopic ACTH production by a tumour (e.g. small cell carcinoma of lung, carcinoid of lung or thymus, pancreatic islet cell carcinoma, ovarian carcinoma) does not usually cause cushingoid clinical features but may present with hyperpigmentation, hypokalaemic alkalosis and hypertension.

Marking criteria table

Criteria	Satisfactory	Unsatisfactory
Introduces self, explains task, obtains consent, washes hands before and after	1	0
Makes a general inspection	2	0–1
Appears to note features of Cushing; including skin changes, weight	2	0–1
Asks to take blood pressure	1	0
Tests for proximal myopathy in arm and lower limbs	2	0–1
Looks for buffalo hump and kyphosis	2	0–1
Asks to look for abdominal scars	1	0
Asks to see urine analysis for glucose	1	0
Knows exogenous steroid use is the most common cause	1	0
Knows tests to investigate for an adrenal versus a pituitary cause	2	0–1

Pass mark: 10

Sudden visual loss

Background

Temporary sudden loss of vision is called amaurosis fugax (fleeting blindness). It is most often the result of an embolus to the retinal artery from the ipsilateral carotid artery or from the heart as a result of atrial fibrillation. Vision will have returned to normal or the blindness cannot be described as fleeting.

Introduction

This woman has experienced sudden loss of vision in her right eye. Please examine her.

Rationale

This is a test of your knowledge of common causes of visual loss. Note that the examiners have told you the loss involved her right eye. This means the problem is not a visual field loss.

Method

1. Introduce yourself and say that you have been asked to examine her eyes and vision. Wash your hands.
2. Ask if she normally wears glasses for reading and get her to put them on. You are not testing for refractive errors.
3. Test each eye for visual acuity using a hand-held eye chart or wall chart if that is available. If visual loss is severe, ask her to count the number of fingers you are holding up. If vision is too poor even for that, ask if she can distinguish hand motion and, if not, if she can tell light from dark in the affected eye.

4. Examine the visual fields by confrontation but remember that visual field loss has different causes from loss of vision in one eye.
5. Assess each pupil's reaction to light and accommodation, and for an afferent pupillary defect (a sensitive test of optic nerve damage).
6. Test eye movement and ask about any pain on movement (optic neuritis, among other causes). Look for limitation of movement, which, if associated with unilateral visual loss, is more likely to be the result of trauma or a space-occupying lesion than a cranial nerve abnormality.
7. Examine the fundi (Fig. 3.57.1).

T&O'C hint box

If the pupils have been dilated for you, there are likely to be important and obvious retinal changes.

It also means that pupillary reaction to light will be absent or reduced, something the examiners should tell you when you attempt to examine pupillary reflexes.

Note whether the disc is swollen and is abnormally pink or white (ischaemic optic neuropathy).
Note any retinal fundal pallor (arterial occlusion), haemorrhages (venous occlusion) or an obvious embolus (at an arterial bifurcation).

8. Feel the temporal arteries for tenderness. (Temporal arteritis is a cause of blindness.)
9. Auscultate for a carotid bruit (stenosis).
10. Take her pulse (irregularly irregular would indicate atrial fibrillation) and blood pressure (hypertension).
11. Ask whether you may test the patient's urine for blood or protein (vasculitis, diabetic nephropathy).

Present your findings

- First say whether vision remains abnormal and how severely, for example 'Corrected visual acuity today seemed normal in each eye' or 'There was only light perception present in the right eye'.

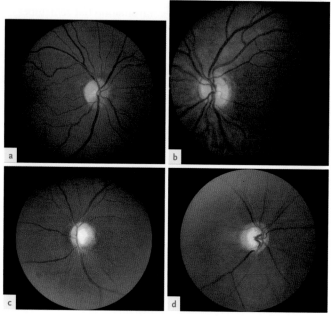

Figure 3.57.1 Patterns of optic atrophy **(a)** Superotemporal sector atrophy in a 59-year-old woman with a supraclinoid internal carotid artery aneurysm compressing the optic nerve **(b)** Band ('bow-tie') atrophy in an 8-year-old boy with a craniopharyngioma compressing the optic chiasm **(c)** Diffuse optic atrophy in a 41-year-old woman with neuromyelitis optica after a severe attack that left her with no light perception **(d)** Glaucomatous cupping with atrophy of the superior and inferior neuroretinal rim appearing as 'notching' of the neuroretinal rim and vertical elongation of the cup (Levin LA, Albert DM (eds). *Ocular Diseases: Mechanisms and management.* Fig. 44.1. Saunders, Elsevier, 2010, with permission.)

- Describe the fundoscopy findings and, especially if vision is now normal, whether an ipsilateral (right) carotid bruit or atrial fibrillation was present.

Examiners' likely questions

- What is the differential diagnosis?

- Note distinguishing sudden monocular vision loss from hemianopia is important as the differential diagnosis is very different (e.g. stroke can cause hemianopia).
- Transient causes of one eye suddenly losing vision (retinal ischaemia, optic neuritis, migraine) differ from causes of prolonged loss (retinal detachment, retinal embolus, temporal arteritis, trauma, diabetes mellitus).

- What treatment would you recommend to this woman, who you have told us now has normal visual acuity and is in atrial fibrillation?
  - Anticoagulation with a novel oral anticoagulant (NOAC) if no brain haemorrhage is seen on CT, unless there are any contraindications

- What relative contraindications to NOAC treatment do you know about?
  - Previous intolerance or significant bleeding in association with these drugs
  - Severe untreated hypertension, severe chronic kidney disease or dialysis, age over 65 years, prior alcohol or drug use, abnormal liver function tests, prior history of stroke.

Marking criteria table		
Criteria	Satisfactory	Unsatisfactory
Introduces self, explains task, obtains consent, washes hands	1	0
Inspects eyes and face	1	0
Tests acuity	2	0–1
Tests visual fields	1	0
Examines fundi	2	0–1
Describes findings	2	0–1
Attempts a plausible differential diagnosis	2	0–1

Pass mark: 6

Background

Examination of the eyes is part of routine examination. If there are symptoms or signs of eye disease, a systematic approach is required.

Introduction

This 40-year-old woman has noticed some changes in her eyes. Please examine her sclerae and conjunctivae.

Rationale

This is likely to be a jaundice (usually from liver disease) or a red eye (e.g. conjunctivitis or uncommonly iritis), or exophthalmos (e.g. hyperthyroidism), but requires a sensible approach to the examination and differential diagnosis.

Method

1. Stand back to look (having washed your hands).
   - Always explain to the patient what you are doing.
   - **Look** for scleral icterus (see Figs 2.10.2, 3.32.1).
   - **Note** the distribution of any redness (e.g. single red eye in iritis). Decide whether conjunctival redness (injection) is central (iritis) (Fig. 3.58.1) or spares the central region (conjunctivitis) (Fig. 3.58.2).
2. If there is conjunctival injection, ask for gloves and explain to the patient, for example 'I need to look under your lower eyelid. I am going to pull it down — let me know if this is at all uncomfortable.' before pulling the lower lid down.
   Note any ocular discharge (conjunctivitis).

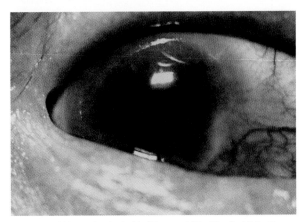

Figure 3.58.1 Iritis and episcleritis (Guerrant DL. *Tropical Infectious Diseases: Principles, pathogens and practice*, 3rd edn. Philadelphia: Saunders, 2011.)

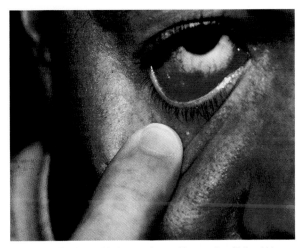

Figure 3.58.2 Conjunctivitis in a patient with measles (Talley NJ, O'Connor S. *Talley and O'Connor's Clinical Examination*. Elsevier Australia, 2017.)

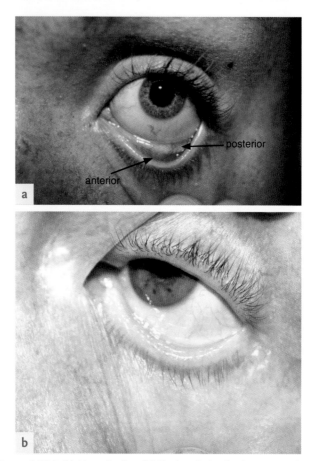

Figure 3.58.3 **(a)** Normal sclera **(b)** Conjunctival pallor in an anaemic patient. Note the contrast between the anterior and posterior parts in the normal eye (Talley NJ, O'Connor S. *Talley and O'Connor's Clinical Examination*. Elsevier Australia, 2017.)

If there is pallor, pull down the lower lid and compare the pearly white posterior part of the conjunctiva with the red anterior part (Fig. 3.58.3).

If there is chemosis, look for proptosis and other signs of thyrotoxicosis.

3. Look at the iris. (Haziness indicates oedema or inflammation.)
4. Look at and test the pupils (e.g. small irregular pupil in iritis, dilated, oval, poorly reactive pupil in acute glaucoma).
5. Assess eye movements. Ask the patient if these movements cause pain (suggests scleritis). Ask if you may perform fundoscopy.
6. Consider other evidence of vasculitis (nail fold, skin and joint changes); ask for the result of urinalysis for protein (nephritis).
7. If there is an obvious spot diagnosis such as scleral icterus, move quickly through the rest of the eye examination and then say that you have found jaundice and would like to examine for signs of liver disease, or if you have found iritis, that you would like to examine for signs of arthritis and vasculitis.

The introduction mentioned specifically the sclerae and conjunctivae. In general this would mean testing for acuity and fundoscopy is not required, but if there is any evidence of iritis it would be prudent to ask if you may do these tests. Even as a routine, it might be sensible to say something like 'I have found evidence of thyroid eye disease and would normally test visual acuity and perform fundoscopy, but I would also like to look for other signs of thyrotoxicosis.' The examiners should tell you what they want you to spend your remaining time on.

Present your findings

- Outline the eye findings first, including the important negatives.
- Then any other findings from your extended examination, if there was one.

T&O'C hint box

Always restrict requests for tests to a modest list and have a reason for each request. A scattergun approach to investigations suggests to the examiners that you have not thought about your findings carefully. It becomes tempting then for the examiner, rather than giving you a useful result to comment on, to ask how your request for a serum selenium level would help you in this case.

- Put the findings together, for example 'I found evidence of thyroid eye disease — exophthalmos and proptosis with some ophthalmoplegia — but the rest of the examination (for tremor, reflexes, thyroid bruits) suggested the patient was euthyroid'.

Examiners' likely questions

- Are there any questions you would like to ask the patient?
    - Depending on your findings, ask about a history of liver, joint or thyroid disease.
- What tests might be useful in the first instance?
    - Think slit lamp examination to assess for supporting features of iritis, fluoresceine to assess for corneal ulcers and tonometer to look for increased pressure predisposing for glaucoma.

Marking criteria table		
Criteria	Satisfactory	Unsatisfactory
Introduces self, explains task, obtains consent, washes hands	1	0
General inspection	1	0
Notes distribution of redness	1	0
After asking permission, pulls down lower lid to look for anaemia	1	0
Examines pupil for haziness	1	0
Tests pupil reactions	1	0
Asks to look at fundi	1	0
Asks to test acuity	1	0
Presents findings	1	0
If asked, asks for a few relevant tests	1	0

Pass mark: 7

Examine for a sore throat

Background

Sore throats are common reasons for patients to visit their doctors. You need to know how to perform this common examination and understand the anatomy involved (Fig. 3.59.1).

Introduction

This patient complains of recurrent sore throat. Please examine her.

Method

1. Introduce yourself, explain what you will be doing and obtain consent. Wash your hands and don gloves.
2. **Ask** the patient if she has dentures and, if so, to remove them for you. Note any drooling or flushing, and whether she appears generally unwell. Also note if there is a cough or not.
3. **Take** a torch and ask the patient to open wide.
4. **Inspect** her mouth and pharynx using a tongue depressor.
5. **Note** tonsillar enlargement and any erythema or other signs of inflammation on the palate. Look for pus on the surface of the tonsils and for unilateral swelling behind a tonsil that may indicate the presence of tonsillar abscess. Note any pooling of secretions.
6. **Note** whether the patient cannot open her mouth fully (trismus) — lockjaw is reduced jaw opening that can occur in tetanus.
7. **Look** at the teeth for decay and at the gums for swelling and inflammation (gingivitis).

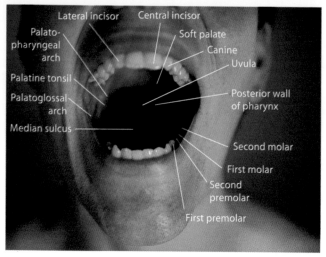

Figure 3.59.1 The mouth and throat (Talley NJ, O'Connor S. *Clinical Examination Essentials: An introduction to clinical skills (and how to pass your clinical exams)*. Elsevier Australia, 2015.)

8. **Look** for ulceration in the oral cavity and signs of candidiasis (white adherent plaques) (Figs 3.59.2 and 3.59.3).
9. **Feel** the oral cavity and tongue gently with a gloved finger.
10. **Ask** if there is tenderness or discomfort anywhere.
11. **Palpate** the submental, submandibular and all cervical lymph nodes carefully (see Fig. 2.16.2a).
12. **Ask if** you may take her temperature (make sure you know how to do this with an electronic or normal thermometer) or see the temperature chart. (fever)
13. Listen for any evidence of stridor (inspiratory wheeze heard without a stethoscope; it may indicate supraglottitis, a medical emergency (so it won't be present in an OSCE!)).
14. **Ask** if you may examine the abdomen to feel for splenomegaly (common in patients with infectious mononucleosis).
15. If there are mouth ulcers or the cervical nodes are enlarged, ask to examine the axillary and inguinal nodes too (e.g. infectious mononucleosis).

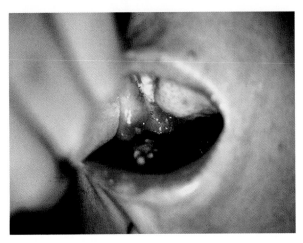

Figure 3.59.2 Buccal ulcer (Courtesy of Dr A Watson, Infectious Diseases Department, The Canberra Hospital.)

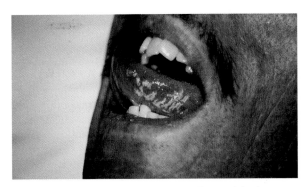

Figure 3.59.3 Candidiasis (Courtesy of Dr A Watson, Infectious Diseases Department, The Canberra Hospital.)

16. Auscultate the heart (acute carditis due to rheumatic fever is rare), other features include arthritis and rash (erythema marginatum) in those at risk.

17. Look for rash (petechiae) and test for neck stiffness (e.g. meningococcal infection) in young adults.

Present your findings

- The examination may be normal. In this case outline the important negatives:
  - no erythema or tonsillar enlargement
  - no lymphadenopathy or splenomegaly
  - normal temperature.
- If there were abnormalities, comment on the severity and any signs of systemic illness.

Examiners' likely questions

- Do you think this sore throat is due to viral or bacterial infection?
  - It is generally not possible to distinguish viral sore throats from bacterial ones clinically.
  - Beta-haemolytic streptococcus pharyngitis is more likely if there is fever, a pharyngeal exudate, anterior cervical lymphadenopathy and NO cough.
  - If there is a tonsillar abscess, a bacterial infection is more likely.
  - If there is splenomegaly, infectious mononucleosis (a viral infection) is likely.
- What findings would make you suspect an immune deficiency disorder?
  - Extensive ulceration and signs of *Candida* infection (a white coating on an ulcer) would make this more likely, or if there are recurrent bacterial infections in the absence of an anatomical abnormality.

Marking criteria table

Criteria	Satisfactory	Unsatisfactory
Introduces self, explains task, obtains consent, washes hands, puts on gloves	2	0–1
General inspection	1	0
Asks about and removes dentures (with permission)	1	0
Uses torch and spatula to inspect mouth, teeth, gums and pharynx, does not make patient vomit	2	0–1
Gets patient to say 'ah'	1	0
Feels oral cavity with gloved hand	1	0
Feels cervical lymph nodes	1	0
Asks to take temperature and feel abdomen	2	0–1
Presents major findings	3	0–2
Answers examiners' questions satisfactorily	2	0–1

Pass mark: 10

Examine a patient with an earache

Background

To examine the ear, remember to inspect both before competently (and safely) using the auriscope, and test hearing.

Introduction

This man complains of a sore ear. Examine his ears.

Method

You need to know how to examine the ear, the normal anatomy and how to use an auriscope (Fig. 3.60.1).

1. Introduce yourself, wash your hands, explain what you have been asked to do.
2. Note whether he looks unwell or feverish.
3. Look at the pinna and external auditory meatus for:
   - gouty tophi
   - dermatitis
   - cellulitis
   - signs of trauma (e.g. haematoma)
   - scars (e.g. surgery)
   - discharge.
   Look at both ears (obviously).
4. **Ask** the patient whether the ear is painful before you use the auriscope to examine the canal and drum.
5. Use the auriscope in the approved manner:
   - Pull the pinna up and backwards to straighten the auditory canal. Insert the auriscope gently into the ear.

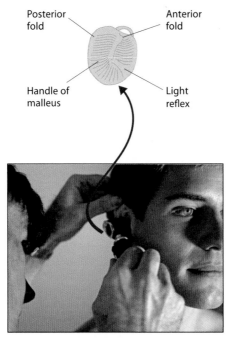

Figure 3.60.1 How to use an auriscope (Talley NJ, O'Connor S. *Clinical Examination Essentials: An introduction to clinical skills (and how to pass your clinical exams)*. Elsevier Australia, 2015.)

Look systematically at the visible structures — the canal itself and the ear drum.

- **Look** for erythema or blisters in the canal, and for wax, pus or discharge from the drum. Is the drum inflamed or is there loss of the normal light reflex — shiny appearance (a sign of inflammation)?
- Now **inspect** the tympanic membrane (ear drum) for perforation, grommets (tympanostomy tubes).

6. **Test** hearing (whispered numbers). Ask if the patient wears hearing aids, then test using whispered numbers.
7. Perform Rinné and Weber tests if hearing is reduced in one or both ears.

- Rinné test: place a vibrating 512 or 256 Hz tuning fork on the mastoid process. When the sound is no longer heard, quickly move the fork close to the auditory meatus (outer ear). Where does it sound louder? No note will be heard if there is CONDUCTION deafness (Rinne negative). If a note is heard this suggests nerve deafness (Rinne positive, as air conduction is better than bone conduction although both are reduced). Test both sides.
- Weber test: place a vibrating 512 or 256 Hz tuning fork at the centre of the patient's forehead. Ask: where is the sound louder? Normal is the centre of the forehead. If there is CONDUCTION deafness, the sound is louder in the ABNORMAL ear. If there is NERVE deafness the sound is louder in the NORMAL ear.

8. Palpate the temporomandibular joint for tenderness and crepitus (referred pain to the ear).
9. **Examine** the throat for inflammation (referred pain to the ear).

Present your findings

Describe the state of the canal and tympanic membrane and any other findings you have made.

Examiner's likely questions

- What might explain the blisters you found in the auditory canal?
  - Consider herpes zoster (can be associated with Bell palsy) or an allergic reaction

Marking criteria table

Criteria	Satisfactory	Unsatisfactory
Introduces self, explains task, obtains consent, washes hands	1	0
Looks at pinnae and external auditory meatus	3	0–2
Appears to know how to use auriscope	1	0
Notes erythema, vesicles, wax and state of drum	3	0–2
Asks to test hearing	1	0
Knows how to perform Weber and Rinne tests	2	0–1
Examines for sites of referred pain to the ear	1	0
Presents important positive and negative findings	2	0–1

Pass mark: 8

Background

The definition of the geriatric patient varies but it is often taken to refer to people over the age of 65. Many 66-year-olds find this somewhat insulting, and indeed physiological age is often not the same as chronological age. The examiners may have found a genuinely elderly patient for you, or you may be faced with an actor trying very hard. In these circumstances, there may be a requirement for even more suspension of disbelief on your part than with other OSCE actors.

Geriatric patients tend to report fewer symptoms but have more numerous chronic diseases. Disease presentation is more likely to be atypical, so spending time taking the history is critical. Patients may have hearing loss, difficulty seeing and cognitive impairment, all of which can hamper history taking here.

Introduction

This woman is now 85 years old. She has come in for a health assessment. Please take a history from her.

Rationale

This can be a complex OSCE as sections of it, such as assessing a patient who has had falls or reviewing an elderly patient's medications, are possible OSCEs in their own right.

Method

This is meant to be a general health assessment but there may be some current presenting symptoms that have precipitated the visit. Falls are a particularly common presenting problem in elderly people.

1. Introduce yourself and explain what you are going to do.
2. Ask: 'Have there been any particular problems that have concerned you recently about your health?'

    If so, go on to ask about these in detail, with particular attention to:
    - the duration of the symptoms
    - whether they are getting better or worse
    - what treatment, if any, has been tried
    - how much they interfere with the patient's life, for example activities of daily living (ADLs), driving, ability to leave the house
    - whether there has been a discussion with the patient's doctor about the prognosis.
3. Inquire about past history.
    - Ask about previous serious illnesses and chronic health problems. 'Have you had to be treated for other medical problems?'
    - Have you had to be admitted to hospital because of these?
    - Have you needed any operations in the past? What were they?
    - Now find out about the immunisation status, especially for pneumococcus, influenza, COVID-19, tetanus and varicella zoster.
4. Ask about medications.
    - A patient's medication list tells much about his or her illnesses (suspected or confirmed). Patients may not remember that they have, for example, hypertension; the presence of an antihypertensive drug on the medication list suggests otherwise.
    The number of medications tends to increase over time unless their need is constantly reviewed. Many patients will be taking multiple medications for several diseases (polypharmacy). They may not really need all of these.
    - Ask what each drug is for, and try to establish whether the original reason for the treatment persists. Ask questions to help find out if the treatment is effective.
    - Has your arthritis been less of a problem since you began taking the arthritis tablets?

Side effects are more common in the elderly:

- Have any of the tablets caused problems?
  You may need to ask specific questions related to the common side effects of the patient's treatment.
- Have the arthritis tablets upset your stomach?
- Do you think you have had problems with dizziness when you stand up since you began the blood pressure tablets?

5. Details about smoking habits should be acquired as usual.
   - Are you a smoker?
   - Have you been a smoker in the past? (Stopping smoking improves lung function, even in patients over the age of 60 years. Furthermore, advice to stop smoking is as successful in older patients as it is in younger ones.)

6. Exercise is generally safe in the elderly and improves flexibility, balance, endurance and strength, which can assist with maintenance of independent function as well as improving quality of life.
   - Are you active? What sorts of things do you do in the way of exercise? For how long each day?

7. Living arrangements: ask whether there is someone to help the patient in the home, if required.
   - Do you have a partner? Is your husband at home with you (if married to a male)? How is his health?

8. Assess vulnerability: abuse and neglect can be problems in this age group. Try to find out whether the patient feels under threat from anyone.
   - Do you feel safe where you live? Have there been any problems that make you feel unsafe that you would like to talk about?

9. Review systems.
   - Vision: Have you had any problems with your eyes? How long is it since you had them tested? Have you had cataract surgery? How well did that work?
   - Hearing: How is your hearing? Have you got hearing aids? Do they help?
   - Eating: Do your teeth (dentures) give you trouble when you eat? Are there certain things you can't eat? How do you manage about that? Have you been to the dentist recently?'

- Weight: Have you lost weight recently? How much? Have you lost your appetite or is it difficult for you to eat?
- Bowels: Have you had problems with constipation or diarrhoea? How difficult does that make things for you?
- Urinary problems: Do you need to wear pads because it is difficult to control your bladder? Do they work? Have you had any tests to look into this problem?' (Ask men about urinary retention and prostatic symptoms.)
- Falls are an important cause of mortality in the elderly and are usually multi-factorial: postural dizziness, poor vision, cognitive impairment, foot problems, and gait problems can all contribute to or exacerbate the problem. A history of falls means that careful enquiry must be made about these associated factors.
  - Have you fallen over when you have been at home? or out?
  - How often has this happened?
  - Have you hurt yourself?
  - Tell me what happens when you fall: do you trip, or lose your balance or feel dizzy when you stand up? Have you blacked out?
- Question about low-trauma fractures or back pain for possible osteoporosis. Impaired bone mineral density means a fracture is more likely to result from a fall.
  - Have you broken any bones when you have fallen, or just out of the blue (spontaneous or minimal trauma fracture)? Have you had any tests to see if your bones are weak?
  - Have you ever had to take cortisone or prednisone treatment? (much increased risk of osteoporosis)
  - Has any treatment been started?
  - Have you been told to use a stick or wheelie-walker? Do you use it or prefer not to?
  - Do you have any six-monthly or yearly injections to prevent osteoporosis — such as denosumab or zolendronic acid?
- Ask about symptoms of depression because this is a common problem in the elderly and needs to be recognised and treated.

SPECIFIC AREAS OF INQUIRY

10. **Physical activities of daily living (ADLs)**: ask the patient how he or she copes with bathing, dressing, toileting and handling money — these can be affected by many different chronic illnesses.

11. **Instrumental activities of daily living (IADLs)**: ask the patient whether he or she has any difficulty using the telephone, shopping, preparing food, housekeeping, doing the laundry, driving and taking medicines.

12. **End-of-life and treatment decisions**: patients generally prefer their clinician to bring up this topic. A general introduction to the question might be, 'If you came into hospital very ill and the doctors thought that you could only make a very limited recovery, would you want to continue with intensive treatment? Have you talked about this sort of thing with your family?'

Report your findings

- Give a summary of the patient's past and present medical problems.
- Emphasise chronic problems and how the patient has been managing. Give examples: 'Despite her arthritis, Mrs X remains active and is able to play golf using a cart. She still drives and has recently passed her driving medical review.'
- Always comment on falls risk and medications.
- Give some indication of her mood and expectations for the future. 'She feels she may not be able to manage at home indefinitely and has made inquiries about aged care residences where she and her husband, who is well but limited by peripheral vascular disease, might move in the future.'
- Report on any end-of-life discussion.

Examiners' likely questions

- Do you think all this woman's current medications are necessary?
    - Go through the list, for example 'She is taking Ramipril for her hypertension. This seems well controlled and

she has had no problems with the drug as far as I can tell. She has not noticed postural dizziness or cough. I feel she should continue with this. She takes low-dose aspirin; she has never had a diagnosis of vascular disease but there is a history of gastric ulceration. I feel this treatment should be reviewed.'

- How much is she at risk of falls and how would you further assess this?
  - Outline the history of or absence of falls. Describe risk factors, for example vision problems, arthritis. Say that you would like to look for postural hypotension and cerebellar problems and get her to walk — describe the get up and go test.

Marking criteria table

Criteria	Satisfactory	Unsatisfactory
Introduces self, explains task, obtains consent	1	0
Possible presenting problems have been asked about and analysed well	2	0–1
Previous health problems have been assessed efficiently	1	0
Medications have been reviewed	1	0
Living circumstances, support etc. have been discussed	2	0–1
Activities of daily living (ADLs) and instrumental activities of daily living (IADLs) have been assessed	2	0–1
Advance care directive planning has been discussed	1	0
There has been a good overall assessment of the patient?	2	0–1

Pass mark: 7, but the student's ability to make a sensible overall assessment is particularly important.

Examination of an older patient

Background

Certain examination abnormalities are more likely in elderly people. These can cause significant problems and some involve risk, such as of falls.

Introduction

This woman is now 86. She has experienced some mild exertional breathlessness but has not had any other symptoms. Please describe the way you would perform a general examination. Tell us what you would be looking for in particular in an elderly patient's screening assessment.

Rationale

The examiners expect you to know how to perform a quick screening examination looking particularly for relevant abnormalities. This is a long OSCE. It would commonly be broken up into shorter OSCE exams, for example:

- This elderly man has had postural dizziness. Please examine his cardiovascular system.
- This woman has had problems with mobility. Please examine her gait.

Method

A complete examination is required as usual, but emphasise the following aspects of the examination.

Begin with a statement such as 'I would wash my hands and ask the patient to undress to her underwear and to put on a hospital gown.' Then go through the following list and explain the purpose as you go.

1. General assessment
   - Introduce yourself and ask about orientation in person, place and time: full name, present location, and the day and date. Disorientation may indicate delirium (acute and reversible) or dementia (chronic and irreversible).
   - Check for postural blood pressure change. This is associated with dizziness and a risk of falls.
   - Assess hydration (dry mucous membranes, reduced skin elasticity — often difficult to assess in elderly patients), which may be impaired in older patients with cognitive dysfunction.
   - Look at the skin carefully for pressure sores (more important if the patient is immobile in hospital or a nursing home) or evidence of bruises from falls or elder abuse. Look at the skin for any evidence of skin cancer.
   - Measure weight and height to calculate the body mass index (BMI). Weight loss is common in the elderly and may be the result of inability to prepare food, eat (dental or swallowing problems), depression or bowel problems including malignancy.

2. Heart
   - Count the pulse. Heart block and bradycardia can be causes of syncope and dizziness. Look for a pacemaker box below the left or right clavicle. If a systolic murmur is heard, consider whether this may be aortic stenosis, which, if severe, is likely to require treatment.
   - Look for ankle swelling, which may indicate venous insufficiency or antihypertensive drug use (e.g. calcium antagonists) rather than congestive cardiac failure. It can interfere with mobility. Ischaemic heart disease is common but often silent in the elderly.

3. Chest
   - Shortness of breath may be due to lung disease or cardiac disease, and these often coexist in the elderly. Look for evidence of chronic obstructive pulmonary disease (COPD) (overinflated lungs, wheeze, and Hoover sign), or interstitial lung disease (fine basal inspiratory crackles).

4. Gastrointestinal system
   - Look at the dentition and check for a dry mouth, which may impair eating.
   - Feel for a palpable abdominal aorta. This may be palpable in the thin elderly patient and be falsely interpreted as an aneurysm but, if the aorta seems significantly enlarged, an aortic aneurysm needs to be excluded.
   - In patients with constipation from hard stool, a mass may be felt in the left lower quadrant: this will clear with treatment for the constipation.
   - Say you would ask to perform a rectal examination to rule out faecal impaction, particularly if there is a history of faecal or urinary incontinence. You won't be allowed.
   - In patients with acute urinary retention, an enlarged bladder may be felt: this problem can present with delirium.

5. Nervous system
   - Evaluation of mental status should be routine in geriatric patients. The mini-mental state examination is useful here. The 3-minute Mini-Cog™ test is as follows:
     - Ask the patient to remember three words (repeat up to three times to make sure the patient understands and can repeat the words).
     - Next ask the patient to draw a clockface with numbers then the hand at a specified times.
     - Finally, ask the patient to repeat the three words. Scoring is out of 5: 1 point for each word remembered and 2 for a correct clock face draw (0 if not fully correct). A score of 0–2 supports a diagnosis of dementia.
   - Test gait with the 'get up and go' test. Ask the patient to stand up out of a chair, walk 3 metres, turn around 180°, return to the chair and sit down (Fig. 3.62.1). Time it (normal 7–10 seconds, abnormal mobility if over 20 seconds). Look for abnormalities in gait, balance and power. You can also grade the test from 1 (normal) to 5 (severely impaired) (subjective!).

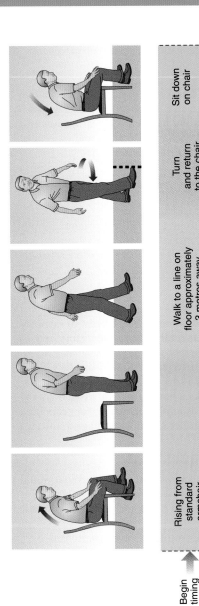

Begin timing

| Rising from standard armchair | Walk to a line on floor approximately 3 metres away | Turn and return to the chair | Sit down on chair |

The normal time to finish the test is between 7–10 seconds.
Patients who cannot complete the task in that time probably have some mobility problems, especially if they take more than 20 seconds.

Figure 3.62.1 Get up and go test: 1. 'Stand up now for me and walk over to here.' 2. 'Now turn around and walk back.' 3. 'Now come and sit down again.' Difficulty in standing up from a chair indicates an increased falls risk (Douglas G, Nicol F, Robertson C. *Macleod's Clinical Examination*, 13th edn. Edinburgh: Churchill Livingstone, © 2013.)

- Performing heel-to-toe walking and Romberg test to assess balance and cerebellar problems or peripheral neuropathy.
6. Eyes and ears
   - Check vision (use a hand-held eye chart and have the patient use her spectacles) and hearing (hearing loss may already be apparent but look for hearing aids and whisper numbers in each ear). Hearing and especially visual loss as may impair independent living.
7. Rheumatological system
   - Examine for deformities and functional disabilities, including the feet.
8. Breasts
   - Ask if there is time to perform a breast examination in women, as the incidence of breast cancer greatly increases with age. This is more likely to be a separate OSCE and there is unlikely to be time.

Present your findings

- In this theoretical examination, it may be best to say that you would correlate your findings with the history and medication list.
- In this case, a murmur or signs of lung disease should be emphasised as there is a history of dyspnoea.
- Say that you would make a make a general assessment of the patient's health, for example whether she appears frail, or younger or older than her chronological age.

Examiners' likely questions

- You found a postural drop in blood pressure. What would you ask the patient to help assess this?
  - Have you felt dizzy when you stand up? Have you fallen or blacked out?
  - What medications do you take? (antihypertensive medications and alpha-blockers (for men with prostatic symptoms))
- How would you assess this woman's mobility?
  - Describe the patient's ability to move around as you examine her and the results of the 'get up and go' test.

Marking criteria

Criteria	Satisfactory	Unsatisfactory
Introduces self, explains task, obtains consent, washes hands before and after	1	0
Indicates the general assessment that would be helpful	2	0–1
Tailors assessment to introduction	1	0
Tests balance, gait and mobility	2	0–1
Knows the get up and go test	2	0–1
Can do a mental state examination	2	0–1
Sensibly answers questions e.g. discusses medications and possibility of polypharmacy	2	0–1

Pass mark: 7

63

Take a history from a patient with a history of falls

Background

Elderly patients and patients on large numbers of medications are at risk of falling and injuring themselves. Many factors contribute to the problem. Falls present a mortality and morbidity risk to elderly people and every effort to understand the cause and prevent injury is most important for these patients.

Introduction

This man, who is now 85, has had a number of falls. Please take a history from him.

Rationale

A good student will take a thorough history that will often help work out the likely causes.

Method

1. Ask if the patient remembers having fallen.
   - How many times?
   - What were the circumstances — tripping, loss of balance, postural, nocturnal? Attempt to obtain as much detail as possible about what happened.
   - Was the patient syncopal? 'Do you think you lost consciousness or do you remember falling?' If so, is there hypotension (including postural), bradycardia or does the patient have a pacemaker?
   - Has the patient had any injuries, fractures?

- Has hospital admission or surgery been required?
- Has drug treatment been recommended or changed?
- Have changes been made around the house, such as removal of loose rugs, installation of rails? Does the patient have an alarm necklace that they wear?
- Does the patient have stool or urinary urgency?
- Have walking aids been recommended?

2. What medications is the patient taking? Ask particularly about:
   - antihypertensive drugs
   - sedatives; for example, sleeping tablets
   - alpha-blockers (often for prostatism)
   - anti-Parkinsonian drugs
   - anticholinergic medications
   - opioid analgesics
   - alcohol
   - anticoagulants (risk of bleeding after a fall, risk of haemorrhagic stroke).

3. Is there a problem with mobility? Ask about:
   - stroke or cerebellar disease
   - muscle weakness
   - arthritis
   - spinal disease
   - inappropriate footwear.

4. What insight does the patient have into the problem?
   - Is there adherence to suggestions about use of aids such as sticks, walking frames?
   - Does the patient undertake risky activities — climbing ladders, clearing gutters etc.?

5. Is there a problem with visual acuity?

6. Has there been a history of vertigo?

7. Has there been a diagnosis of osteoporosis? (increased risk of fracture caused by a fall)

8. Has the patient lost confidence as a result of falls and is this affecting his or her ability to leave the house, drive, shop etc.? Is the rest of the family affected?

Present your findings

List the most likely causes of the episodes and indicate how severe a risk they pose to the patient's health and independence.

Examiners' likely questions

- What changes to the patient's medications might be helpful?
  - Discuss cessation of any of the drugs you have recorded that may be increasing the risk of falls and say in what way they can increase risk.
- Do you think this patient can continue to live at home? What assistance might be needed to enable him to stay at home?
  - This is an opportunity to talk about the patient's insight into the problem and whether he is realistic about what he can do. Talk about help at home and also about his likely acceptance or otherwise of this.
- How is *this* patient coping with these falls?
  - Talk here about the patient's mood and psychological response to his problem and particularly about how he is coping with possible or real loss of independence.

Marking criteria table

Criteria	Satisfactory	Unsatisfactory
Introduces self, explains task, obtains consent	1	0
Asks what the patient remembers of the fall or falls	1	0
Asks for details of the episodes	1	0
Asks about injuries	1	0
Asks about precautions now used or lack thereof	2	0–1
Asks about medications	1	0
Asks about risk factors for falls	3	0–2
Asks about effects on patient's confidence about doing things	1	0
Asks about walking and balance aids	1	0
Presents findings	1	0
Comments on the risk to the patient's independence	1	0

Pass mark: 10

Examination of a patient with a history of falls

Background

Falls are often multifactorial in the elderly. Develop a systematic method for examination, remembering the common causes. If there is a history of two or more falls, a comprehensive falls assessment is critical.

Introduction

Please examine this 85-year-old man, who has had several serious falls in the last 3 months. He has been admitted to hospital after 2 of these.

Rationale

The history will often indicate the most likely cause of falls but the examination, when directed appropriately, can help confirm this or uncover unexpected problems.

Method

1. Look for walking aids: sticks, walkers, orthotics, footwear.
2. Is the patient obese? frail?
3. Does the patient seem confused or disorientated?
4. Take the pulse. Atrial fibrillation?
5. Measure the blood pressure; lying and standing if possible. Is there a postural drop? Is the patient symptomatic when standing?
6. Ask the patient to walk. Look for unsteadiness. Note any gait abnormalities. Try heel-to-toe walking.

7. If the patient looks Parkinsonian, test for other evidence of this syndrome (resting tremor, tone at the wrists, bradykinesia by finger tapping, glabellar tap).

8. Perform the Romberg test. Ask the patient to stand with the feet together and eyes open. Then once stable, ask them to close their eyes, reassuring them you won't let them fall (hold your hands around the upper arms to do so). Marked unsteadiness is abnormal and if it increases on closing the eyes, the Romberg sign is positive and suggests proprioception loss.

9. Test visual acuity.

10. Perform a get up and go test if possible.

11. With the patient back in bed, perform a lower limb neurological examination including cerebellar testing and assess for peripheral neuropathy. Note muscle strength.

Present your findings

Give a general appraisal of the patient's frailty and mobility. Indicate whether you think you have found an explanation for the falls, such as severe postural hypotension or peripheral neuropathy.

Examiners' likely questions

- What investigations might be helpful?
  - If there are focal neurological or cerebellar signs, CT or MRI scanning may be useful. (focal lesion, normal pressure hydrocephalus)
  - Full blood count and electrolytes (anaemia, hyponatraemia)
  - If syncope is suspected, an electrocardiogram (ECG) and Holter monitor may be useful. (conduction system disease)
- What would be the management options?
  - Review medications that may be causing problems
  - Can antihypertensives be stopped or changed?
  - Are anti-Parkinsonian drugs optimal?
  - Should sedatives be stopped?
  - Are alternative analgesics possible?
  - Correct electrolytes or haemoglobin

- Recommend more appropriate footwear, prostheses and walking aids
- Consider rehabilitation and physiotherapy
- Evaluation for new spectacles
- Assessment of house; removal of loose rugs and installation of ramps, bars etc.
- Consider whether possible syncope needs further investigation or treatment.
- Is the patient's response to the episodes appropriate and how might this be improved?

Marking criteria table

Criteria	Satisfactory	Unsatisfactory
Introduces self, explains task, obtains consent, washes hands	1	0
Scans room for walking aids etc.	1	0
Conducts general inspection of patient	1	0
Takes pulse and postural blood pressure	1	0
Asks patient to walk	1	0
Tests for Romberg sign	1	0
Conducts get up and go test	1	0
Offers to perform a neurological examination for peripheral neuropathy and cerebellar signs	1	0
Presents findings and if possible most likely causes of the problem	2	0–1
Proposes sensible answers to examiners' questions	2	0–1

Pass mark: 7

Background

Any patient with a history of confusion or who is suspected of having dementia or a major psychiatric illness should undergo a mental state examination. Test for orientation, memory and attention. Even gross disturbances of these functions may not be obvious unless they are formally tested.

Introduction

This man (likely to be an actor) has had some memory problems. Please assess his mental state.

Rationale

This is a test of your ability rapidly to test for confusion or dementia.

Method

1. Introduce yourself. Then say something like, 'I have been asked to ask you some questions about your memory if that is all right.'
2. Then, first some orientation questions.
   - Do you know where you are now?
   - What day of the week is it?
   - What month and year?
   - Do you know the name of the prime minister, the queen?
   - Do you think you have had memory problems?
   - How long for?
   - Have other people commented on this?

- Do you think they are exaggerating the problem?
- Give me an example of a time when your memory has failed you. (If necessary, give possible examples.)
  - Do you forget the names of people you know well?
  - Do you have trouble working out money and change at the shop?
  - Do you get lost if you go out or even around the house?
- Do you think the problem is getting worse?
- What do you do to cope? (e.g. write lists and notes)
- Have you had any tests or treatment for the problem?
3. Then use a screening tool for cognitive impairment. The Mini-Cog™ test (3 steps, 3 minutes) is one of these:
   - Ask the patient to remember three words (and repeat these up to three times to ensure they have been captured by the patient).
   - Ask the patient to draw a clock face with all the numbers then draw the hands at a specific time, for example 10 past 11 o'clock.
   - Ask the patient to repeat the three original words. Scoring is out of 5 (0–2 suggests formal testing for dementia is indicated): 1 point for each correct word and 2 points for a fully correct clock face (0 if not fully correct).

Present your findings

Give the history of the problem and the results of the screening test. Try to estimate the severity of the problem.

Examiners' likely questions

- What insight has this man into his problem?
  - Describe the severity of the abnormality, the patient's coping mechanisms and if he feels those around him are exaggerating the problem.

Marking criteria table

Criteria	Satisfactory	Unsatisfactory
Introduces self, explains task, obtains consent	1	0
Tests orientation: person, place, time	2	0–1
Asks sympathetic questions about memory problems	1	0
Makes an assessment of the patient's insight	1	0
Performs a Mini-Cog™ test or similar	3	0–2
Gives an assessment of the severity of the problem and how the patient copes	2	0–1

Pass mark: 5

Assess a patient with depression

Background

Depression is prevalent and the most common psychometric disorder. The majority presenting to primary care with depression complain of somatic symptoms such as headache, backache or chronic pain, insomnia or fatigue.

Introduction

This woman has been having problems with depression. Please take a history from her.

Rationale

The patient in this type of OSCE is likely to be an actor well rehearsed in giving appropriate answers to your questions. A case of this sort requires a particularly sympathetic approach. Questions must not be rushed and the patient given time to consider her answers.

Method

1. Introduce yourself.
2. Explain that you have been asked to ask some questions about her mood but that she must not feel she has to answer any questions she finds very upsetting.
3. If the patient seems withdrawn, it might be useful to begin with some general remarks about being involved in student exams or the surroundings or even the weather.
4. Ask her the following:

- Have you been feeling sad or blue or depressed? For how long?
- Have you felt depressed or lost interest in things daily for 2 or more weeks in the past?
- Has there been any particular problem that brought this on — at work, at home? Have you had similar episodes in the past?
- How have you been sleeping? Do you wake early in the mornings?
- Do you suffer from loss of appetite or weight?
- What are your thoughts about the future?
- Are you able to concentrate?
- Do you have guilty thoughts?
- Have you experienced loss of interest in things you usually enjoy?
- Have you had little need for sleep? Have you felt especially good about yourself? Have you gone on big spending sprees? Do you feel you are special or have special powers? (possible mania)
- Do you have a history of major medical health problems like cancer or stroke (which can cause depression)?
- Have you thought that your life is not worth living? Have you ever thought of killing yourself? Have you thought how you might do this? Have you made any plans to do this? Are there people or places you feel you can think about or turn to if these thoughts occur?
- Have you got pets at home that you look after and enjoy being with when you are sad?
- What treatment have you had?
- Ask about drug therapy and psychotherapy. Has this been helpful? Have there been any side effects of drug treatment?
- Who is at home with you? How have the rest of the family been affected by this, do you think? Are they as helpful as they might be?
- Ask the examiners if you may perform a mental state examination.

Report your findings

List the answers the patient has given that suggest depression.

Examiners' likely questions

- How severe do you think the problem is at the moment?
  - Discuss the effect the depression has had on the patient; for example, loss of appetite, loss of interest in things.
  - Try to grade the severity of the depression. Outline the length of the disease and what has happened with previous episodes. Talk about the effectiveness of drug treatment.
- Do you think there is a risk of suicide?
  - Any thinking about suicide on the part of the patient is worrying, and ideas about how it might be carried out are even more so.
- What medical conditions may mimic depression?
  - Mention hypothyroidism, Parkinson disease, multiple sclerosis, menopause, chronic disease (e.g. heart failure), medications (e.g. cancer therapy).

Marking criteria table

Criteria	Satisfactory	Unsatisfactory
Introduces self, explains task, obtains consent	1	0
The student's ability to tailor the timing and tone of questions is very important.	2	0–1
Good screening questions for depression	2	0–1
Asks about possible mania	1	0
Have possible causes of the illness been assessed?	1	0
Has treatment been discussed in terms of effectiveness and side effects?	1	0
Has the patient's insight into the condition been analysed?	1	0
What effect has the illness had on the patient's life, work, friends and ability to function?	2	0–1
Does suicide or self-harm seem a real risk?	2	0

Pass mark: 7, but an unsatisfactory approach to the patient would make passing difficult. You will be judged in this type of case on your approach to the patient and the way you ask your questions — this needs to be sympathetic but still objective.

Pigmented skin lesion examination

Background

Skin cancers are very common in Australia. Early diagnosis makes a difference to prognosis and students must know what features of skin lesions suggest malignancy (Fig. 3.67.1).

Introduction

This man has noticed a pigmented lesion on his face. Please ask a few relevant questions and then examine him.

Method

QUESTIONS

1. Did you have much sun exposure when you were a child? Did you get sunburnt often? To the point of blistering? Do you work outside in the sun? What sun protection do you use?
2. Is there any history of melanoma in your family? (10% of melanomas have such a history.)
3. When did you first notice the lesion? Is it new?
4. Has the lesion changed in appearance? Is it in only one place
5. Has there been any itching or bleeding?
6. Have you ever had a melanoma? (increases risk of subsequent melanoma threefold)
7. Has this lesion or any other pigmented lesion been biopsied or excised?

EXAMINATION

1. Inspect the lesion. Note the ABCDE checklist:
   - whether it is **a**symmetrical or not

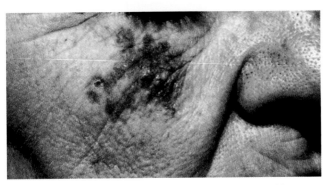

Figure 3.67.1 Malignant melanoma on the face (Zenith, Corinthian Colleges, Inc. *Medical Assistant: Integumentary, Sensory Systems, Patient Care and Communication—Module A.* Elsevier Inc., 2016.)

- regular or irregular **b**order
- **c**olour: whether the pigmentation is uniform or variable and
- **e**levated (raised or not)
2. Measure its **d**iameter. Over 6 mm is concerning for melanoma.
3. Note if there is any ulceration or inflammation.
4. Ask if you may perform an examination of the draining lymph nodes and a general inspection of the entire skin surface.

Present your findings

- For any pigmented lesion, consider the melanoma ABCDE checklist:
    - **A**symmetrical (typically)
    - **B**order irregular
    - **C**olour variation
    - **D**iameter large
    - **E**levated above the skin
- Mention other high risk features, such as:
    - ulceration
    - loss of normal skin markings around the lesion, such as creases
    - satellite lesions
    - bleeding
    - a ring of paler pigment around the lesion.

Examiners' likely questions

- Do you think this might be a melanoma? Why?
- What would you recommend to the patient?
  - Biopsy and complete excision if you suspect a melanoma
- What might make this difficult in this case?
  - Comment on the position on the face and proximity to other structures such as the eye that might make excision difficult, especially when it is vital to achieve an adequate margin around the tumour.
- Is there a differential diagnosis?
  Obviously the answer must be 'yes':
  - A pigmented naevus
  - A pigmented seborrhoeic keratosis
  - A pigmented basal cell carcinoma
  - A dark freckle.

Marking criteria table

Criteria	Satisfactory	Unsatisfactory
Introduces self, explains task, obtains consent, washes hands	1	0
Asks about sun exposure	1	0
Asks about family history of melanoma	1	0
Obtains history of the lesion	1	0
Asks whether it is itchy or has bled or changed colour	1	0
Asks about past history of melanoma	1	0
Examines lesions for features suggestive of melanoma	2	0–1
Knows or demonstrates ABCDE checklist	2	0–1
Examines draining lymph nodes	1	0
Asks to examine all the skin	1	0
Describes characteristics of the history and examination consistent with melanoma	2	0–1

Pass mark: 9

Elbow rash examination

Background

Psoriasis is a common chronic skin condition. (See Fig. 3.68.1.) It can be associated with serious arthritis.

Introduction

This man has had a rash on his elbows for some years. Please examine him.

Method

The psoriatic rash is usually a simple spot diagnosis. Note the often bright red, scaly plaque with silvery scale over the joints.

1. Ask to examine the other commonly affected parts of the skin:
   - the other elbow
   - the extensor surfaces of the knees
   - the umbilicus
   - the scalp (look in the hairline).
2. Look for the lesions of pustular psoriasis on the hands and feet. Ask if these are painful (and ask to take the temperature for fever).
3. Look at the nails for onycholysis and for pitting, which is associated with seronegative psoriatic arthritis. The presence of pitting should prompt you to ask if you may examine the joints of the hands and feet.

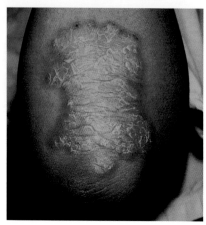

Figure 3.68.1 A well-demarcated, irregularly shaped plaque of psoriasis with silvery scales on the elbow (Goldbloom RB. *Pediatric Clinical Skills*, 4th edn. Elsevier Inc., 2011.)

Present your findings

Describe the features that suggest psoriasis — scaly silver rash with underlying erythema — and the areas involved. Indicate whether there is nail involvement.

Examiners' likely question

- Is the lesion likely to be pruritic?
  - No.

Marking criteria table		
Criteria	Satisfactory	Unsatisfactory
Introduces self, explains task, obtains consent, washes hands	1	0
Recognises psoriasis	2	0–1
Asks to examine relevant parts of the skin	2	0–1
Asks to look at nails	1	0
Knows of association with seronegative arthritis	1	0

Pass mark: 4

Rash on the trunk examination

Background

Dermatological examination depends on description. Students need to understand the common dermatological terms.

Introduction

Mrs Tran has noticed a rash on her trunk. Would you have a look at it and describe what you see?

Method

1. Wash hands, introduce yourself.
2. Ask if you may uncover the affected area.
3. Look at the rash and compare it mentally with the descriptions in Box 3.69.1.

Present your findings

- Describe what you have seen to the examiners.
- Try to give them a differential diagnosis.

Examiners' likely questions

- Will depend on what you have been shown. They may ask what further examination you would like to perform.
  - The rest of the skin
  - Joints
  - Lymph nodes
- What investigations might help?
  - Biopsy
  - Blood tests for inflammatory disorders, autoimmune diseases

Box 3.69.1
Terms used to describe skin conditions

Annular: Ring-shaped (hollow centre; e.g. tinea infection)
Arcuate: Curved (e.g. secondary syphilis)
Atrophy: Thinning of the epidermis with loss of normal skin markings
Bulla: A large collection of fluid below the epidermis
Circinate: Circular
Confluent: Lesions that have run together (e.g. measles)
Crust: Dried serum and exudate
Discoid: Circular without a hollow centre (e.g. lupus)
Ecchymoses: Bruises
Excoriations: Lesions caused by scratching that results in loss of the epidermis
Eczematous: Inflamed and crusted (e.g. allergic eczema)
Keloid: Hypertrophic scarring (see Fig. 3.69.1)
Keratotic: Thickened from increased keratin (e.g. psoriasis)
Lichenified: Thickened and roughened in association with accentuated markings of the epidermis
Linear: In lines (e.g. contact dermatitis)
Macule: A circumscribed alteration of skin colour
Nodule: A circumscribed palpable mass, greater than 1 cm in diameter
Papule: A circumscribed palpable elevation, less than 1 cm in diameter (e.g. erythema nodosum)
Papulosquamous: Plaques associated with scaling
Petechiae: Red, non-blanching spots <5 mm
Pigment alteration: Change in pigmentation, either increased (hyperpigmentation) or decreased (hypopigmentation)
Plaque: A palpable disc-shaped lesion
Purpura: Red, non-blanching spots >5 mm
Pustule: A visible collection of pus
Reticulated: In a network pattern (e.g. cutaneous parasite)
Scale: An accumulation of excess keratin
Sclerosis: Induration of subcutaneous tissues, which may involve the dermis
Serpiginous: Sinuous
Ulcer: A circumscribed loss of tissue
Vesicle: A small collection of fluid below the epidermis
Wheal: An area of dermal oedema
Zosteriform: Following a nerve distribution

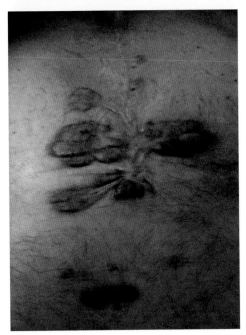

Figure 3.69.1 Hypertrophic (keloid) scarring (Talley NJ, O'Connor S. *Talley and O'Connor's Clinical Examination*. Elsevier Australia, 2017.)

Marking criteria table

Criteria	Satisfactory	Unsatisfactory
Introduces self, explains task, obtains consent, washes hands, undresses patient correctly	1	0
Can describe the rash and its distribution	2	0–1
Uses approved dermatological terms to describe lesions	1	0
Gives a differential diagnosis	2	0–1
Suggests investigations	1	0
Suggests treatment	1	0

Pass mark: 5

Take a history from a patient with pruritic rash

Background

Pruritis means itching. A pruritic rash can be due to skin disease or systemic conditions, especially if localised (Fig. 3.70.1). Look for scratch marks and their distribution when assessing.

Introduction

Mr Miles is 45-year-old man who has developed a pruritic rash. Please take a dermatological history from him.

Method

1. Introduce yourself.
2. Keep in mind the important causes of pruritis:
   - Asteotosis (dry skin)
   - Atopic dermatitis
   - Urticaria
   - Scabies
   - Dermatitis herpetiformis
   - Bullous pemphigoid
   - Systemic causes include cholestasis (e.g. primary biliary cholangitis), chronic kidney disease, pregnancy and lymphoma.
3. Ask:
   - How long have you had the rash?
   - Have you ever had it before?
   - Is it getting worse?
   - What parts of your skin are affected (e.g. sun-exposed areas, areas in contact with clothing or chemicals)?

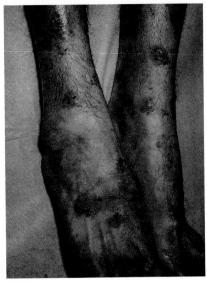

Figure 3.70.1 Nummular eczema—typical scattered coin-like lesions of indolent dermatitis (Reeves JT, Maibach H. *Clinical Dermatology Illustrated: A regional approach*, 2nd edn. Sydney: MacLennan & Petty Pty Ltd, ©1991, with permission)

- Was the rash flat or raised to begin with, or was it blistered?
- Is the area still itchy?
- Has your diet changed recently?
- Does anything seem to make it better?
- What treatment have you tried for it?
- Have you had any problems with joint pains? (autoimmune or inflammatory disorder)
- Have you had allergies in the past?
- Are you taking any tablets or medicines? Are any of these new?
- Have you changed your soap, deodorant or washing powder recently? (Rashes are often the result of chemical sensitivities or allergies and detective work is needed to discover the offending substance.)

- What sort of work do you do? Do you come into contact with chemicals at work or with any of your hobbies?
- Have you travelled recently? Where to?
- Has anyone you know got a similar rash?
- Has it made it difficult for you to work or sleep? (It is important to find out how badly the problem affects the patient's life.)
- Have you had any other problems with your health? A history of asthma may indicate atopic problems.

Present your findings

Make a point of outlining:
- the extent of the rash
- the duration
- the severity of its effect
- any associated symptoms
- any possible causes that might have emerged from the history.

Examiners' likely questions

- How serious is the problem?
  - You have probably already told them, but describe the symptom severity and impact on the patients life if necessary.
- What would you do next?
  - Examine the patient — assessment of the full skin surface.
- What investigations or treatment would you suggest?
  - This will depend on the history. Suggest a trial of elimination of new drugs, soaps etc.
  - Blood tests for inflammatory or autoimmune conditions
  - A biopsy of the rash
  - Topical steroids (know the indications)

Marking criteria table

Criteria	Satisfactory	Unsatisfactory
Introduces self, explains task, obtains consent	1	0
Asks about nature and duration of rash	1	0
Asks about associated features, including pruritis	1	0
Asks about treatment tried	1	0
Finds out about success or otherwise of treatment	1	0
Asks about systemic symptoms	1	0
Asks about effect of condition on life, work etc.	1	0
Tries to establish cause: occupation, use of detergents, soaps etc.	2	0–1
Asks about other atopic problems	1	0
Presents summary of findings	2	0–1
Suggests treatment	1	0

Pass mark: 9

Demonstrate a systematic approach to skin examination

Background

A systemic approach to skin examination is helpful in determining the likely differential diagnosis. In undergraduate examinations, only common skin disease is likely to be encountered.

Introduction

- Describe how you would perform a general examination of the skin.
- Please perform a general examination of the skin for this 60-year-old man. He has no symptoms but has a history of sun exposure.

Rationale

Students need to have a general approach to examination of the skin. This needs to be comprehensive and systematic. You may be asked to examine a patient or model or to describe your technique to the examiners and explain what you are doing as you go along.

Method

1. Even if the patient shows the examiner only a small single area of abnormality, proceed to examine all the skin. Men should be asked to leave their underpants on and women underpants and bra to begin with. A hospital gown might be available that allows exposure of parts of the skin in turn. Ask for more light if necessary.

2. Begin by looking at the **nails and hands**. Paronychia is an infection of the skin surrounding the nails. Other changes to note include:
   - pitting (psoriasis, fungal infections)
   - onycholysis (e.g. thyrotoxicosis, psoriasis)
   - dark staining under the nail that may indicate a subungual melanoma
   - linear splinter haemorrhages (e.g. vasculitis) or telangiectasias (e.g. systemic lupus erythematosus) that may be seen in the nail bed
   - a purplish discolouration in streaks over the knuckles that may indicate dermatomyositis.

3. Also look at the backs of the hands and forearms for the characteristic blisters of porphyria, which occur on the exposed skin.
   - Papules and scratch marks on the backs of the hands, between the fingers and around the wrists may indicate scabies.
   - Viral warts are common on the hands.

4. Look at the palms for Dupuytren contracture and
   - pigmented flat junctional moles (which have a high risk of becoming malignant) and
   - xanthomata in the palmar creases.

5. Next look at the arms, where lichen planus (characterised by small shiny, purple-coloured papules) may occur on the flexor surfaces of the forearms and for:
   - psoriasis, which may be present on the extensor surfaces around the elbows
   - palpable purpura — raised bruising that indicates bleeding into the skin — that may be seen on the arms, indicating vasculitis
   - acanthosis nigricans, which can occur in the axillae.

6. Inspect the patient's hair and scalp. Decide whether or not the hair is dry and whether the distribution is normal.
   - Alopecia may be due to male pattern baldness, recent severe illness, hypothyroidism or thyrotoxicosis.
   - Patches of alopecia occur in the disease alopecia areata.
   - Short broken-off hairs occur typically in systemic lupus erythematosus.
   - In psoriasis there are silvery scales, which may be seen on the skin of the scalp.

- Metastatic deposits may rarely be felt as firm nodules within the skin of the scalp.
- Sebaceous cysts are common.
- The unfortunate examiner may find nits sticking to the head hairs.

7. Move down now to the **eyebrows** and look for scaling and greasiness, which are found in seborrhoeic dermatitis.
   - A purplish erythema occurs around the eyelids in dermatomyositis.
   - Xanthelasmata are seen near the eyelid.

8. Look at the **face** for rosacea, which causes bright erythema of the nose, cheeks, forehead and chin, and occasionally pustules and rhinophyma (disfiguring swelling of the nose).
   - Acne causes papules, pustules and scars involving the face, neck and upper trunk.
   - The butterfly rash of systemic lupus erythematosus occurs across the cheeks, but is rare.
   - Spider naevi may be present.
   - Ulcerating lesions on the face may include basal cell carcinoma, squamous cell carcinoma or, rarely, tuberculosis (lupus vulgaris).
   - Benign tumours of the face include kerato-acanthoma (a volcano-like lesion from a sebaceous gland) and congenital haemangiomas.
   - Look for the blisters of herpes zoster, which may occur strictly in the distribution of one of the divisions of the trigeminal nerve.

9. Inspect the **neck**, which is prone to many of the lesions that occur on the face.
   - Rarely, the redundant loose skin of pseudoxanthoma elasticum will be seen around the neck.

10. Go on to inspect the **trunk**, where any of the childhood exanthems produce their characteristic rashes. Look for spider naevi.
    - Campbell de Morgan spots are commonly found on the abdomen (and chest), as are
    - flat, greasy, yellow-coloured seborrhoeic warts. In addition,
    - erythema marginatum (rheumatic fever) occurs on the chest and abdomen

- herpes zoster may be seen overlying any of the dermatome distributions
- metastases from internal malignancies may rarely occur anywhere on the skin
- neurofibromas are soft flesh-coloured tumours; when associated with more than five 'café-au-lait' spots (brownish, irregular lesions) they suggest neurofibromatosis (von Recklinghausen disease)
- pigmented moles are seen on the trunk and evidence of malignancy must be looked for with these
- the patient's buttocks and sacrum must be examined for bedsores (with the permission of the patient and examiners), and
- the abdomen and thighs may have areas of fat atrophy or hypertrophy from insulin injections.

11. Go to the **legs**, where erythema nodosum or erythema multiforme may be seen on the shins.
    - Necrobiosis lipoidica diabeticorum affects the skin over the tibia in people with diabetes.
    - Pretibial myxoedema also occurs over the shins.
    - Look for ulcers on either side of the lower part of the leg.
    - Livedo reticularis is a net-like, red reticular rash that occurs in vasculitis, the antiphospholipid syndrome and with atheroembolism.

12. Inspect the **feet** for the characteristic lesion of Reiter disease (reactive arthritis) called keratoderma blennorrhagica, where crusted lesions spread across the sole because of the fusion of vesicles and pustules.
    - Look at the foot for signs of ischaemia, associated with wasting of the skin and skin appendages.
    - Trophic ulcers may be seen in patients with peripheral neuropathy (e.g. diabetes mellitus).
    - Always separate the toes to look for melanomas.

Present your findings

You may have described what you are looking for as you go along, but if there are abnormalities describe them again to the examiners. A selection of the many possible skin abnormalities is shown in Figs 3.71.1–3.71.17.

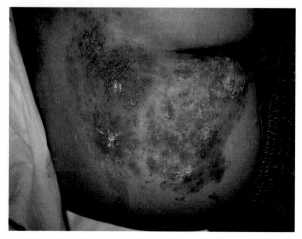

Figure 3.71.1 Zosteriform rash of the left buttock (Courtesy of Dr A Watson, Infectious Diseases Department, The Canberra Hospital.)

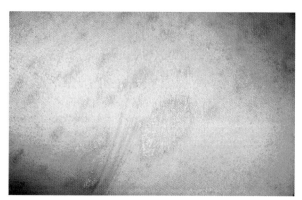

Figure 3.71.2 Pityriasis rosea, with scattered scaly oval lesions on the trunk and a larger 'herald' patch (Reeves JT, Maibach H. *Clinical Dermatology Illustrated: A regional approach*, 2nd edn. Oxford University Press, 1991.)

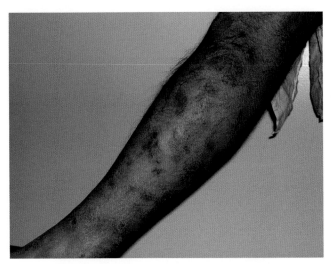

Figure 3.71.3 Nummular eczema — pink oval scaling, slightly crusted patches (Miller JJ, Marks JG. *Lookingbill and Marks' Principles of Dermatology*, 6th edn. Philadelphia: Elsevier, 2018.)

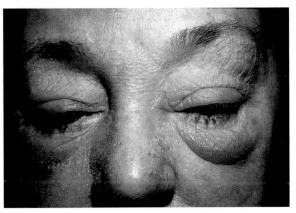

Figure 3.71.4 Allergic contact dermatitis from over-the-counter topical medication rubbed over congested sinuses (Courtesy of Dr A Watson, Infectious Diseases Department, The Canberra Hospital.)

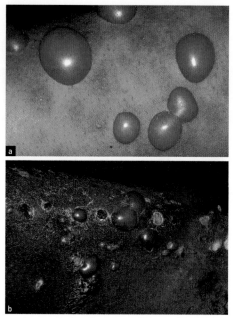

Figure 3.71.5 Bullous pemphigoid (Schwarzenberger K. *General Dermatology*. Philadelphia: Saunders, 2008.)

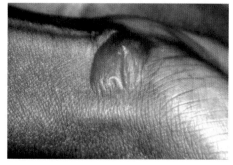

Figure 3.71.6 Pemphigus vulgaris (Reeves JT, *Clinical Dermatology Illustrated: A regional approach*, 2nd edn. Oxford University Press, 1991.)

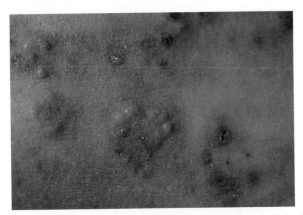

Figure 3.71.7 Dermatitis herpetiformis (Talley NJ, O'Connor S. *Talley & O'Connor's Clinical Examination Essentials: An introduction to clinical skills (and how to pass your clinical exams)*. Elsevier Australia, 2020.)

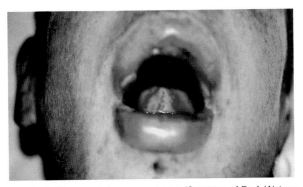

Figure 3.71.8 Stevens–Johnson syndrome (Courtesy of Dr A Watson, Infectious Diseases Department, The Canberra Hospital.)

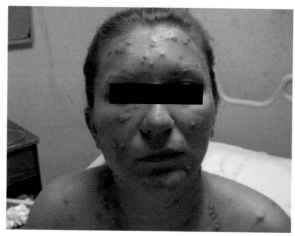

Figure 3.71.9 Sweet syndrome (acute febrile neutrophilic dermatosis) characterised by painful red plaques and nodules and often fever (Fazili T, Duncan D, Wani L. Sweet's syndrome. *American Journal of Medicine* 2010; 123(8):694–696.)

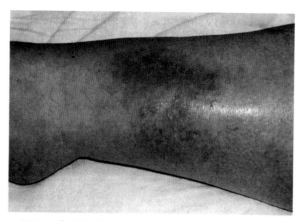

Figure 3.71.10 Cellulitis (Courtesy of Dr A Watson, Infectious Diseases Department, The Canberra Hospital.)

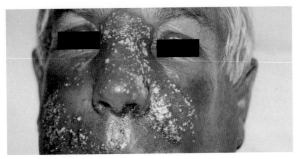

Figure 3.71.11 Erysipelas (Courtesy of Dr A Watson, Infectious Diseases Department, The Canberra Hospital.)

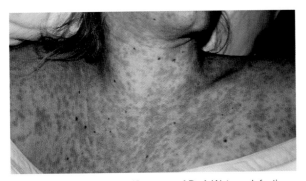

Figure 3.71.12 Viral exanthem (Courtesy of Dr A Watson, Infectious Diseases Department, The Canberra Hospital.)

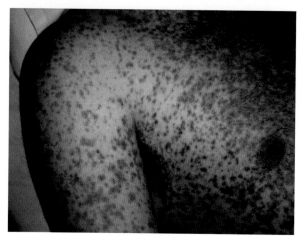

Figure 3.71.13 Epstein–Barr virus infection after amoxicillin (Courtesy of Dr A Watson, Infectious Diseases Department, The Canberra Hospital.)

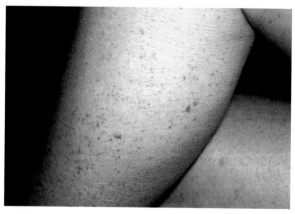

Figure 3.71.14 Petechial rash (Marks J, Miller J. *Lookingbill & Marks' Principles of Dermatology*, 4th edn. Philadelphia: Saunders, 2006.)

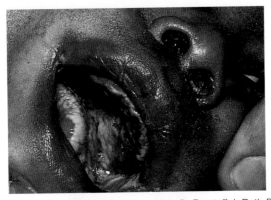

Figure 3.71.15 *Candida albicans* (From Male D, Brostoff J, Roth D, Roitt I. *Immunology*, 8th edn. Philadelphia: Saunders, 2012.)

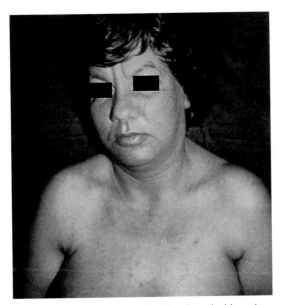

Figure 3.71.16 Patient with lung carcinoid and carcinoid syndrome with severe, long-standing flushing, lacrimation and a swollen face (Talley NJ, O'Connor S. *Talley & O'Connor's Clinical Examination Essentials: An introduction to clinical skills (and how to pass your clinical exams)*. Elsevier Australia, 2020.)

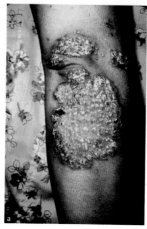

Figure 3.71.17 Psoriasis — typical bright red, scaly plaque with silvery scale over a joint (Paller AS, Mancini AJ. *Hurwitz Clinical Pediatric Dermatology: A textbook of skin disorders of children and adolescence*, 5th edn. Philadelphia: Elsevier, 2016.)

Examiners' likely questions

There may be none if the examination was routine, but any abnormalities must be given a differential diagnosis.

Marking criteria table

Criteria	Satisfactory	Unsatisfactory
Introduces self, explains task, obtains consent, washes hands, undresses patient appropriately	1	0
Conducts systematic examination	1	0
Examines nails and hands	2	0–1
Examines palms and forearms	2	0–1
Examines axillae	1	0
Examines face	2	0–1
Examines hair and scalp	2	0–1
Examines trunk	2	0–1
Examines legs	1	0
Examines feet	1	0
Summarises findings or important negatives in each part of the body	4	0–3

Pass mark: 14

Examining a tremor

Background

Tremor is a rhythmical movement. Tremor can be slow or rapid. Determine if the tremor is at rest (e.g. Parkinson disease), postural or with deliberate movement (action tremor in cerebellar disease).

Introduction

This 65-year-old man complains of a tremor in his right hand at rest. Please assess him.

Rationale

Think Parkinson disease but remember other possibilities. You will be doing a focused neurological examination. If your examination of the tremor suggests Parkinson disease, you will want to move on to examine for other manifestations of this disease, including function testing. Expect a real patient with signs.

Method

1. Introduce yourself. Confirm the patient details (name, date of birth). Ask if he is right- or left-handed. Ask permission to proceed. Note any speech abnormality (monotonous, soft, poorly articulated and faint in Parkinson). Wash your hands!
2. Take a step back and do a general inspection. Look for any lack of facial expression (mask-like facies) and any obvious tremor of the head (titubation in essential tremor), hands or feet. Examine the voice for microphonia (Parkinson) and voice tremor (essential tremor), (e.g ask the patient how was the trip to hospital today).

3. Ask him to stretch out his hands in front of him and look for the resting tremor, typically 'pill rolling' and often unilateral in Parkinson.

4. Next do a finger–nose test: a resting tremor will decrease or disappear, but an action tremor will become apparent (e.g. thyrotoxicosis, anxiety, familial or idiopathic).

5. Assuming a resting tremor, examine the upper limbs next, focusing on tone first. Assess if there is cogwheel or lead-pipe rigidity at rest or on reinforcement (patient turning his head from side to side). Note if power and reflexes are normal.

6. Test for abnormal rapid alternating movements — ask the patient to rapidly tap index and thumb together and note any progressive diminution in magnitude (bradykinesia).

7. Go to the face. Look for lack of expression (Fig. 3.72.1).
   - Do a glabellar tap (positive when patient continues to blink).

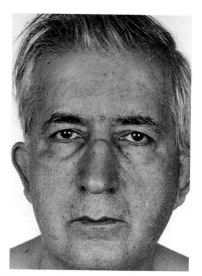

Figure 3.72.1 The mask-like facial expression typical of patients with Parkinson disease (Heimgartner NM, Workman ML, Rebar CR, Ignatavicius DD. *Medical-Surgical Nursing: Concepts for interprofessional collaborative care*, 10th edn. Elsevier Inc., 2021.)

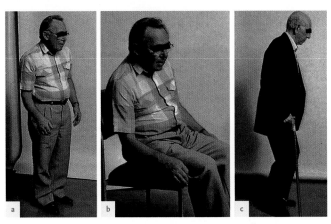

Figure 3.72.2 Parkinson disease. Posture and gait can give important clues to neurological diagnosis (Page CP, Hoffman BB, Curtis MJ, Walker MJA. *Integrated Pharmacology*, 3rd edn. Elsevier Ltd, 2006.)

- Test ocular movements for progressive supranuclear palsy (causes truncal rigidity and falls).
8. Examine gait (Fig. 3.72.2). Ask him to walk, turn quickly and stop, and restart. Note any difficulties, shuffling or freezing.
9. Ask the patient to write (micrographia).
10. Additional assessments to complete the examination include screening for dementia (Mini-Cog™) and testing for postural hypotension.
11. Check on patient's comfort and address any questions he may have.

T&O'C hint box

- Don't confuse an intention tremor in cerebellar disease or an action tremor with a resting tremor in Parkinson disease.
- Always examine gait if you suspect Parkinson disease.
- Parkinson plus syndromes should be recognised — progressive supranuclear palsy (test gaze), dementia with Lewy bodies (offer to test higher centres), and multiple systems atrophy (take the blood pressure lying and standing — autonomic neuropathy with postural hypotension).

Present your findings

- Be prepared to describe relevant normal and any abnormal findings step by step (in the order you performed the examination).
- Provide a provisional diagnosis and a short differential diagnosis if there are any abnormalities.

Examiners' likely questions

- What may be the cause this man's tremor and why?
  - A resting tremor is characteristic of Parkinson disease.
- Could it be due to any other cause?
  - A familial tremor is a consideration. An action tremor is present throughout movement (e.g. thyrotoxicosis). A cerebellar tremor increases towards the target.
- What are the major causes of Parkinson disease?
  - Usually idiopathic (may first present with a REM sleep disorder — abnormal movements during dreams — and no other features). Drugs may be a cause (e.g. phenothiazines). Rarely a structural lesion or Wilson disease.
- How would you treat this man? (senior students)
- Would treatment be the same if he has progressive supranuclear palsy?
  - This does not respond to levodopa.

Marking criteria table		
Criteria	Satisfactory	Unsatisfactory
Introduces self, confirms details, explains task	1	0
Examines tremor	2	0–1
Conducts finger–nose test	1	0
Examines face	1	0
Tests gait	2	0–1
Examines speech	1	0
Tests writing	1	0
Tests ocular movements	1	0
Asks to measure blood pressure sitting and standing	1	0
Summarises findings adequately	2	0–1
Offers differential diagnosis	2	0–1

Pass mark: 10

Suspected sexually transmitted disease

Background

A sexual history is a sensitive assessment, so seek permission as part of your assessment and explain why you need to ask the questions.

Introduction

A 19-year-old male presents to you with urethral discharge for the past week. He is a new patient and you have not met him before.

Please take a history.

Rationale

This is a communication and history-taking station. There is a growing incidence of sexually transmitted infections in Australia. The ability to take a thorough sexual history is an important skill. It is important to be non-judgmental and respectful throughout the consultation.

Method

1. Introduce yourself. Seek permission to ask some sensitive questions.
2. Explain the need to discuss a sexual history. It is essential that you reassure the patient that their conversation will be confidential; however, if there was risk of significant harm to the patient or others, this confidentiality may need to be broken.

3. Ask for permission to take a sexual history.
4. Take a history of the presenting complaint. Important questions to ask males in regard to symptoms including:
    - urethral discharge
    - testicular pain
    - skin lesions
    - dysuria
    - systemic symptoms.
      For each of these symptoms it is important to take a complete symptoms history, this includes questions about onset, duration, severity, exacerbating factors, relieving factors and any previous episodes.
5. Following this, ask a more general sexual history.
    - When did you last have sex?
    - Who have you been having sex with? Was this a regular sexual partner, or a casual sexual encounter?
    - Clarify the sex of the partner(s).
    - You should clarify what type of sexual contact, e.g. genital, anal, oral, and digital.
    - Ask about use of contraception, including type or consistency.
    - Do you regularly wear a condom (or does your partner)?
    - Seek past history of sexually transmitted infections (STIs): Have you ever been tested for an STI? Do you know if any of your partners have been diagnosed with or tested for STIs?
    - In the past 6 months, how many sexual partners have you had?
6. Screen for high-risk activities:
    - overseas travel
    - human immunodeficiency virus (HIV) positive partner
    - intravenous drug use
    - sex work.
7. Do not forget to ask routine questions!
    - Past medical history
    - Medications, e.g. to prevent HIV
    - Drug allergies
    - Smoking
    - Alcohol
    - Drugs

- Occupation
- Social support
- Vaccinations

8. Praise any protective practices.
9. Thank the patient for being open and honest.

> **T&O'C hint box**
>
> This is a communication station. It is important to be non-judgmental and respectful.

> **T&O'C hint box**
>
> It is important to be comfortable when discussing a patient's sexual history. The OSCE station "patient" is likely to be an actor.

Present your findings

- Present the results of your history.
- Ensure you include relevant positive and negative findings.
- Highlight any high-risk behaviours or concerns you may have.

Examiners' likely questions

How would you advise the patient about contact tracing? What options are available?

Marking criteria table

Criteria	Satisfactory	Unsatisfactory
Sympathetic and matter of fact manner	1	0
Asks permission for questions	1	0
Questions about symptoms	2	0–1
Questions about sexual practices	2	0–1
Questions about contacts	1	0
Questions about high risk activities	1	0

Pass mark: 4

Breast examination

Background

Breast examination is a sensitive examination, so always seek permission and explain why it is necessary before commencing.

Introduction

This 59-year-old woman reports feeling a lump in her left breast. Please conduct a breast examination.

Rationale

A lump in the breast raises the strong suspicion of cancer and engenders great anxiety. Sensitive examinations require an empathetic, tactful approach with explanation, consent and, where possible, a chaperone. You will be expected to know how to inspect and palpate the breasts. You will also be expected to examine the draining lymph nodes (axillary and supraclavicular). In an OSCE, if there is a lump it's likely to be benign.

Method

1. Introduce yourself. Wash your hands.
2. Confirm the patient details (name, date of birth) — you don't want to perform a breast exam on someone who doesn't need (or want) it.
3. Explain why you want to perform the examination. (In this case, to assess a lump.) Explain exactly what you are going to do (see steps below).
4. Ask the patient for permission to proceed. Ask about a chaperone. Make the area private (or ask to do so).

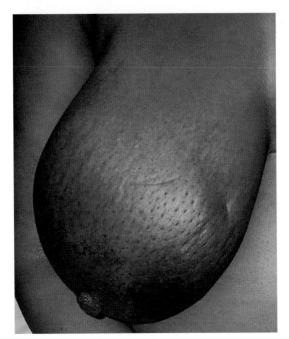

Figure 3.74.1 Paget disease of breast. Sharply marginated plaque with a slightly raised edge and an irregular outline. If the crusts are removed, a red, glazed and moist surface is revealed (Khanna N. *Illustrated Synopsis of Dermatology and Sexually Transmitted Diseases*, 5th edn. Elsevier Inc., 2016.)

5. Expose the chest with the patient sitting up.
6. Inspect the nipples (e.g. retraction, or any red scaling or bleeding area suggestive of Paget's disease). Then inspect the rest of the skin, noting visible veins, dimpling, or rarely peau d'orange skin (Figs 3.74.1–3.74.3). Inspect both breasts, including underneath (abnormal side first, if known).
7. Ask the patient to elevate her left then right arm above her head and look for tethering or a mass. Ask the patient to then rest her hands on her hips and press her hands onto her hips to look for increased dimpling or fixation of skin.

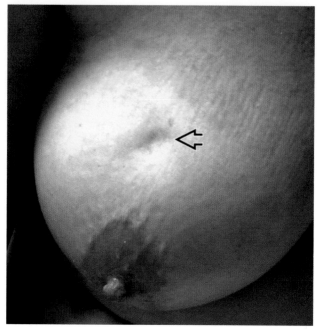

Figure 3.74.2 This 35-year-old woman self-palpated a right breast lump with overlying skin dimpling. Her mother and two aunts had breast cancer in their 50s, as did her maternal grandmother in her 60s (Berg WA, Leung JWT. *Diagnostic Imaging: Breast*, 3rd edn. Elsevier Inc., 2019.)

8. Ask the patient to lie flat and, after placing her arm behind her head, palpate each breast systematically with your flattened three middle fingers. Feel each area of the breast — think of the breast as a clock face and go to each hour of the clock, covering all four quadrants and the axillary tail. Then palpate behind the nipple in the areolar area. Note any discharge. You may only be allowed to examine the abnormal breast in an OSCE, but ask to examine both as in real-life practice.

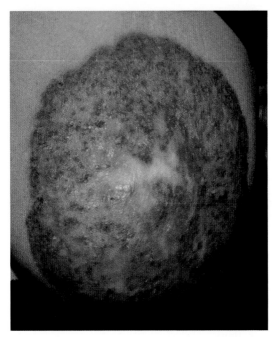

Figure 3.74.3 Breast lymphoedema and peau d'orange skin in advanced breast cancer (Skirven TM, Feldscher SB, Amadio PC et al. *Rehabilitation of the Hand and Upper Extremity*, 7th edn. Elsevier Inc., 2021.)

9. If you feel a lump, you must characterise it like any lump on the body — site, size, shape and consistency, tenderness, and fixation. Is there more than one lump?
10. Examine the draining lymph nodes (axillary, supraclavicular). If you suspect malignancy, you can search elsewhere for cancer spread — hard enlarged liver, vertebral tenderness, pleural effusion, focal neurological signs (e.g. localised weakness).
11. Cover her chest, check on patient's comfort and address any questions she may have.

Present your findings

- Be prepared to describe relevant normal and any abnormal findings step by step (in the order you performed the examination).
- Provide a provisional diagnosis and a short differential diagnosis if there are any abnormalities.

Examiners' likely questions

- How would you differentiate a benign from malignant breast lump?
  - Tethering, not tender, lymph nodes palpable, bloody discharge from nipple
- What would be your next initial investigation? (Depends on the introduction and findings).

Marking criteria table

Criteria	Satisfactory	Unsatisfactory
Introduces self, confirms details, suggests chaperone	1	0
Explains why/what	1	0
Consent obtained	1	0
Patient set up/exposure	1	0
Inspects breasts, including manoeuvres	2	0–1
Palpates breasts adequately	2	0–1
Assesses lump satisfactorily	3	0–2
Palpates draining lymph nodes	2	0–1
Summarises findings adequately	2	0–1
Offers sensible differential diagnosis	2	0–1

Pass mark: 12

Background

Assessment of the urine can provide insights into underlying renal disease, as well as diabetes mellitus.

Introduction

- You are a junior medical officer working in the emergency department. You are reviewing Mrs Cecilia Greer, a 58-year-old female who has presented with a 2-day history of dysuria and increased urinary frequency. You suspect a urinary tract infection and perform urinalysis. Please explain the steps you would perform in conducting this and answer the examiners' questions.

- You are a junior medical officer working in the emergency department. You are reviewing Miss Amanda Young, a 32-year-old female who has presented with dark urine. Her last menstrual period started 11 days prior and a pregnancy test is negative. She reports having a sore throat 3 weeks earlier. You suspect post-streptococcal glomerulonephritis. What would you expect to find on urinalysis?

Rationale

Urinalysis is a very useful tool in clinical practice. There are three main aspects — gross assessment, dipstick assessment and microscopy and culture — that can provide a range of information to aid in interpretation of the clinical picture.

Method

GROSS ASSESSMENT

1. Assess **turbidity**. (Turbid urine may reflect infection, crystals or chyluria.)
2. Assess **colour**.
   - Light — dilute
   - Darker — concentrated — dehydrated
   - Red
     - haematuria (indicates red blood cells)
     - haemoglobinuria (indicates haemolysis)
     - myoglobinuria (indicates rhabdomyolysis)
     - medications — rifampicin, phenytoin, senna
     - foods — dyes, beetroot, rhubarb
     - acute intermittent porphyria
   - White — phosphate crystals, chyluria, propofol
   - Pink — uric acid crystals
   - Green — methylene blue, propofol, amitriptyline
   - Black — haemoglobinuria, myoglobinuria, melanuria
   - Purple — bacteriuria, urinary catheters

URINE DIPSTICK

1. Interpret readings from urine dipstick.
   - **Haem** — haemoglobin, red blood cells, myoglobin
   - **Leukocyte esterase** — released by lysed neutrophils and macrophages, marker for presence of white blood cells
   - **Nitrite** — many Enterobacteriaceae species release an enzyme that converts the nitrate present in urine to nitrite
   - **Protein** — detects macroalbuminuria (>300 mg/day), detection is affected by dilution of urine
   - **pH** — 4.5–8, low in response to systemic acidaemia, high in renal tubular acidosis
   - **Specific gravity** — compares weight of urine to weight of water, determined by number and size of particles in urine; can be used to infer information about urine osmolality (number of molecules (regardless of size) per kg of water), increasing with increased osmolality
   - **Glucose** — inability of glucose reabsorption (proximal tubule dysfunction), increased plasma glucose

MICROSCOPY

1. Consider microscopy findings.
   - Red blood cells (haematuria)
     - transient — post exercise or sexual intercourse
     - malignancy
     - urinary tract infection
     - kidney stones
     - glomerular disease — suggested by dysmorphic red blood cells (e.g. acanthocytes — red blood cells that have membrane protrusions — glomerulonephritis)
   - White blood cells
     - neutrophils — bacteriuria, interstitial nephritis, renal tuberculosis, nephrolithiasis
     - eosinophils — acute interstitial nephritis
   - **Epithelial cells** — shed from anywhere along genitourinary tract
   - **Casts** — cylindrical structures formed in the tubular lumen
     - formed with urine stasis, low pH, concentrated urine
     - **red blood cell casts** — proliferative glomerulonephritis
     - **white blood cell casts** — interstitial or glomerular inflammation
     - **renal tubular epithelial cell casts** — acute tubular necrosis, acute interstitial nephritis, proliferative glomerulonephritis
     - **granular casts** — dark and coarse casts — acute tubular necrosis, ischaemic or toxic injury to tubular epithelial cells
     - **hyaline** casts — concentrated urine, diuretic therapy
     - **waxy casts** — degenerated granular casts, non-specific
     - **broad casts** — associated with advanced chronic kidney disease

- Crystals
  - **uric acid** — acidic urine, tumour lysis syndrome
  - **calcium oxalate** — risk factor for kidney stone formation; ethylene glycol ingestion
  - **calcium phosphate** — only in alkaline urine
  - **cysteine crystals** — cystinuria, risk factor for kidney stone formation
  - **magnesium ammonium phosphate crystals** — *Proteus* or *Klebsiella* urinary tract infection
- Microorganisms
  - **bacteria** — clinical significance guided by clinical features
  - fungi
- **Lipuria** — glomerular disease, polycystic kidney disease

Present your findings

- For Mrs Greer, if this is a urinary tract infection, the urinalysis would show an elevated urine white cell count, elevated urinary nitrites, red cells and occasionally a small amount of protein if acute. Most are due to *E. coli* or occasionally *Staphyloccoccus saprophyticus* or *Proteus mirabilis*. Flank pain and fever would suggest pyelonephritis.
- For Miss Young, in post-streptococcal glomerulonephritis, expect fragmented red cells (and red cell casts), there may be increased protein (worse prognosis). If asked about symptoms, remember a presentation with back pain, haematuria and reduced urine output (oliguria or even anuria). It would be advisable to check the blood pressure.

Examiners' likely questions

- Is there anything you would look for in the sample before performing tests on it?
  - Gross examination.
- Is there a way you could quickly get more information?
  - Dipstick
- Are there any further tests you would like to send the sample off for?
  - Microscopy and culture

- – Renal function and electrolytes
- – Microscopy for casts
- Do patients with bacteriuria always require antibiotic therapy?
  - – No! Justify your answer.
- What is the most common organism responsible for urinary tract infections?
  - – See above.
- What are the typical findings on urinalysis in glomerulonephritis?
  - – See above.

Marking criteria table

Criteria	Satisfactory	Unsatisfactory
Undertakes a gross assessment	1	0
Dipstick readings	2	0–1
Interprets Microscopy/Culture findings	1	0
Knows when to treat bacteriuria	1	0
Knows most common organisms causing urinary infection	2	0–1
Knows typical findings of glomerulonephritis	1	0
Knows causes of glomerulonephritis	2	0–1

Pass mark: 6

Peak flow and spirometry

Background

Peak flow meters measure the amount and the rate of air expelled during expiration; they do not directly measure airflow obstruction. The measurements are most useful when performed serially on an individual. This can be used together with symptoms to monitor worsening of asthma. Bedside assessment of lung function with spirometry is an extension of the physical examination and can demonstrate airflow obstruction and evidence of significant restrictive lung disease.

Introduction

You are performing a routine health check on a 60-year-old female patient. During the consult the patient laments she is struggling to walk the same distances she used to without getting quite puffed. The patient is an ex-smoker, having ceased 10 years prior, but before then had smoked 10 cigarettes a day since she was 20 years of age. As part of the work-up for breathlessness, you decide to perform spirometry. Please tell us how you would explain this test to the patient, perform the test and interpret the results.

Rationale

Spirometry is a measure of the forced expiratory flow a patient is able to achieve after maximal inspiration. It allows differentiation between restrictive and obstructive patterns. It can also be used to quantify disease severity and then as a marker of progression or response to therapy. When performed before and after a short-acting beta agonist (salbutamol/albuterol) it can be used to demonstrate variable airflow obstruction and assist in the diagnosis of asthma.

Method

1. Explain the purpose of spirometry to the patient.
   - The speed air moves in and out of our lungs is affected by many factors. This test will measure how well your lungs are able to inflate with air and how quickly you can breathe the air out of your lungs. Diseases that affect the flow of air, such as asthma and chronic obstructive pulmonary disease (COPD) will affect how quickly you can breathe air out. Other conditions may make the lungs stiff and they do not fill with air as well.
   - Spirometry is important in the diagnosis of asthma and COPD. It helps the doctor determine the severity of these and other lung diseases.
2. Explain the spirometry procedure to the patient.
   - This is a spirometer (point). (See Fig. 3.76.1.) It is used to measure how quickly the air can move out of your lungs and calculate how much air your lungs can hold. It then compares the information to what we would expect other people in a similar age and gender bracket to perform.

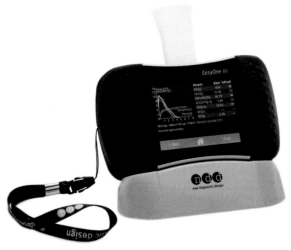

3.76.1 Spirometer (© NDD Medical Technologies.)

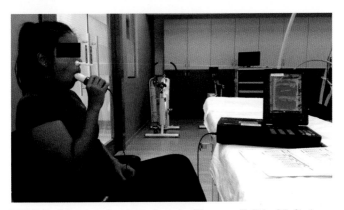

3.76.2 Participant performing spirometry (Choezom T, Raja GP, Shah SG. Comparison of respiratory parameters in participants with and without chronic low back pain. *Journal of Bodywork and Movement Therapies* 2019; 23(4).)

- We'll have a practice first as we talk through this (Fig. 3.76.2). Once you understand, we will do three attempts to get an accurate result and take the best attempt as your final result.
- First, we'll apply a nose clip to help stop air escaping.
- Sit up tall or stand as straight as possible, take the biggest breath you can and hold it (while facing away from the device). Put the tube in your mouth and form a tight seal with your teeth and lips, so that no air can escape other than through the tube. Next, exhale as forcefully as you can, breathing all of your breath out. Try to make your breath out last for as long as you can, even if you feel there is no air flowing — it will feel like a very long time. That's the first attempt complete. Take a moment to recover and then we will try again.
3. Interpreting spirometry results
   - Tables 3.76.1–3.76.3 list the results you will be given. Note that total lung capacity (TLC) is not included in spirometry readouts but requires lung volume measurement. Regardless, you may be given these results!

TABLE 3.76.1

Test	Predicted	Best	% of predicted	Post bronchodilator % change
FVC (L)	4.39	4.32	102	-1
FEV1 (L)	3.20	3.37	95	7
FEV1/FVC (%)	73	78		8
TLC (L)	6.86	6.09	113	

TABLE 3.76.2

Test	Predicted	Best	% of Predicted	Post bronc-hodilator	
				Actual	Per-centage
FVC (L)	4.22	3.19	76	4.00	25
FEV1 (L)	3.39	2.18	64	2.83	30
FEV1/ FVC (%)	80	68		71	4

TABLE 3.76.3

Test	Predicted	Best	% of Predicted
FVC (L)	1.73	4.37	40
FEV1 (L)	1.57	3.65	43
FEV1/FVC (%)	91	84	
TLC (L)	2.68	6.12	44

- The FEV1 (the forced expiratory volume in 1 second) is the volume forcefully exhaled in 1 second after maximal inspiration.
- The FVC (forced vital capacity) is the total volume of air a person can forcibly exhale after taking a maximum breath in. This can take as long as necessary during spirometry.

This does not include the residual volume, which when added to the FVC gives you the total lung capacity.

- The ratio FEV1/FVC is expressed as a percentage.
  All of the results are given in litre and as a percentage. This is compared to what is considered 'normal' for a population matched in age, sex, and height.
- An FVC over 80% predicted indicates no evidence of restriction. If the FEV1 > 80% predicted and the FEV1/FVC ratio is over 70%, this is a 'normal' result.
- If the FVC is less than 80%, the patient is displaying a restrictive pattern or an obstructive pattern with air trapping. To differentiate these two, you will need to measure lung volumes by plethysmography to obtain the total lung capacity (TLC). If the TLC is over 80%, these combined results indicate obstruction; if they are both low, it indicates restriction.
- FEV1 is used to further classify an obstructive pattern when combined with an FEV1/FVC ratio <0.7. If the FEV1/FVC is reduced, FEV1 ≥80% predicted indicates mild obstructive disease, 50–79% FEV1 indicates moderate obstruction and 30–49% severe obstruction.
  The last step is to determine if reversible airflow obstruction can be detected. This is done by comparing results of spirometry pre and post bronchodilator therapy. If a patient normalises or significantly improves their spirometry results (improvement in FEV1 by >12% or FVC by 200 mL) it is considered there is some reversibility of airflow obstruction. In the correct clinical context this can be used to confirm a diagnosis of asthma.

Present your findings

- Table 3.76.1 is an example of normal spirometry.
- Table 3.76.2 shows a moderate airflow obstruction.
  Following bronchodilator there is a 220 mL or 25% increase in FEV1, consistent with variable airflow obstruction.
- Table 3.76.3 demonstrates severe restriction.

Examiners' likely questions

- Why is spirometry a useful test to perform?
  - Readily available

- Takes a short amount of time to perform
- Bedside
- Carries minimal risk (occasionally dizziness and syncope)
- It is essential in the diagnosis of asthma and COPD.
- When should you not use spirometry?
  - In the COVID-19 pandemic spirometry will increase the risk of coughing and the forced expiratory manoeuvre will increase the risk of spreading infectious particles. Thus it should only be used in a person not complaining of acute respiratory symptoms and in a setting where the risk of transmission of infection is reduced, with the person perfoming the maneouvre wearing correct personal protective equipment (PPE).
  - Patients who have had abdominal, intracranial, or eye surgery, or a pneumothorax in the 6 weeks before testing are advised not to participate due to the increased pressures generated during the procedure.
- What can make spirometry unreliable?
  - An inability to complete the FVC
  - Being unable to achieve the FEV1 and FVC 0.1 L on at least two (preferably three) attempts
  - Additional breaths taken during expiration
  - Any coughing that occurs during expiration
  - Slow start to expiration
  - Poor effort

Marking criteria table

Criteria	Satisfactory	Unsatisfactory
Introduction	1	0
Explanation of spirometry	2	0–1
Performing of spirometry	2	0–1
Interpretation of results	2	0–1
Describing results to patient	2	0–1
Indication for testing	1	0

Pass mark: 7

Cannulation

Background

Any doctor graduating must be able to competently insert a cannula for intravenous access.

Introduction

Mr Moore is a 40-year-old man who has been admitted to hospital for pneumonia, requiring intravenous antibiotics. You have been requested to insert an intravenous cannula (IVC). Please proceed.

Rationale

Intravenous cannulation is a procedure often performed in the hospital. It involves inserting a plastic tube into a patient's vein that then can be used to infuse fluids, medication and blood products, for example. This is a show-and-tell station.

Method

There are two parts to this station:
1. Preparation
2. Insertion of the cannula

PREPARATION

1. Wash your hands.
2. Introduce yourself to the patient. Explain the procedure (in layman's terms) and make sure you gain consent.
3. Gather equipment. Invest some time in this step and make sure you have a sharps bin close by.

4. Sanitise your hands and position the patient's arm so that it is comfortable and you are able to identify a vein.
   - You should ask the patient if they have a preference for which arm to use.
   - Pre-existing conditions, for example arteriovenous dialysis fistula or lymphoedema, will prevent a particular limb from being used. Also avoid areas of swelling, bruising or broken skin.
5. Apply the tourniquet and confirm the position of an appropriate vein. The tourniquet should be applied approximately 4–5 finger widths above the planned cannulation site.
   Once you have identified a suitable vein you may need to temporarily release the tourniquet, as it should not be left on for more than 1–2 minutes.

INSERTION OF THE CANNULA

1. Wash your hands and put on gloves. Clean the optimal insertion site with alcohol wipe. Start cleaning from the centre of the cannulation site and work outwards to approximately 5 cm.
2. Re-apply the tourniquet if you have removed it previously.
3. Remove the cannula cap.
4. Stretch the skin distally and inform the patient prior to inserting the IVC.
5. Insert the cannula directly above the vein, through the skin at ~30° with the bevel facing upwards.
6. Advance the cannula until you observe flashback of blood into the cannula chamber, which confirms the needle is in the vein.
7. Lower the cannula and then advance a further 2 mm and then fix the needle. Continue to advance the plastic cannula until the cannula is fully inserted.
8. Release the tourniquet. Apply pressure to the vein at the tip of the cannula and remove the needle fully.
9. Carefully dispose of the needles into the sharps bin.
10. Apply a bung to the end of the cannula and flush with 5 mL of normal saline to ensure it is patent.
11. Apply the dressing to the cannula to fix it in place.

12. Dispose of your gloves and equipment appropriately and ensure the patient is comfortable.
13. Thank the patient and ensure you complete the IVC sticker in the notes.

Examiners' likely questions

- What are the potential risks of IVC insertion?
  - These include:
    - phlebitis and thrombophlebitis
    - haematoma
    - extravasation
    - insertion site infection
    - bacteraemia
    - needle stick injury.

Marking criteria table

Criteria	Satisfactory	Unsatisfactory
Washes hands	1	0
Obtains consent	1	0
Explains adequately to patient	1	0
Prepares injection arm	2	0–1
Injects correctly	2	0–1
Disposes of sharps	1	0
Completes sticker	1	0
Knows potential risks	2	0–1

Pass mark: 7

Male catheter insertion

Background

Indwelling catheters (IDCs) are used for many reasons:
- Management of urinary retention
- Strict fluid balance in severe illness
- During surgery for fluid status monitoring and prevention of bladder distention
- To facilitate certain operations, for example surrounding the genitourinary tract or adjunct regions
- Bladder irrigation, for example in cases of haematuria and clot retention
- Management of immobile patients, such as a NOF or pelvic fracture, stroke
- Neurogenic bladder
- Management of wounds aggravated by a patient's incontinence, such as broken down perineal skin that has become cellulitic
- Bladder instillation (where medications are placed directly in the bladder)
- Patient comfort at end of life
  IDCs carry risks:
- Urinary tract infection (UTI)
- Pain on insertion, discomfort while in place
- Bleeding
- Incontinence
- Bladder perforation
- Urethra or bladder fistula (creating a false passage)
- Bladder stone formation
- Retained balloon fragments
- Traumatic self-extraction in demented or delirious patients

IDCs should be avoided in patients with urethral injury, which could have occurred during a traumatic insertion or from pelvic trauma. A catheter should be placed by an urologist when there is a urethral stricture, recent surgery to the genitourinary area or after multiple failed attempts by other clinicians.

Alternative options include sheath catheters (urodome), suprapubic catheters, intermittent catheterisation and incontinence management with absorbent and protective garments.

Introduction

You are a 5th year medical student assisting the surgical team in theatres. The next case is an 81-year-old man who has fallen and fractured his neck of femur (NOF). A catheter is necessary for monitoring throughout the operation but also because he will be immobile for a period postoperatively. You will need to obtain the patient's consent and then place the catheter.

Rationale

Interns are required to be able to successfully and safely catheterise a male.

Method

1. Wash your hands.
2. Introduce yourself to the patient, explain what you have been asked to do and why a catheter is necessary. The patient may be a manikin or you may just be asked to describe the procedure details.
3. Discuss the risks of catheterisation with the patient and confirm that you have their consent to place the catheter in theatre.
4. In theatre, the wonderful scrub nurse will probably already have a sterile catheter pack waiting. You should scrub up and join her or him.
5. Expose the supine patient, then open the sterile drape so that only his penis remains visible.
6. Using one hand as your 'dirty' hand, hold the patient's penis firmly.
7. Using tongs, clean the head of the penis with wet gauze, at least three times.

Some packs contain chlorhexidine solution, others contain sterile saline. Each site will have different preferences and protocols, which you should follow.

8. Next, insert the local anaesthetic gel. The goal will be to try to keep the gel inside the patient's urethra for 30 seconds. This can be achieved by firmly holding the meatus closed or by leaving the syringe tip in situ as a plug (carefully).

9. Next the catheter (usually somewhere between a 14 and 20 gauge Foley catheter) will be inserted into the meatus, while holding the penis perpendicular to your supine patient.

10. Gently guide the catheter through the urethra. There may be a point of resistance as you pass the prostate; this is common, and with gentle pressure is easily bypassed. If this causes considerable pain to the patient or requires excessive pressure to pass, abort the catheter insertion rather than risk causing a false lumen. Calling for a senior's help is always preferable to causing trauma. A senior may be there guiding you, however, and sometimes more force than you would expect is required to bypass an enlarged prostate.

T&O'C hint box

Ways to bypass an enlarged prostate
- Ask the patient to relax, concentrate on wiggling toes or coughing.
- Change the angle of the IDC or gently twist it.
- Use a larger catheter (they are firmer, which gives you more push power).
- A Coude or Tieman tipped catheter may be required. If you have never used these before it is best to do so under the guidance of the urology team.

---

11. Continue advancing the IDC until it is inserted all the way to the hilt. Wait until urine comes out of the catheter before inflating the balloon.

T&O'C hint box

This is the stage to collect a urine sample if required.

12. Once the balloon inflated with 10 mL of sterile water, attach the leg bag to the catheter.
     Only use water, as saline can precipitate out. The crystals can then prevent the balloon deflating for removal.
13. Gently retract the IDC until the balloon is resting against the internal urethral opening.

T&O'C hint box

If you had to retract patient's foreskin to clean it, remember to replace it. Retracted foreskins become painful and oedematous after only a short time.

T&O'C hint box

Managing an oedematous foreskin is similar to managing a prolapsed and oedematous stoma: cold compresses, firm pressure and sometimes glucose can be applied to shrink the foreskin and return it to its correct location (exclude signs of ischemia or necrosis).

---

14. Secure the IDC to the patient's leg.

Present your findings

This will likely be a demonstration of the above methodology on a manikin.

Examiners' likely questions

- How would you respond to a call about new haematuria found in a draining catheter bag?
  - Look for a history of traumatic insertion, either by discussion with the person responsible for the IDC or in the notes. It would be safe to assume that if multiple attempts were required, there is trauma.
  - Check a full blood count, coagulation studies and observations — is the patient stable or deteriorating as a consequence of the blood loss?
  - Is the patient on antiplatelet or anticoagulant agents that should be withheld until the haematuria has resolved?

- Has the patient gone into retention (a bladder scan would help you find out) — there could be a clot that requires three-way irrigation.
- If there are concerning answers to the questions above, it is a good idea to speak to the urology team for guidance.
- What should you do if a catheter that was previously draining urine stops?
  - Check there are no obvious kinks in the IDC. Check the location of the catheter bag; it is gravity fed to a point so must be below the level of the bladder.
  - Flush 10 mL of water into the IDC. It should go in without resistance and return via the IDC. If it does not, it suggests obstruction and the IDC needs to be replaced. If the patient is experiencing haematuria and there is suspected clot retention, it is likely you will need a three-way catheter and irrigation. This should first be discussed with urology.
  - Deflate the balloon and then advance the catheter to the hilt again to see if urine comes out.
  - Bladder scan to ensure the patient is not anuric.

Marking criteria table

Criteria	Satisfactory	Unsatisfactory
Introduces self	1	0
Explains benefits	2	0–1
Obtains consent	1	0
Step-by-step approach understood	3	0–2
Knows what to do if drainage stops	2	0–1

Pass mark: 6

Background

A stoma is a temporary or permanent connection from any hollow viscus to the skin, including the colon (colostomy), ileum (ileostomy) or the stomach (gastrostomy). A urostomy looks like an ileostomy but the connection is to the ureter (so the effluent is urine, not loose stool or green small bowel fluid). These are associated with a number of complications, including infection, hernias, necrosis and obstruction.

Introduction

The nurse has called you to assess this 39-year-old man because of a reduced output from his stoma. Please examine him.

Rationale

You need to know about the different stoma types, how to differentiate an ileostomy from a colostomy, and what are abnormal findings (e.g. skin changes, bleeding, prolapse, and luminal obstruction). Proper inspection of the stoma in an OSCE is a critical step, but an abdominal examination is also part of the evaluation.

METHOD

1. Introduce yourself. Confirm the patient details (name, date of birth).
2. Explain why you want to perform the examination and explain exactly what you are going to do (see steps below) and obtain consent.
3. Ask the patient if he is in pain anywhere in the abdomen, and ask for permission to proceed.
4. Wash your hands and don gloves. Make the area private (or ask to do so).
5. Expose the abdomen fully. Inspect the abdomen and stoma area. Note any abdominal scars or other abnormalities. There may be a scar at the same level on the other side of the abdomen from re-siting the stoma.
6. Check the stoma is fully exposed. Typically the bag will be see-through so you can inspect the stoma. Do **not** ask the patient to remove the stoma bag because the effluent cannot be controlled and may pour all over the student and examiner (not helpful). Is the stoma new (incompletely healed), or old?
7. Observe the location of the stoma (this may be anywhere, and is now less often in the right or left iliac fossa because many patients have a high body mass index), the surface (spout or not), one lumen or two, one or two stomas (two may be present), any skin changes (normally red or pink, and moist) and note the stoma contents (volume, colour, consistency— stool, small bowel green effluent, or urine).
8. Ask if you may palpate the stoma. You usually won't be allowed in an OSCE. Be ready to describe what you would do and what you would be looking for. (tenderness, mass, luminal narrowing at the opening)

9. Move on to palpating the abdomen for masses and complete a proper abdominal examination (palpate, percuss, auscultate).

10. Look for a parastomal hernia, preferably by asking the patient to stand. Note any localised protrusion. A parastomal hernia is usually large and falls forward so the stoma may no longer be seen. A hint is the patient wearing a belt or corset to support his or her abdomen.

11. Assess hydration — skin turgor reduced on the arms, tongue dry, pulse rate (tachycardia), blood pressure (hypotension), urine concentrated (dehydration may explain low output or follow high output).

12. Ask to see a chart of the stoma output over the previous days, Look for high volume output.

13. Cover the patient. Ask about any pain or other distress, and wash your hands.

Be ready to describe the stoma, offer your summary of the findings and differential diagnosis, plus next steps in management.

T&O'C hint box

Stoma examination
- A stoma examination is an intimate body part examination.
- A stoma may cause psychological distress and stigma — be a sensitive, caring examiner and do not cause pain.
- An ileostomy has a spout, and usually produces green liquid stool when mature.
- A colostomy is sutured next to the skin but may have a spout. It usually produces brown, formed stool when mature.
- Look for skin changes around the stoma (e.g. rash from stool irritating the skin, fungal infection or allergy to stoma product used; peristomal pyoderma gangrenosum in Crohn disease, which is rare), fissures or bleeding, retraction or prolapse, parastomal hernias, and narrowing of the stomal lumen. See Figs 4.79.1-4.79.3.

Present your findings

Summarise your findings. Comment on the type of stoma and why.

Examiners' likely questions

- What type of stoma do you think this is, and why?
- What may explain the decreased output? Discuss local factors (e.g. stomal obstruction) and systematic explanations (e.g. dehydration).

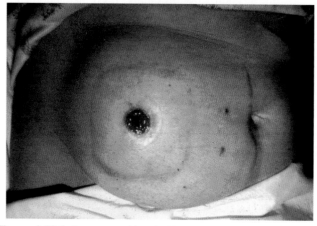

Figure 4.79.1 A parastomal hernia. Note stomal retraction and likely an ileostomy, but the case is complex as it has at least one, possibly two other lumens in view. This may be Crohn disease with an ileostomy and mature fistulae (Frantzides CT, Carlson MA. *Video Atlas of Advanced Minimally Invasive Surgery*. Philadelphia: Elsevier, 2012.)

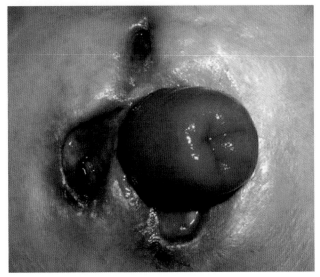

Figure 4.79.2 Stomal retraction (Ramirez PT, Frumovitz M, Abu-Rustum NR *Principles of Gynecologic Oncology Surgery*. Philadelphia: Elsevier, 2018.)

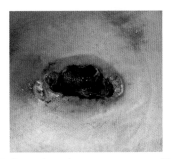

Figure 4.79.3 Peristomal pyoderma gangrenosum. The differential diagnosis is stomal retraction. Pyoderma is rare (Radbruch L, Foley KM, Fainsinger R, Caraceni AT, Walsh T, Olarte JN, Lloyd-Williams M, Goh C, Glare P. *Palliative Medicine*. Philadelphia: Elsevier, 2009.)

Marking criteria table

Criteria	Satisfactory	Unsatisfactory
Introduces self, confirms details	1	0
Explains why/what	1	0
Obtains consent	1	0
Patient set up, washes hands, dons gloves	1	0
Asks about pain/sensitive examination	1	0
Asks to palpate, knows relevance	2	0–1
Abdominal examination	1	0
Abdominal scars identified	1	0
Describes type of stoma: site, spout, retracted, 1 or 2 lumens, new (not healed) / old, effluent type	3	0–2
Assesses for parastomal hernia	1	0
Assesses hydration	1	0

Pass mark: 10

Handover of a patient

Background

ISBAR is an acronym for Introduction, Situation, Background, Assessment and Recommendation, and is an example of a framework for communication. This structure is designed to convey clinical information concisely and thoroughly.

Communication and handover happens numerous times throughout the day. Examples of when effective communication is required include change of shift, requesting a test or procedure, transferring patients from facilities or wards, discussing patients with other speciality teams and at multidisciplinary team meetings.

Unfortunately the data shows poor communication during these scenarios leads to patient harm by omission or misunderstanding. Without a structured approach, handovers are often unpredictable and unreliable.

Introduction

This station is likely to give you an example situation that requires you to make a clinical handover, such as:

- calling the registrar after reviewing an unwell patient
- handing a patient over to the after-hours staff so they know what the team's plan is and what to look out for
- transferring a patient to another facility.

Here is a stem overabundant with information. Determine what information is key and how you would plan to call a senior for help.

You are the evening junior medical officer (JMO) at the hospital. Mr Cook is a 76-year-old man who presented to hospital 4 days ago with fevers and a hot, swollen left leg. He has been treated with intravenous (IV) antibiotics for cellulitis. He has a background of ischaemic heart disease, chronic obstructive pulmonary disease (COPD), prostate cancer treated surgically, and type 2 diabetes mellitus requiring insulin.

The nursing staff call you, the evening JMO covering their ward, to review him because he is very breathless after having his shower. His observations are: respiratory rate 23 per minute (trending up), 96% saturation on room air, heart rate is 95 beats/minute, blood pressure is 140/80 mmHg and temperature is 37°C.

On examination you find he is warm and well perfused, regular heart rate, heart sounds dual with no murmurs, slightly elevated jugular venous pressure (JVP), visible 1–2 cm above the base of his neck, pitting oedema to his knees. Respiratory examination — the patient is taking a breath mid-sentence, does not appear cyanosed centrally or peripherally; you can hear breath sounds throughout but there are crackles in both lung bases. His abdomen is soft. His calves are non-tender and the cellulitis leg is much improved according to the patient.

The bedside investigations include an electrocardiogram (ECG) in sinus rhythm, no ST depression or elevation. He has some Q waves that are similar to a previous ECG. His mobile chest X-ray (CXR) shows some air space opacification bilaterally around his hilum, and Kerley B lines.

Rationale

ISBAR is straightforward to use; it is easy for all clinical staff to remember and is structured logically to help a situation make sense in order to best convey information from person to person.

Method

1. **Introduction:** Explain who you are, your role and location in the hospital. This can be adapted slightly according to

---

T&O'C hint box

Include your request here so that the person listening knows what to listen for. For example, 'My name is Bob Jones, I'm the junior medical officer working on the wards of Hospital X. I'm calling because I've completed a review on a patient and I would like to run my plan through with you.'

with whom you are conversing. For example, a nurse requesting a clinical review will inform you of the floor and bed number, but the neurosurgical advanced trainee may need only the hospital you are calling from.

2. **Situation:** What is the problem? Why have you been called to review this patient? What symptoms is the patient experiencing? This is a good place to discuss a patient's observations (both current and the trend), the stability of the patient and your level of concern.

T&O'C hint box

As a junior doctor, managing reviews for 'clinical concern' can be difficult, especially when there is no overt problem. In the ISBAR handover to a senior, even though you may be unconcerned, it is worth mentioning how concerned the nurse or allied health worker is. Experienced hospital staff can have a sixth sense that is worth respecting.

---

3. **Background:** The history of this patient's presentation, what factors led to this situation occurring, pertinent past medical history. A patient's history of childhood eczema is not relevant when he is hypotensive postoperatively.

4. **Assessment:** In your opinion, what is the problem? What are your differential diagnoses?

T&O'C hint box

It is OK not to know the diagnosis — sometimes this is why you are calling for help. The fact that you are concerned is enough. However, giving a clear ISBAR with your findings will help your senior guide your next steps so that you can work together to best manage the patient.

---

5. **Recommendations:** What do you want from the person you are handing over to? Do you want guidance, a second opinion, for him or her to take over care of your patient? Discuss treatment and investigations that are underway or that you would like to do. Does this patient need review by

a senior doctor or another speciality or intensive care? A plan for what needs to occur once the immediate investigations or treatments have taken effect?

Present your findings

SAMPLE ANSWER

Hello, my name is Sally Green, I'm the evening junior medical officer at Hospital X.

I was asked to review Mr Cook, Level 4 Room 8, because he told the nursing staff he was feeling really short of breath after coming back from his shower. His observations are within the flags but his respiratory rate is now sitting at 23 when it is usually 16. He is talking in broken sentences. When I listened to his lungs, I could hear bibasal crackles. He has pitting oedema to his knees and a JVP visible at the base of his neck. His ECG has no new ischaemic changes, sinus rhythm. His CXR looks most like fluid overload.

Mr Cook was admitted to hospital with cellulitis and has a past medical history that includes ischaemic heart disease (IHD) and COPD.

My top differential is fluid overload, but he might also have a new pneumonia, or less likely a pulmonary embolus.

I've taken a set of bloods including a venous blood gas and stopped his fluids.

Would you be able to have a look at Mr Cook's CXR and venous blood gas results to help me decide on the next best step in management?

Examiners' likely questions

- If the patient had deteriorated during your review and you had needed to call a rapid response, can you think of a more succinct ISBAR you would give the critical care team as they arrive to the patient's bedside?
  - Hi, I'm Sally Green, ward junior medical officer. I called this rapid response for tachypnoea and hypoxia, with saturations down to 80% before we put on the non-rebreather. He has a history of chronic obstructive pulmonary disease and ischaemic heart disease and is currently being treated with IV antibiotics for cellulitis.

– He appeared fluid overloaded when I first reviewed him and he deteriorated while I was prescribing him diuretics. I worried he may need non-invasive ventilation (NIV) and transfer to the intensive care unit (ICU).

Marking criteria table

Criteria	Satisfactory	Unsatisfactory
Introduces self	1	0
Describes situation	1	0
Describes background	1	0
Identifies problem	1	0
Offers differential diagnosis	1	0
Describes main reason for handover	2	0–1

Pass mark: 4

Background

Communication failure is a major source of error in the health system. A difficult patient interaction tends to require a disproportionate amount of time and emotional intelligence for a doctor.

Anger is a common and natural part of being human. Patients and their families are vulnerable when unwell. Emotions tend to be kept consistently raw, fuelled by fear, frustration and insecurity.

COMMON SITUATIONS WHERE ANGER MAY BE PROVOKED

- Expectations that are let down
- Emergencies
- Unexpected events
- Bad news, for example a new diagnosis that will lead to significant morbidity or mortality, and the grief surrounding that
- Medical error or misdiagnosis
- Financial stress
- Long waits for clinician review
- Inappropriate clinician behaviour, such as poor bedside manner

Introduction

You have been asked to see one of your patients. He is a 45-year-old man who was seen yelling at other clinical staff because he believed there had been a medication error.

He has been generally unhappy with lack of a definite diagnosis. He feels the medical staff have dismissed what he sees as the likely diagnosis.

Rationale

Anger is an important emotion that medical staff must recognise to keep themselves and others safe. Although uncommon, there have been extreme instances where a patient or family member has become physically violent, resulting in the death of the medical practitioner. The 'patient' is almost certainly an actor but you must respond as if the situation is real.

Method

1. Do not mirror the patient's anger (though it may feel natural to do so). It will damage your relationship with the patient and possibly any future doctor–patient interaction, and is likely to inflame the problem.
2. Remain calm, be patient and still, establish eye contact.
3. Try to analyse what is happening — try to understand the patient's motives.
4. Ask the patient to sit down. Avoid aggressive posturing.
   - Have yourself closest to the door to help with escape if there is concern the situation may turn violent.
   - In a potentially violent situation in the real world, it is a good idea to wear a duress alarm and have security nearby. Your top priority is always your own safety. Sometimes it is best to leave the situation and wait for senior help.
5. Using the patient's correct name and title, begin to converse calmly with the patient to find out the concerns. Appear comfortable, controlled, and concerned about the problems.
6. Listen intently; it can help to allow a patient to vent.
7. Respond to the patient's anger with empathy.
   - Acknowledge the person's grievance and frustration.
   - Give reassurance where possible and appropriate.
   - Shift the focus of the conversation to problem solving.
   - Your response is key in building rapport with the patient, defusing the situation and helping the patient and family to feel comfortable to raise their concerns openly.
8. Acknowledge and apologise if an error has occurred. Take care in how this is phrased, however, as it is not about blame or assuming responsibility (if you have not directly

caused the error). It can be helpful to explain the process by which medical errors are managed to try to avoid a second occurrence.

9. Arrange follow-up for the patient so that any further concerns can be addressed.

10. Encourage the patient to ask any residual questions he may have.

Present your findings

Summarise that patient's key concerns and how you tried to address them.

Examiners' likely questions

- What are some signs that may signal your de-escalation attempt is not working?
  - Increasingly agitated body language, closing in on your personal space
  - A change in speech pattern — becoming more quiet or more pressured with a higher volume
  - The patient may be becoming more red in the face
  - Loss of eye contact
- What are the differential diagnoses for anger?
  - Pain, insomnia, traumatic brain injury, delirium, Alzheimer disease, hypoglycaemia, temporal lobe epilepsy etc. Delirium is often not recognised in hospital patients but must always be considered and the cause (e.g. a urinary tract infection) corrected if possible.
  - Medication side effect — steroids, methamphetamine, alcohol intoxication
  - Psychological — grief, post-traumatic stress disorder, mania, depression
- If verbal de-escalation fails, what options are left?
  - Physical and chemical restraint is a last resort and you would call a senior to assess first
  - However, hospital policy requires regular review of physical restraint and it is considered to be a last-line

option. The patient needs vigorous monitoring while physically restrained.

– There can be substantial pressure to sedate chemically or restrain a patient. It is important to recognise that there are many potentially dangerous side effects to the patient associated with administering these medications. Although verbal de-escalation is the more difficult and time-consuming route, it is always preferred. It can help to bring a patient's family member in, or have a family member on the phone, to help settle the patient.

Marking criteria table

Criteria	Satisfactory	Unsatisfactory
Introduces self	1	0
Professional approach	1	0
Positions self in safe place	1	0
Shows awareness of patient's body language	1	0
Calm questioning to ask about patient's concerns	2	0–1
Acknowledges patient's problems	1	0
Reassures where possible	1	0
Attempts to negotiate a solution calmly	1	0
Has an approach to examiners' questions	3	0–2

Pass mark: 6

Breaking bad news

Background

Good communication skills are essential in medicine when you find yourself the bearer of bad news. Having a systematic approach to these situations helps in ensuring you and the patient feel as comfortable as possible and you get the message approach clearly.

Introduction

- Mrs Benness is a 41-year-old woman who is currently seeing you as her general practiner (GP) for antenatal care in her first pregnancy. She has just had her nuchal translucency test and the result has come back as high risk (1 : 12 chance of chromosomal abnormality). She has come in today to receive the results of this test. Please explain this result to her and answer any questions she may have.

This station is designed to test your communication skills and not your knowledge of early pregnancy testing.

Rationale

- When giving bad news, take a structured approach. Find a quiet area, and ask if the presence of a partner or relative is wanted for the discussion.
- Next, introduce yourself. Summarise. Check what the patient knows.
- Formally seek an invitation to talk about the results.
- Warn the patient that you have some bad news. Provide the information in short bursts to aid comprehension and understanding. Keep it simple and check for understanding with each burst of information.

- Monitor the patient's emotions and be empathetic.
- To conclude, offer a plan and follow-up appointments.
- Summarise and recheck understanding before concluding the discussion.

METHOD (SPIKES)

1. Introduce yourself.
2. Setting
   - Ensure you have the conversation in appropriate an place.
   - Ensure enough space and no barriers to communication.
   - Ensure you have allowed sufficient time.
   - Ensure you have all the relevant people involved — find out who the patient wants (relatives/friends/other supports), ensure all the appropriate healthcare professionals are involved.
3. Perception: Begin the conversation by finding out what the patient's current understanding is.
4. Invitation: Find out how much the patient wants to know.
5. Knowledge
   - Let the patient know you are going to deliver the news.
   - Speak clearly.
   - Avoid medical jargon.
   - Deliver small amounts of information and check in with the patient frequently.
6. Emotions
   - Be prepared for any kind of emotional response from the patient.
   - Have tissues present.
   - Demonstrate empathy.
7. Strategy/summarise
   - Organise a plan with the patient — for follow-up, and for anything else that may need to occur.
   - Summarise, ensuring the patient has his or her questions answered and a good understanding of everything you've discussed.

Present your findings

You may be asked to present your findings. This may include a summary statement for the patient at the end of the consultation.

For example, 'You are currently 13 weeks pregnant. You recently had your early pregnancy ultrasound scan and are visiting your GP today for a check-up and to discuss the result. You are aware that this investigation is looking for chromosomal abnormalities such as Down syndrome and that you are at an increased risk due to your age, but you are hoping for reassuring test results. If offered, you would like some pamphlets regarding options for further investigation, but you would like to think about it and come back in next week with your partner to discuss the findings.'

Examiners' likely questions

- In clinical practice, what would you do to ensure the setting was appropriate for this discussion?
- What would you like to organise at present in terms of follow-up for Sarah?

Marking criteria table

Criteria	Satisfactory	Unsatisfactory
Introduces self to patient	1	0
Explains confidentiality	1	0
Asks for consent	1	0
Provides appropriate setting, or addresses how they would ensure this	1	0
Addresses patient's perception at outset	1	0
Gains invitation from patient to discuss news	1	0
Ascertains level of detail the patient wishes to know	1	0
Provides knowledge	1	0
Demonstrates empathy	1	0
Arranges appropriate follow-up plan	1	0
Summarises discussion	1	0
Demonstrates appropriate and professional behaviour throughout	1	0

Pass mark: 7

Cross-cultural communication

Background

Patients of Aboriginal and Torres Strait Islander descent come from a wide range of communities whose communication needs may require cultural sensitivity.

These communication needs can be influenced by differences in health literacy, beliefs, values and lived experiences.

Aboriginal and Torres Strait peoples experience higher rates of social disadvantage and health conditions than the general population in Australia. Although chronic disease and comorbidities may be more common for Aboriginal patients, it is important to assess and manage every patient as an individual, based on their presentation, healthcare needs and preferences.

Introduction

Mrs Smith is a 46-year-old Aboriginal female who has presented to the practice with urinary urgency and burning.

You notice that she has not yet returned to discuss the results of blood tests from 5 months ago, despite several calls from the practice nurse. The results showed hypercholesterolaemia and an HbA1c of 10.4%. She has a 2-year history of type 2 diabetes and also has hypertension, gastro-oesophageal reflux and gout.

She works as a machine operator and is married with three children. She lives 45 minutes from the nearest medical facility. She is a non-smoker and has stated that she drinks approximately 2 standard drinks of alcohol per day.

Rationale

It is important to be aware of the lived experiences of each Aboriginal and Torres Strait Islander patient. Ensuring that communication is effective and respectful will optimise interactions and health outcomes.

Method

1. Before you start the consultation, introduce yourself and offer the patient an Aboriginal liaison officer or translator, if she would prefer to speak in her native Indigenous language Also ask if the patient would like a family member to be present.

2. Ask if she would like an Aboriginal staff member or Aboriginal health worker to be present during the consultation.

3. **Rapport:** It is important to build a rapport with your patient. Be warm and friendly. Spend a few moments getting to know the patient, finding topics of mutual interest. Find out which country the patient is from.

4. Take a history of the presenting complaint.

5. Pay attention to **language**.
   - It is important to appreciate that Aboriginal culture has many different languages, and for some Aboriginal and Torres Strait Islander patients English may not be their first language.
   - Avoid using jargon. Explain why you need to ask so many questions.
   - Always check that both you and the patient have understood the meanings of words used.
   - Use diagrams and models to explain concepts and instructions.
   - Be friendly in your approach and ask informally what is going on, rather than rapidly firing questions.

6. Listen and ask questions, rather than talking at the patient. Explore and understand her situation. Be accommodating and flexible.

7. Discuss with the patient the importance of diabetes management and her need to engage with services and why you feel it is important for her to engage with services. Ask whether she has any concerns about using health services; listen with genuine interest to any concerns.

This needs to be done in a non-confrontational, non-judgmental manner.

8. Assess body language and non-verbal communication for alignment with verbal responses.

9. **Time** is perceived differently in Aboriginal and Torres Strait Islander cultures; more value is placed on family and community relationships.
   - It is important to consider flexible consultation times and to take the time to explain without rushing the patient.

10. **Listen** to your patient.
    - Ensure you are actively listening.
    - Paraphrase by summarising and repeating what the patient said. This helps clarify and signal that you are listening.
    - Be attentive, and avoid continually interrupting or speaking over the patient.

11. **Questioning** needs to be handled with care.
    - Use indirect approaches, giving the patient time to answer.
    - Avoid compound questions (as with all patient interviews).
    - Avoid hypothetical examples.
    - Allow the patient to ask you questions.

12. Aim for yourself and Mrs Smith to come to a mutual understanding and management strategy that is cognisant of her current situation.

13. **Clear instructions** are essential.
    - Give clear and full instructions. Offer these in writing.
    - Provide options for care.
    - Ensure these options are practical and accessible

14. Options to ensure ongoing engagement include:
    - Ask the patient if she would to liaise and consult with her family regarding the plan.
    - Familiarise yourself with the local Aboriginal medical services. Explore what local options are available for linking with these services.
    - Engage with the local Aboriginal community health worker.
    - Discuss options such as a GP management plan or nurse support.

15. Consider the option of undertaking cultural mentoring with an Aboriginal Elder.

T&O'C hint boxes

- Silence plays an important role in Indigenous cultures. It is important not to compensate by filling a patient's silence with conversation. Pause and allow the patient time to think.
- Do not rush the consultation. Take the time to chat.
- Aboriginal culture is diverse. Never assume knowledge of the Aboriginal culture. Be led by your patient.

Present your findings

Summarise the discussion and planned outcomes.

Examiners' likely questions

- Discuss what communication tools help when communicating cross-culturally.
    - Participating in cultural awareness training
    - Interpreter services
    - Ensuring pamphlets and information sheets are available and provided in the patient's language
    - Offering a liaison officer
    - Being patient and flexible, taking the time to listen and understand the other's cultural beliefs
    - Booking longer appointments, to prevent both yourself and the patient from feeling rushed
    - Looking for culturally meaningful analogies that make sense within the patient's lived experience and worldview
    - Benefits of involving trusted family members in consultations.

Marking criteria table

Criteria	Satisfactory	Unsatisfactory
Introduction made	1	0
Offers language service	1	0
Establishes rapport	1	0
Active listening	1	0
Prompts discussion	1	0
Mutual understanding checked	1	0
Instructions clear	1	0
Discusses follow-up	1	0
Sensitive communication issues understood	2	0–1

Pass mark: 6

Consenting for a procedure — blood transfusion

Background

Patients have the autonomy to make their own informed decisions as certain risks may be more acceptable to some than to others.

Introduction

An 85-year-old female presents with haematemesis and melaena. She is identified to have a haemoglobin of 55 grams/litre (lower limit of normal for a female 115 grams/litre). You are asked by your consultant to gain her consent for a blood transfusion.

Rationale

It is important to always gain a patient's consent before any procedure or treatment. This is because all treatments and procedures carry a risk of potentially serious adverse outcomes.

Method

1. Introduce yourself to the patient.
2. Ensure the patient has capacity to consent and ensure the patient does not require a translator. Ask if she has any religious objection to transfusion (e.g. as a Jehovah's Witness).
3. First, explain to the patient the cause of the bleeding and why a transfusion is recommended. It is often worth saying to the patient that all treatment involves risk and benefit. A transfusion has been recommended in her case because the benefit is thought to be much greater than the risk.
4. Explain the nature of the blood transfusion and the expected benefits. For the above lady, explain 'Red blood

cells are needed to replace the blood you have lost from your bowel. The transfusion is to prevent life-threatening blood loss.' After gastrointestinal bleeding, blood transfusion is considered if the haemoglobin is under 70 grams/litre.

5. It is important to explain the procedure. 'A cannula will be inserted into one of your veins and you will receive the blood through this. It takes about 1–4 hours to complete, during which time you will be monitored for any reactions.'

6. Next, it is important to explain the risks associated with a blood transfusion. It is essential to explain both common risks and rare but serious risks. It is also vital to explore risks that may be important to the patient. These need to be communicated in the patient's own words so they can understand the risk.

It is important to reassure patients that the Blood Bank has a vigorous process of ensuring that risks are minimised and blood transfusions are safe, and that reactions due to issues with donor blood have significantly reduced.

7. Once you have explained the risks, be sure to explain to the patient the risk of doing nothing.

8. When gaining consent from a patient, be sure to give the patient an option to ask any further questions and a chance to clarify any questions she may have. (Box 4.84.1)

Box 4.84.1
Risks of blood transfusion explained in the patient's own words[a]

Common risks
- Temperature rise
- Rash, hives and itching
- Feeling unwell

Rare risks and complications
- Having too much blood can give you shortness of breath
- Haemolysis — an abnormal breakdown of red blood cells
- Antibodies may develop — this may complicate future blood transfusions and future organ or tissue transplants
- Lung injury can occur, resulting in shortness of breath
- Spread of infections, both viral and bacterial, from the blood of donors
- There is a very rare chance that these reactions can result in severe harm or even death.

[a] From the State of Queensland (Queensland Health), 2016.

TABLE 4.84.2 Definitions of risk

Risk description	Percentage	Fraction
High	1	More than 1 in 100
Moderate	0.1	1 in 100 to 1 in 1000
Low	0.01	1 in 1000 to 1 in 10 000
Very Low	0.001	1 in 10 000 to 1 in 100 000
Minimal	0.0001	1 in 100 000 to 1 in 1 000 000
Negligible	0.000 01	Less than 1 in 1 000 000

It is useful to offer the patient some written information, which can easily be found on the Australian Red Cross website, for them to do some further reading.

Examiners' likely questions

- How do you explain risks in common language?
- What is meant by 'high' or 'low' risk?
  - See Table 4.84.2.
- What are the acute risk associated with blood transfusions?
  - These risks can be seen as either immune or non-immune reactions (Box 4.84.2).

Box 4.84.2
Acute risks associated with blood transfusion

Immunological reactions (<24 h)
- Acute haemolytic transfusion reaction: this is often due to blood group incompatibility
- Febrile non-haemolytic transfusion reaction: this is an isolated temperature rise with transfusions
- Mild allergic reactions
- Anaphylaxis
- Transfusion related acute lung injury

Non-immune acute (<24 h)
- Non-immune mediated haemolysis: these are usually due to issues with blood storage and how the blood is given.
- Transfusion of transmitted bacterial infection*
- Transfusion-related circulatory overload*: this occurs in the context of heart failure when a patient develops pulmonary oedema from either rapid infusion or large volumes.

*Are associated with the highest mortality.

- Explain how you will check the patient is receiving the correct transfusion.
    - Note that giving a patient the wrong bottle of blood (because you fail to check carefully who the patient is, including their hospital number, and exactly how the bottle is labelled) is a medicolegal disaster. This serious error must always be avoided.

Marking criteria table

Criteria	Satisfactory	Unsatisfactory
Introduces self, explains task, obtains consent	1	0
Ensures patient is able to understand the process — language, deafness etc.	2	0–1
Asks about religious or other objections to transfusion	1	0
Outlines reason for and benefits of transfusion	2	0–1
Explains process	1	0
Offers patient an opportunity to ask questions	1	0
Explains important risks, tailored to patient's situation	2	0–1

Pass mark: 5

References

1. Fresh blood and blood products transfusion consent [Internet]. Health.qld. gov.au. 2019 [sighted 10 November 2019]. Available from: https://www. health.qld.gov.au/__data/assets/pdf_file/0014/150134/shared_file_03.pdf.
2. Understanding risk — BMJ Best Practice [Internet]. Bestpractice.bmj.com. 2019 [sighted 10 November 2019]. Available from: https://bestpractice.bmj. com/info/toolkit/practise-ebm/understanding-risk/.

Interpreting
an electrocardiogram

Introduction

- Would you mind interpreting this 12 lead electrocardiogram (ECG) for us? See Figs 4.85.1–4.85.13.

The examiners may add some history to give you help. Possibilities include (see Fig. 4.85.1):

- This is the ECG of 54-year-old man who has had an episode of severe chest pain. Look for previous infarction or ischaemic changes. (Fig. 4.85.1)
- This 87-year-old woman has rapid and irregular palpitations. Look for atrial fibrillation. (Fig. 4.85.2)
- This 20-year-old woman has a history of the sudden onset of very rapid and regular palpitations. Look for supraventricular tachycardia (heart rate 180 or more and narrow complexes) or a short PR interval.
- This elderly man has had recurrent syncope. Look for conduction abnormalities — bradycardia and heart block or right bundle branch block and left anterior hemiblock or atrial fibrillation (AF) with a slow ventricular response rate and pauses. (Fig. 4.85.3)
- This man has had recurrent syncope until recent treatment. Look for paced rhythm. (Fig. 4.85.4)
- This man has recurrent palpitations; he feels his heart miss and jump, especially when he is resting. Look for atrial or ventricular ectopic beats. (Figs 4.85.5, 4.85.6)
- This man has had uncontrolled hypertension for many years. Look for changes of left ventricular hypertrophy. (Fig. 4.85.7)

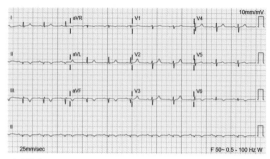

Figure 4.85.1 Inferior infarct. Note Q waves in leads II, III and aVF and T wave inversion in these leads (Figure reproduced courtesy of The Canberra Hospital.)

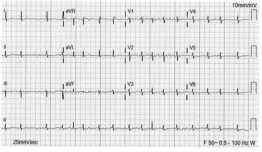

Figure 4.85.2 Atrial fibrillation. Note the irregular ventricular rhythm and absence of P waves (Figure reproduced courtesy of The Canberra Hospital.)

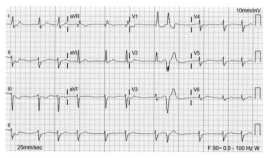

Figure 4.85.3 Atrial fibrillation with a slow ventricular response rate, right bundle branch block, left anterior hemi-block and a ventricular ectopic beat (Figure reproduced courtesy of The Canberra Hospital.)

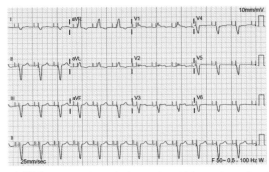

Figure 4.85.4 Atrial and ventricular pacing. Note pacing spikes before atrial and ventricular complexes (Figure reproduced courtesy of The Canberra Hospital.)

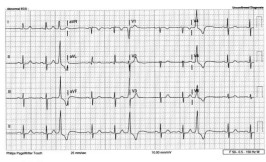

Figure 4.85.5 Ventricular ectopic beats. Every third beat is an ectopic — ventricular trigeminy (Figure reproduced courtesy of The Canberra Hospital.)

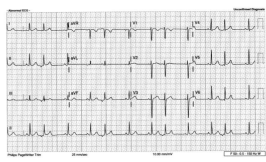

Figure 4.85.6 Atrial ectopic beats. The atrial ectopics are not wide but occur early (Figure reproduced courtesy of The Canberra Hospital.)

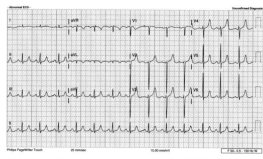

Figure 4.85.7 Left ventricular hypertrophy (LVH) (Figure reproduced courtesy of The Canberra Hospital.)

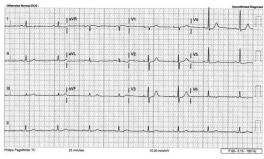

Figure 4.85.8 Sinus bradycardia (Figure reproduced courtesy of The Canberra Hospital.)

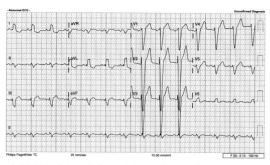

Figure 4.85.9 Left bundle branch block (LBBB) (Figure reproduced courtesy of The Canberra Hospital.)

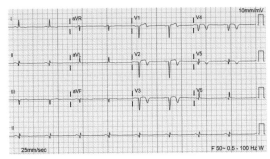

Figure 4.85.10 Old inferior and anterior infarcts. Q waves are present in leads II, III and aVF. Q waves are also present in the anterior leads and the T waves are biphasic (Figure reproduced courtesy of The Canberra Hospital.)

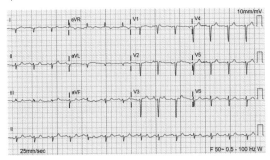

Figure 4.85.11 Reduced R wave progression. There are no anterior R waves until V6 (Figure reproduced courtesy of The Canberra Hospital.)

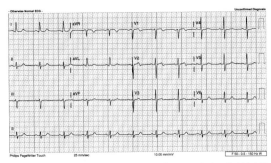

Figure 4.85.12 Biphasic T waves. The T waves in leads V1–V3 are positive and then negative (Figure reproduced courtesy of The Canberra Hospital.)

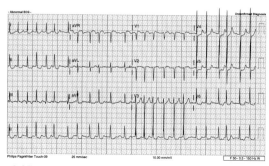

Figure 4.85.13 Atrial fibrillation with a rapid ventricular response rate and lateral ST changes associated with the tachycardia (Figure reproduced courtesy of The Canberra Hospital.)

Rationale

Obviously students should be able to interpret common ECG abnormalities. Although most ECG machines now offer an interpretation, this should always be approached with some scepticism. It is best to think of it as a way of checking your own interpretation.

Method

Have a system for interpreting ECGs and practise it. This is a suggested method.

1. Check the date of the ECG and name of the patient. (These may have been removed for an OSCE exam.)
2. Look for the paper speed (should be 25 mm/s) and calibration marks (1 cm = 1 mV).
3. Look at the lead II rhythm strip, which is usually at the bottom.
4. Does it seem regular? What is the heart rate? Count the number of large squares between complexes and divide into 300; for example 5 squares = 60 beats per minute. (Fig. 4.85.8)
5. Try to decide if the patient is in sinus rhythm — P waves followed by QRS complexes. Are all P waves conducted,

does the PR interval look normal (up to one large square from start of P wave to start of QRS)?

6. If not sinus rhythm, is it atrial fibrillation (AF) — irregular, no P waves, or is sinus rhythm interrupted by wide or narrow complexes (VEBs or AEBs)?

7. If AF, give the average heart rate or range of rates, for example 50 to 100 beats per minute.

8. Look at QRS complexes. Are they wide >3 small squares? (Fig. 4.85.9)

9. If wide, consider common possibilities — bundle branch block, paced rhythm ventricular ectopics, ventricular tachycardia.

10. Is it left bundle branch block (Fig. 4.85.9)? Further interpretation of the ECG is not usually possible and you are off the hook.

11. What is the electrical axis? Look at Leads I and II. If both are positive (R waves taller than S wave), say confidently 'The axis is normal'. If Lead II is negative, this is usually left axis deviation and usually left anterior hemiblock can be diagnosed. If LI is negative, this is usually right axis deviation. If both are negative, this is usually a result or reversed limb leads. In this case, L aVR will have positive complexes instead of negative ones.

12. Are there pathological Q waves? If so, are they in the inferior, anterior or lateral leads, or some combination of these? This usually means a previous myocardial infarction. (Fig. 4.85.10)

13. Look at the R wave progression. R waves usually become taller from V1 to V5. If not, this is usually called 'poor R wave progression'. It is mostly the result of rotation of the heart but can indicate a previous anterior infarction. (Fig. 4.85.11)

14. Are the lateral R waves very tall and the septal S waves deep? This may mean left ventricular hypertrophy, especially if the ST segments and T waves are down-sloping in V5 and V6 (strain pattern).

15. Is there ST depression or T wave inversion anywhere? This suggests ischaemia, but you must learn where T wave inversion is normal (e.g. aVR and V1). (Fig. 4.85.12)

16. If you are feeling confident, look at the QT interval (from beginning of Q wave to end of T wave). Prolongation (generally more than 400 ms but depends on the heart rate) is associated with ventricular arrhythmias.

17. Are pacemaker spikes visible? Are they before the P waves (atrial pacing) or before the QRS complexes (right ventricular pacing) or both? Ventricular paced beats look like left bundle branch block.

18. Is the ECG of poor quality? Look for artifact or missing leads (see Figs 3.25.2–3.25.6).

The examiners' introduction about the patient is meant to help you. Try to tie it in with the ECG findings.

Present your findings

If you are confident, you can make a good impression by summarising the important findings, rather than giving a blow-by-blow description. Examples include:

- This ECG shows atrial fibrillation with a rapid ventricular response rate. This is consistent with the patient's awareness of a rapid palpitations (Fig. 4.85.13) and inferolateral ST depression.
- Fig. 4.85.4 shows ventricular paced rhythm. This suggests the patient's syncopal episodes were a result of bradycardia, now treated with a pacemaker.
- Fig. 4.85.5 shows frequent ventricular ectopic beats. This is consistent with the patient's awareness of missed beats.

Examiners' likely questions

- What symptoms might this patient have noticed? (Fig. 4.85.5)
- Does this patient need admission to hospital? Or cardiac monitoring? (Fig. 4.85.5)
- Do you think this patient's pacemaker is working? (Fig. 4.85.4)

Marking criteria table

Criteria	Satisfactory	Unsatisfactory
Notes date, name etc.	1	0
Interprets rhythm and rate	2	0–1
Asks about waist circumference	1	0
Notes axis correctly	2	0–1
Detects normal or abnormal QRS duration	1	0
Detects presence or absence of abnormal Q waves	1	0
Presence or absence of ischaemic changes	1	0
Notes other significant abnormalities, present or absent	2	0–1

Pass mark: 6

Interpreting a chest X-ray

Background

The chest X-ray (CXR) is one of the most frequently performed radiological investigations. As such, it is important to have a consistent framework to ensure for reliable interpretation. Chest X-rays help with diagnosis in a broad range of acuities; they are also useful for gauging progress and resolution.

Introduction

A 60-year-old man presented to his local emergency department after experiencing fevers, rigors, and flu-like symptoms for 3 days. He chose to present today because he developed a new, non-radiating, right-sided chest pain that was worse whenever he coughed or took a deep breath.

To aid in his diagnosis, he has had a chest X-ray.

Rationale

This station is assessing the following:

- Do you have a system of approach to reading a chest X-ray?
- Are you able to identify significant abnormalities?

Method

1. Always begin with identification and quality of the chest X-ray, the name, age, location, date and type of image. Is it a view of the chest or another region? Lateral, anteroposterior (AP) or posteroanterior (PA)? Is the quality and exposure acceptable? Try to decide if there is rotation of the patient, whether a reasonable inspiratory effort was made, and the penetration of the X-ray. See Box 4.86.1.

Box 4.86.1 Hints on how to read a chest X-ray
(Fig. 4.86.1)

The chest X-ray is a valuable investigation and some even consider it as an extension of the physical examination. It is essential to be familiar with the various radiographic appearances. As a doctor, you should feel personally responsible for viewing all the patient's radiographs.

1. When first viewing the chest radiograph, check:
   a. date, to ensure that it is current
   b. type of X-ray — posteroanterior or anteroposterior; the latter (which may be labelled 'portable') magnifies heart size, making assessment of cardiac diameter difficult
   c. correct orientation — the left side is most reliably determined by the position of stomach gas
   d. image 'centring' — the medial ends of each clavicle should be equidistant from the spines of the vertebrae; rotation affects the mediastinal and hilar shadows, causing undue prominence on the side opposite that to which the patient was turned

2. Next, systematically examine the PA, comparing right and left sides carefully for abnormalities of:
   a. soft tissues (e.g. mastectomy, subcutaneous emphysema) and bony skeleton (e.g. rib fractures, malignant deposits)
   b. tracheal displacement, paratracheal masses
   c. heart size, borders and retrocardiac density
   d. aorta and upper mediastinum (count the ribs, look for mediastinal shift, mediastinal masses — see Figs 4.86.1 and 4.86.2)
   e. diaphragm (right higher than left by 1–3 cm normally), cardiophrenic and costophrenic angles
   f. lung hila (left normally above right by up to 3 cm, usually no larger than an average thumb)
   g. lung fields — upper zone (to lower border of second rib), mid zone (from upper zone to lower border of fourth rib) and lower zone (from midzone to diaphragm)
   h. pleura
   i. gastric bubble (normally there should be no opacity >0.5 cm above the air bubble)
   j. the presence of monitoring leads, a permanent or temporary pacemaker, central lines or other 'hardware'. Learn to do all this rapidly and accurately.

3. Finally, always ask to look at a lateral X-ray. Examine it just as carefully. The lateral image is used to help decide the exact anatomical site of an abnormality.

continued

> **Box 4.86.1**
> **Hints on how to read a chest X-ray (Fig. 4.86.1)** *continued*
>
> Know the normal position of the fissures (the horizontal fissure, seen sometimes on the PA and lateral image, is a fine horizontal line at the level of the fourth costal cartilage, whereas the oblique fissure is seen only sometimes on the lateral, beginning at the level of the fifth thoracic vertebra and running downwards to the diaphragm at the junction of its anterior and middle thirds).
>
> Learn to recognise the lung lobes. Students do not need to know the lung segments but they are useful to help localise pathology.
>
> Remember: abnormalities in the lung fields are described by terms such as 'mottling', 'opacity' or 'shadow' — it is usually unwise to attempt to make a precise diagnosis of the underlying pathology in your initial assessment of the chest X-ray (Box 4.86.2).

Adapted from https://radiopaedia.org/articles/chest-X-ray-summary?lang=gb.

> **T&O'C hint box**
>
> The clavicles should be equidistant from the spinous process. Regarding penetration; the mid-thoracic vertebrae should be clear. This is particularly important to note when comparing chest X-rays to one another, as the interstitial markings may be correspondingly brighter or dull, misleading you when comparing old and new findings.

2. Note whether there are any tubes, lines or devices such as nasogastric (NG) tubes, central venous catheters, chest drains or pacemakers.
3. A – Airway. Follow the trachea through to the carina. Comment on whether the trachea is midline, straight or narrowed. Look for foreign bodies or stenoses as you track down to both main bronchi.
4. B – Breathing. Looking at the lungs and pleural spaces, you should note how well expanded both lungs are and if expansion is equal. How many posterior ribs can you see? Ideally there should be 9–10; if there are more the lungs may be hyperexpanded. When looking at the lobes, look for changes in density compared to each other. When looking at the lung vessels, note whether they branch out

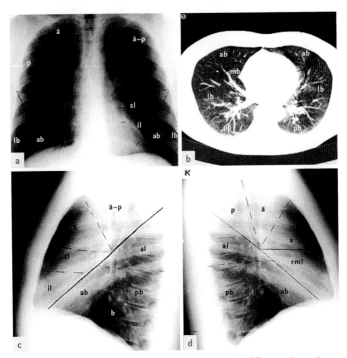

Figure 4.86.1 The lung segments. (a) PA view. (b) CT scan through lung bases. (c) Left lateral view. (d) Right lateral view. Right upper lobe: ä = apical segment; a = anterior segment; p = posterior segment. Left upper lobe: ä–p = apico-posterior segment; a = anterior segment; sl = superior lingular segment; il = inferior lingular segment. Right lower lobe: äl = apical segment; mb = medial basal segment; lb = lateral basal segment; ab = anterior basal segment; rml = right middle lobe; pb = posterior basal segment. Left lower lobe: äl = apical segment; lb = lateral basal segment; ab = anterior basal segment; pb = posterior basal segment (The Canberra Hospital X-Ray Library, reproduced with permission.)

uniformly right to the edges of the lung windows. Are there visible vessels retrocardiac and retro-diaphragmatically? Is there an area where the lung vessels aren't visible but they normally would be?

5.   Looking at the hemidiaphragms, note whether the costo- and cardiophrenic angles are crisp, or if there is opacity

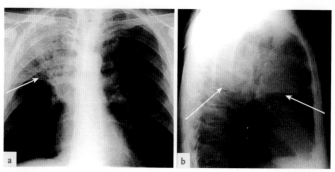

Figure 4.86.2 (a) PA, **(b)** lateral. Lateral, right upper lobe consolidation. The right upper lobe is opacified and is limited inferiorly by the horizontal fissure (arrows). There must be some collapse as well, as the fissure shows some elevation (Figures reproduced courtesy of The Canberra Hospital.)

obscuring them. Trace the cardiac silhouette and descending aorta — are they clear?

> **T&O'C hint box**
>
> Be careful to describe what you see without commenting on the cause. It can be tempting to say an area of opacity is the same as an area of consolidation, but the latter is not an objective observation but your subjective opinion on the cause.

6. **C – Circulation**. Looking at the cardiac outline, measure the heart size. Is the cardiothoracic ratio less than 50% of the chest width? The heart should also be situated approximately one-third to the right and two-thirds to the left of the mediastinum. Looking for the size and position of the aortic arch and pulmonary trunk, is there enlargement?

7. **D – Density**. Look at the bones. Look for obvious fracture or malignancy. To ensure thoroughness, painstakingly trace the outlines of each bone, looking for disruptions. Check anterior and posterior ribs, visible vertebrae, humorus and scapula.

When looking at vertebrae, check they look rectangular and are of a similar height. Are there two pedicles per vertebra, are the disc spaces preserved and equal?

BOX 4.86.2
Differential diagnosis of radiological appearances in chest X-ray

Homogeneous opacity
Pneumonia — lobar or segmental
collapse
Effusion (see Fig. 4.86.3)

Localised non-homogeneous opacity
Pneumonia (see Fig. 4.86.2)
Pulmonary infarct
Carcinoma (see Fig. 4.86.4a and e)
Tuberculosis (see Fig. 4.86.5)

Diffuse opacities
Miliary (<2 mm):
- miliary tuberculosis
- miliary metastases (especially breast, thyroid, melanoma, pancreas)
- sarcoidosis
- pneumoconiosis
- lymphoma, often with prominent hilar lymph nodes (see Fig. 4.86.6b)
- lymphangitis
- viral pneumonia
- vasculitis (e.g. polyarteritis, granulomatosis with polyangitis — see Fig. 4.86.7)
- pulmonary haemorrhage (see Fig. 4.86.8)
Nodular (3–10 mm):
- pneumonia
- pneumoconiosis
- tuberculosis
- metastatic carcinoma (see Fig. 4.86.9)
- sarcoidosis (see Fig. 4.86.6a)

Reticular (linear opacities)
Fibrosis (see Fig. 4.86.10)
Bronchiectasis (thickened bronchial walls – see Fig. 4.86.11)

continued

BOX 4.86.2
Differential diagnosis of radiological appearances in chest X-ray *continued*

Cavitated lesion
Lung abscess
Carcinoma (usually squamous cell) or Hodgkin lymphoma
Tuberculosis
Fungi (e.g. coccidioidomycosis)

Calcified lesions in the lung fields
Tuberculosis
Pneumoconiosis

Miliary calcification
Post-chickenpox pneumonia
Histoplasmosis
Coccidioidomycosis
Eptopic calcification in renal failure, hyperparathyroidism

Coin lesion
Carcinoma (primary or metastatic — look closely for any rib lesion)
Tuberculoma
Hamartoma
Granuloma (e.g. fungus)
Arteriovenous fistula
Rheumatoid nodule
Lung abscess
Hydatid cyst

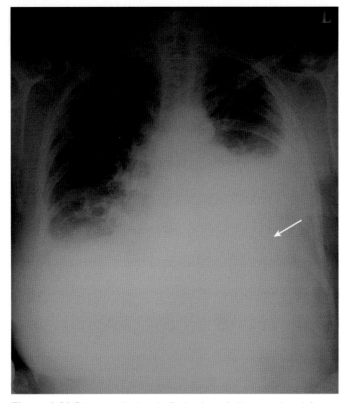

Figure 4.86.3 Large left pleural effusion (arrow). Note previous left mastectomy (Figure reproduced courtesy of The Canberra Hospital.)

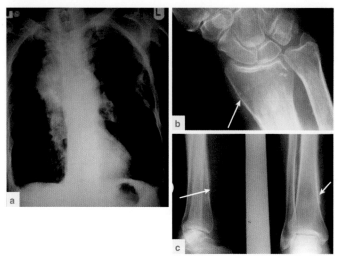

Figure 4.86.4 **(a)** Recurrent carcinoma of the lung following right upper lobectomy. Note mass and rib destruction **(b)** Hypertophic pulmonary osteoarthropathy (HPOA) of the ulna in the same patient as in (a) (arrow) **(c)** HPOA of the tibia in the same patient as in (a) (arrows) (Figures reproduced courtesy of The Canberra Hospital.)

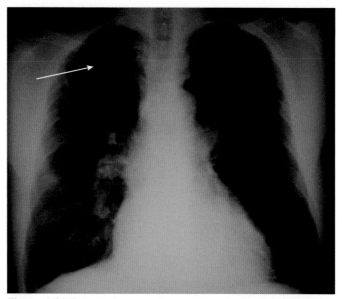

Figure 4.86.5 Right upper lobe scarring; old TB infection (arrow)
(Figure reproduced courtesy of The Canberra Hospital.)

8. **E – Everything else**. Review the other areas in the chest
   X-ray, including the upper abdominal region. Is there gas
   under the diaphragms? Any subcutaneous emphysema? Is
   the gastric bubble on the left side and below the lung fields,
   or is there a hiatus hernia? If there is a hiatus hernia, make
   note of how large the defect appears (a raised diaphragm
   compared to a portion of small bowel sitting in the chest
   cavity). Are there two breast shadows? Surgical clips?

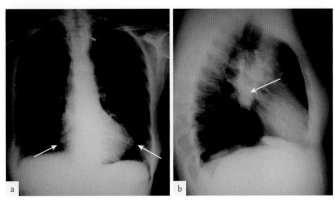

Figure 4.86.6 **(a)** Sarcoidosis basal infiltrate (arrows) **(b)** Hilar lymphadenopathy (arrow) (Figures reproduced courtesy of The Canberra Hospital.)

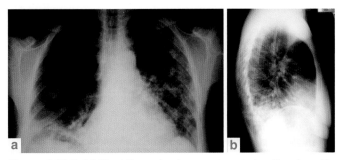

Figure 4.86.7 **(a)** Chest X-ray showing granulomatosis with polyangiitis (GPA, or Wegener granulomatosis). Note infiltrates and destructive changes **(b)** Lateral view. Note infiltrates and destructive changes (Figures reproduced courtesy of The Canberra Hospital.)

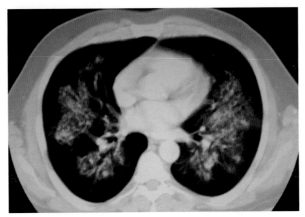

Figure 4.86.8 CT scan of chest showing pulmonary haemorrhage in a patient with Goodpasture syndrome (Figure reproduced courtesy of The Canberra Hospital.)

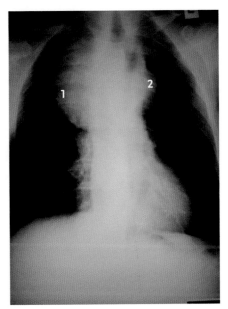

Figure 4.86.9 Retrosternal mass thoracic aortic aneurysm (1) and pulmonary metastases (2) (Figure reproduced courtesy of The Canberra Hospital.)

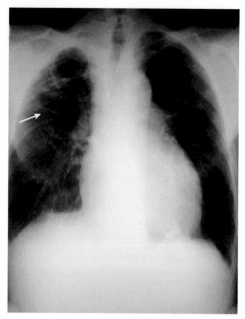

Figure 4.86.10 Right upper lobe fibrosis. Note the loss of volume and increased lung markings (arrow) (Figure reproduced courtesy of The Canberra Hospital.)

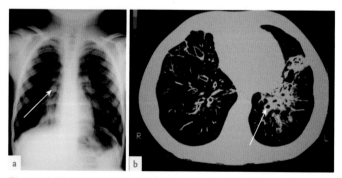

Figure 4.86.11 (a) Right middle lobe bronchiectasis. Note the increased lung markings and the thickened bronchial walls (arrow) **(b)** CT scan of the chest of a patient with bronchiectasis. Note the thickened bronchial walls (arrow) (Figures reproduced courtesy of The Canberra Hospital.)

Present your findings

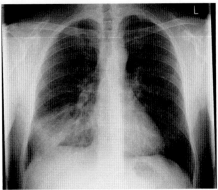

Right lower lobe consolidation (Figure reproduced courtesy of The Canberra Hospital.)

- Identity not provided. Likely AP.
- Good exposure, slightly rotated.
- A — Trachea midline, no stenosis
- B — Area of increased opacity in the right middle lobe. Costophrenic angles are clear. Good lung expansion
- C — No cardiomegaly, mediastinum is not widened
- D — No obvious fracture or bony abnormality
- E — No pneumoperitoneum or hiatus hernia, no clips, tubes or devices

EXAMINERS' LIKELY QUESTIONS

The examiners are likely to question you on your findings and what pathology you suspect it represents. In this case the discussion may revolve around pneumonia as a diagnosis.

Marking criteria table		
Criteria	Satisfactory	Unsatisfactory
Differentiates PA from AP	1	0
Checks identity	1	0
Assesses trachea position	2	0–1
Assesses lung fields	2	0–1
Assesses heart	1	0
Assesses bones	1	0
Differential covered	2	0–1

Pass mark: 6

Arterial blood gas interpretation

Background

Arterial blood gas (ABG) interpretation is a key skill in the assessment of both respiratory and renal disease. Identification of an abnormality and the common differential diagnoses will be tested.

Introduction

Remember the normal readings (Table 4.87.1).

Remember also how to interpret the results (Table 4.87.2).

TABLE 4.87.1 Normal ranges for arterial blood gases at sea level	
Parameter	Range
pH	7.35–7.45
$PaCO_2$	35–45 mmHg
PaO_2	80–100 mmHg
Bicarbonate	22–28 mmol/L
Anion gap	7–17 mmol/L depends on albumin level
A–a gradient	5–15 mmHg
Base excess	–2 to +2 mEq/L

Anion gap = Na+ – Cl– – HCO3–.
A–a gradient increases with age

TABLE 4.87.2 Acid–base disturbance

	Metabolic acidosis	Metabolic alkalosis	Respiratory acidosis	Respiratory alkalosis
pH	↓	↑	↓	↑
$PaCO_2$	↓ (compensatory)	↑ (compensatory)	↑	↓
HCO_3^-	↓	↑	Normal OR ↑ (compensatory)	Normal OR ↓ (compensatory)

Rationale

1. What does the pH tell us? Acidotic or alkalotic?
2. What does the CO_2 tell us? Respiratory acidosis, alkalosis or neutral?
3. What does the HCO_3^- tell us? Metabolic acidosis, alkalosis or neutral?

And remember, you can have a mixed picture (i.e. respiratory acidosis and metabolic acidosis, metabolic acidosis and respiratory alkalosis, etc.). See Boxes 4.87.1, 4.87.2.

Box 4.87.1
Four-step method to assess acid–base disorders

1. Look at the pH. What is the *primary* acid–base problem: acidosis (arterial pH < 7.35) or alkalosis (arterial pH > 7.45)?
2. Next look at the bicarbonate (HCO_3^-). A HCO_3^- < 22 mmol/L = metabolic acidosis. A HCO_3^- > 28 mol/L = metabolic alkalosis.
3. Look at the $PaCO_2$. In an acidosis or alkalosis there will normally be respiratory compensation (blowing off or retaining CO_2). Calculate if the $PaCO_2$ is higher or lower than expected with compensation (see below).
   - To work out if lung disease is contributing to the pH change (respiratory acidosis or alkalosis), calculate the **actual** $PaCO_2$ versus the **expected**:
   - Metabolic acidosis: expected $PaCO_2$ = 15 (as the normal $PaCO_2$ = 40 mmHg and normal HCO_3^- = 25 mmol/L: difference 15) **plus** measured HCO_3^- from the electrolytes.
   - Metabolic alkalosis: expected $PaCO_2$ increases by 0.7 mmHg for every 1 mol/L increase in HCO_3^-.

continued

Box 4.87.1
Four-step method to assess acid–base disorders *continued*

- – If the actual $PaCO_2$ is higher than expected, a respiratory acidosis is present.
- – If the actual $PaCO_2$ is lower than expected, a respiratory alkalosis is present.

4. Calculate the anion gap from the electrolyte results (or it may be provided in the results for you).
   - – A *high* anion gap metabolic acidosis (HAGMA, typically >18) has a different differential diagnosis from a normal anion gap metabolic acidosis (NAGMA).
   - – Advanced students can calculate if there is a *mixed* acid–base disorder using the HCO_3^- and anion gap numbers. For example, high anion gap, metabolic acidosis, normal HCO_3^- = HAGMA **plus** a metabolic alkalosis.

Box 4.87.2
Consider the causes

Metabolic acidosis

High anion gap metabolic acidosis (HAGMA)
Common causes include:
- Ketoacidosis (diabetes mellitus, alcohol, starvation)
- Toxins (salicylate, methanol, ethylene glycol, paraldehyde, toluene)
- Lactic acidosis (hypotensive collapse, drugs)
- Renal failure (decreased secretion of H^+ ions and reduced reabsorption of HCO_3^- ions)
- Metformin

Normal anion gap metabolic acidosis (NAGMA)
Common causes include:
- Renal tubular acidosis (usually hyperchloraemic acidosis, Cl^- ions are absorbed instead of HCO_3^- that are lost)
- Diarrhoea (loss of HCO_3^-, serum chloride likely low)
- Medications.

Metabolic alkalosis
- Vomiting
- Hyperadrenocorticism
  - – Cushing syndrome
  - – Conn syndrome
  - – Steroid therapy
- Severe potassium depletion

> **Box 4.87.2**
> **Consider the causes** *continued*
>
> **Respiratory acidosis**
> - Hypoventilation, impaired central respiratory drive, from either sedation or central nervous system impairment or respiratory muscle weakness that may be acute or chronic
> - Severely impaired ventilation perfusion mismatch
>
> **Respiratory alkalosis**
> - Hyperventilation, for example from anxiety
> - Pulmonary embolism
> - Sepsis
> - Toxins — salicylates

OXYGENATION

When determining oxygenation, the fraction of inspired oxygen (FiO_2) needs to be taken into consideration. Room air has a FiO_2 of 21% or 0.21. Disorders in oxygenation can be the result of either hypoventilation or ventilation : perfusion mismatch. Ventilation : perfusion mismatch results in an increased alveolar–arterial (A–a) gradient.

$$P(A{-}a)O_2 = PAO_2 - PaO_2 \text{(normal range } - 5{-}15\,mmHg)$$

where
  PAO_2 = Alveolar partial pressure of oxygen
  PaO_2 = arterial partial pressure of oxygen

$$PAO_2 = FiO_2 \times (P_{atmos} - P_{H2O}) - (PaCO_2)\,/\,R$$

  where
  $R = 0.8$
  P_{atmos} = 760 mmHg at sea level
  P_{H2O} = 47 mmHg at 37°C

4. Ask yourself: considering FiO_2, is oxygenation adequate?
  The normal A–a gradient value increases with age: the normal value is approximately age (in years) /4.

Method

Interpret the following ABG results then answer the questions asked by the examiner. For the purposes of these questions, all

ABGs can be assumed to be taken from a patient with a temperature measuring 37°C at sea level.

Case 1
pH = 7.32
$PaCO_2$ = 30 mmHg
PaO_2 = 102 mmHg
HCO_3^- = 15 mmol/L
FiO_2 = 0.21

Case 2
pH = 7.52
$PaCO_2$ = 57 mmHg
PaO_2 = 101 mmHg
HCO_2- = 33 mmol/L
FiO_2 = 0.21

Case 3
pH = 7.21
$PaCO_2$ = 20 mmHg
PaO_2 = 80 mmHg
HCO_3^- = 8 mmol/L
FiO_2 = 0.5

Case 4
pH = 7.22
$PaCO_2$ = 55 mmHg
PaO_2 = 63 mmHg
HCO_3^- = 26 mmol/L
FiO_2 = 0.21

Case 5
pH = 7.12
$PaCO_2$ = 58 mmHg
PaO_2 = 70 mmHg
HCO_3^- = 18 mmol/L
FiO_2 = 0.21

Examiners' likely questions
- Please comment on the acid–base disturbance.
- Is there evidence of compensation?
- Please comment on the oxygenation.
- What could be causing this disturbance?

For the examples above:
1. Metabolic acidosis with respiratory compensation.
2. Metabolic alkalosis with partial respiratory compensation.
3. Metabolic acidosis with partial respiratory compensation.
   Hypoxaemia with increased A–a gradient —
   ventilation : perfusion mismatch.
4. Respiratory acidosis.
   Hypoxaemia with increased A–a gradient —
   ventilation : perfusion mismatch.
5. Mixed metabolic and respiratory acidosis.
   Hypoxaemia with normal A–a gradient — hypoventilation.
You would need to be able to justify your answers.

Marking criteria table

Criteria	Satisfactory	Unsatisfactory
Interprets values correctly	2	0–1
Correctly identifies primary abnormality	2	0–1
Talks sensibly about the differential diagnosis	3	0–2

Pass mark: 3

The septic patient: a rapid assessment

Background

Sepsis can be life threatening. If left untreated it will rapidly lead to multi-organ failure and death. It is caused by an infection coupled with a dysregulated host response. Septic shock is defined as organ dysfunction, persistent hypotension requiring vasopressors and a raised serum lactate.

Introduction

You have been called to review a patient on an evening shift. The nurse informs you the patient has spiked a fever of 39°C with associated tachycardia. This 70-year-old patient is recovering from an elective surgical procedure (day 3 post), and has a background of chronic obstructive pulmonary disease (COPD).

Rationale

Best practice guidelines for antibiotic and fluid resuscitation state that in a patient with severe sepsis or septic shock, fluids and antibiotics need to be commenced within 60 minutes of recognition. There is a slightly longer window (2 hours) for sepsis without shock.

Method

1. Take a targeted history particularly focused on signs and symptoms of an infective source, such as fevers and chills.
   • If a patient had an existing source of infection, has this changed or worsened?

- When you're struggling to find a clear source, it can help to complete a systems review:
  - new headache, photophobia, neck stiffness, dizziness, confusion
  - new or changed productive cough, cold, runny nose
  - chest pain, palpitations, shortness of breath
  - abdominal pain or distension, diarrhoea or vomiting
  - itching, burning, stinging or increased frequency urinating
  - new rash or wound (including infection or inflammation around a cannula)
  - new joint swelling.

2. Perform relevant examinations (wash hands and wear a mask).
   - The patient in the Introduction requires cardiac, respiratory and gastrointestinal assessment at a minimum. The surgical site should be examined as best as possible. Check what is draining — purulent or frank blood?

3. Management
   - Hospitals usually have a procedural guideline for sepsis management. If this applies, follow it.
   - Call for help from the senior doctor or rapid response team, depending on the patient's risk and clinical picture.
   - Gain vascular access.
   - Begin aggressive fluid resuscitation, while monitoring for signs of fluid overload and pulmonary oedema.
   - Chart and give antibiotics. (Know the antibiotic guidelines for sepsis.)
   - Keep a strict fluid balance with or without the use of an indwelling urinary catheter.

Present your findings

- Summarise the patient's relevant background and current issues.
- Highlight pertinent examination findings.
- Explain whether you believe the patient is septic.
- What are your most likely differentials?
- Outline your management plan.

Examiners' likely questions

- What are some of the red flags for sepsis?

- Re-presentation within 48 hours
- Recent wound or surgery
- Indwelling medical device
- Immunocompromised
- >65 years of age
- Recent fall
- Pregnant or within 6 weeks of delivery

- To help decide how urgently this patient needs treatment or when to call for help, what factors would help you stratify this patients risk for sepsis?
  - High risk — any red zone observation: systolic blood pressure <90 mmHg, lactate ≥4, or base excess <−5.0
  - Moderate risk — 2 or more yellow zone criteria: respirations ≤10 or ≥25 per minute, systolic blood pressure <100 mmHg, heart rate ≤50 or ≥120/minute, temperature <35.5 or >38.5 degrees C, SpO$_2$ <95%, altered level of consciousness, lactate ≥2 mmol/L
  - Low risk — no more than one yellow zone observation
- What investigations would you like to perform?
  - Bloods — 2–3 sets of cultures, full blood count (FBC), electrolytes, urea and creatinine (EUC), liver function tests (LFTs), C-reactive protein (CRP), glucose, lactate, venous blood gases
  - Beside tests — mobile chest X-ray (CXR), electrocardiogram (ECG), wound swab, urine + stool, microscopy, culture and sensitivity (MCS)
  - Other more targeted investigations depending on history and examination findings — CT brain, chest or abdomen

Marking criteria table

Criteria	Satisfactory	Unsatisfactory
Appears to appreciate the importance of the problem	1	0
Correctly targeted history	3	0–2
Systems review	3	0–2
Outlines examination that is required, including vital signs	3	0–2
Sensible approach to investigations	2	0–1
Knows when to ask for help	1	0

Pass mark: 8

Explaining a disease — asthma

Background

Asthma is a complex and usually chronic disease with varied, recurring symptoms caused by bronchial hyperreactivity and underlying inflammation that result in airflow obstruction. The airways of a person with asthma narrow excessively when exposed to certain stimuli. These stimuli provoke little to no bronchoconstriction in a non-burdened population. Asthma can be distinguished from other obstructive airways diseases such as chronic obstructive pulmonary disease (COPD) or bronchiolitis by its reversibility with bronchodilators, the age range and exposure history. Unfortunately, there are exceptions to every rule, and thus there is a recognised asthma–COPD overlap.

Introduction

Mr Major is a 28-year-old male presenting to his local general practitioner (GP). He's noticed increasing shortness of breath, wheezing and coughing episodes, particularly while he's at work. It used to improve on the weekends but, worryingly, he's experiencing symptoms on his weekends off now too. He's a non-smoker and doesn't have a history of childhood asthma, but he does have hay fever. He works as a carpenter.

After some investigations he is given a new diagnosis of asthma.

Rationale

Adult-onset asthma is often misdiagnosed. It is often more difficult to control and carries a poorer prognosis regarding lung function than does childhood asthma. Risk factors associated in development of adult-onset asthma include obesity, environmental and occupational exposures, respiratory tract infections, rhinitis, and psychological stress.

This station aims not only for you to understand asthma but also to be able to gauge a patient's understanding and explain it to them in a clear and systematic way.

Method

When explaining a disease such as asthma to a person or patient, it is important to avoid medical jargon. There are a few key areas that should be explained, such as covering the population likely to experience the condition, the prevalence and the basic pathophysiology. Linking the pathophysiology to the symptoms a person experiences can really help with understanding. In regards to asthma, causes and triggers should also be discussed, followed by the treatment aims and some of the regimens available.

T&O'C hint box

It may feel like you're being excessively brief; however, when someone is learning about a new disease that is affecting the patient or someone he or she cares about, it is very difficult to absorb every fact. If you have the resources, a patient information booklet or just a pen and paper can be exceptionally useful.

It is always better to start simply. Answering questions and creating depth later is easier than repairing the damage after overwhelming and intimidating your patient.

A large portion of failed treatment regimens is due to poor technique. It is particularly important to demonstrate the correct use of an inhaler and spacer. There are three basic types of inhaler: soft mist inhalers (SMIs) or Respimat inhalers, dry powder inhalers (DPIs), and metered dose inhalers (MDIs). MDIs require timing of a breath with release of the medication. If timing is difficult, the addition of a spacer is often all that is required. A DPI does not require a timed breath with medication release, as the dry powder is simply released when the cannister is pressed. However, with a DPI, a more forceful inhalation is required to deliver the medication to the lungs. This may be difficult for the elderly or patients with respiratory muscle weakness.

The aerosols created by SMIs come out more slowly and last longer than MDIs; it is also produced without a propellant. SMIs come with some user-friendly functions such as a dose counter that turns red when the canister is nearly empty, and the device also locks itself after a dose is administered so that it is not possible to overdose.

Present your findings
EXAMPLE EXPLANATION

Asthma is a common disease that affects people of all ages. Nearly 3 million people in Australia have asthma. It causes airway narrowing in a few ways. When a person is exposed to a trigger, the muscles constrict, there can be inflammation or swelling, and the airways themselves can start to fill with mucus.

When this occurs, people can experience symptoms such as wheeze, cough, and shortness of breath and chest tightness. The more narrowed someone's airways become, the more intense these symptoms become.

Each person is different, but there are some common triggers for asthma which include a viral illness (a cold), allergens such as dust mites or pet hair, exercise, medication side effects, or something in your environment (tobacco or petrol fumes etc.).

The two aims of asthma treatment to prevent asthma attacks and relieve symptoms if they occur. Other components of asthma management include an 'emergency plan', trigger avoidance and monitoring (keeping track of how often you require your puffers, number of attacks). All of this information is helpful for your GP or respiratory doctor to determine if your treatment is sufficient or if there is more they need to do.

It is important to use puffers correctly. When they are used poorly, the medication doesn't get to its target location in your lungs and you do not experience any benefit, just a nasty taste in your mouth.

Salbutamol is a commonly used medication in asthma. It is used for quick relief to dilate the airways. To use a new puffer (MDI), there are a couple of easy steps to follow. To start (or when you haven't used your puffer in over 2 weeks), the puffer will need to be primed. Shake the puffer for 5 seconds, press down on the canister with your index finger while pointing the inhaler away from your eyes. This should be repeated four times before administering Ventolin to yourself.

Next, remove the cap from the mouthpiece, and insert the mouthpiece into your mouth. Keep your tongue under the mouthpiece so the opening is not blocked. The aim will be to inhale through your mouth, not your nose. Take a slow deep breath through your mouth when you press down on the canister and hold that breath as long as possible before exhaling, giving the medication most time to work. If timing is a real challenge, the addition of a spacer is helpful. Spacers allow the propellant in the MDI to evaporate, slowing the particles of medication down and allowing time for it to be breathed in without coating your mouth and throat and being absorbed by the stomach.

Examiners' likely questions

- Please look at this spirometry (Table 4.89.1) — what do you think?
  - The ratio of forced expiratory volume to forced vital capacity (FEV1/FVC) is under 70% and the FVC is normal, indicating obstruction. There was a 23% increase in FEV1 with bronchodilators, indicating reversibility defined as an FEV1 increase post bronchodilator >12% and >200 mL. This spirometry indicates suboptimally controlled asthma.
- What would be a standard action plan?
  - An action plan includes instructions for symptom monitoring and management to be implemented when symptoms occur. In general they are broken into a traffic light system: green when a person is essentially asymptomatic and well controlled, amber when asthma symptoms become more frequent and severe. This would usually result in a short-term increase in medication or change in medication. Finally, at the red light stage, the symptoms are severe and potentially life-threatening. A patient will often require multiple medications in a stepwise fashion. There is usually an established point where a patient needs to call an ambulance.

TABLE 4.89.1   Patient spirometry

Spirometry	Predicted	Pre broncho-dilator	% predicted	Post broncho-dilator	% change
FEV1 (L)	2.62	3.00	92	3.70	+23%
FVC (L)	3.13	4.51	114	4.85	+8%
FEV1/FVC	71%	67%	80	76%	

Marking criteria table

Criteria	Satisfactory	Unsatisfactory
Introduces self, confirms details	1	0
Asks patient what he knows	1	0
Explains disease	2	0–1
Identifies current symptoms	1	0
Covers complications of the disease	2	0–1
Covers background health	1	0
Identifies patient concerns	2	0–1
Provides guidance on education resources	2	0–1

Pass mark: 7

Background

Type 2 diabetes mellitus is a common condition that is encountered in all areas of medicine. It is important to be able to explain a new diagnosis to a patient as this is a significant moment for the patient. It is important to explain what the disease is, how it will affect the patient and what the patient is required to do to manage it.

Introduction

Mrs Jones, aged 48, has just been found to have an elevated fasting blood sugar (10.1 mmol/L) by her general practitioner (GP). The diagnosis of diabetes mellitus has been confirmed by an HbA1c measurement. You are now required to explain the diagnosis to the patient.

Rationale

The patient may be real or an actor who has been well briefed. The patient may be surprised and upset about the new diagnosis. She may be worried about why she now has developed the disease, and she may have a number of concerns (e.g. impact on work or family, need to take medications or insulin, long-term effects of the disease). Be prepared for the more difficult encounter where the patient is not keen to be compliant with medical advice.

Method

1. Introduce yourself and state that you are here to explain the new diagnosis of diabetes mellitus.

2. Ask what she knows or understands about diabetes. Briefly explain what diabetes mellitus is and the different types after listening to the response and, if needed, correcting any misunderstandings (which you will likely hear).

3. You will want to confirm this is most likely type 2 diabetes mellitus, remembering use of insulin is common in end-stage type 2 disease. Ask about current age (age of onset), current therapy (including diet) if any, recent weight change and family history.

4. Find out about current symptoms of diabetes (e.g. polydipsia, polyuria).

5. Ask if there are any particular concerns or expectations.

6. Check if the patient can recognise hypoglycaemic episodes and if any have occurred.

7. You will need to ascertain if there are any diabetic complications — ask about atherosclerotic diseases (e.g. heart attacks, angina, stroke, intermittent claudication), kidney disease (blood pressure, protein in the urine, abnormal creatinine), neuropathy (pins and needles in the feet, foot ulcers (Fig. 4.90.1)), retinopathy (loss of vision, ophthalmic screening), recurrent infections, or dizziness on standing (postural hypotension from autonomic neuropathy), or weight loss, early satiety and vomiting (gastroparesis).

8. Ask about other background risk factors for atherosclerosis and any therapy for them at present — especially ask about smoking, high cholesterol or hypertension. If these are present ask, if she has tried to stop smoking and describe the high importance of treating these risk factors in the setting of diabetes to prevent multiple complications.

9. Ask about symptoms of depression, for example, 'Have you been feeling sad, down or blue? Have you felt depressed or lost interest in things daily for 2 or more weeks recently?' Depression may coexist with any chronic disease and may need therapy. Ask the patient about any social support and how she is coping with her disease.

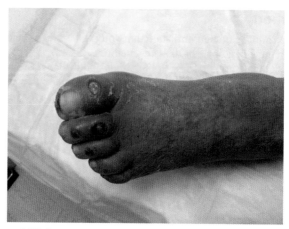

Figure 4.90.1 Diabetic foot with multiple skin ulcers caused by toe deformity and skin-friction trauma due to ill-footing shoes (Bandyk DF, Setacci C. The diabetic foot: Pathophysiology, evaluation, and treatment. *Seminars in Vascular Surgery* 2018; 31(2–4):43–48.)

10. Provide guidance on where to seek accurate disease information, such as through the Diabetes Australia website, or via patient leaflets (may be some in the room).
11. Be prepared for the patient who does not want dietary or medical treatment, where you will need to further explain the risks and offer options for further discussion and counselling.
12. Thank the patient at the end, but ask again if they have any final questions or concerns. Address any that arise.

- Before explaining the disease, find out what the patient knows and understands.
- Check the patient's understanding at each stage of the discussion and ask if there are any questions (and answer them).
- General health promotion and lifestyle change (e.g. stopping smoking) is part of the counselling process and a key part of any explanation of chronic disease.
- Avoid medical jargon (gobbledegook, a common error) when explaining a disease in an OSCE.

Present your findings

Be prepared if asked to sum up your assessment of the patient's understanding and the next steps in counselling.

Examiners' likely questions

- Why do you think this is type 2 and not type 1 diabetes mellitus? Remember type 2 diabetes can occur in obese adolescents.
  - Type 2 diabetes mellitus is usually diagnosed later in life (after 45 years of age), may run in first-degree relatives and is more common in those who are obese.
- What routine screening and lifestyle changes would you recommend for this particular patient?
  - Optometry review and podiatry review annually is recommended. Check the albumin : creatinine ratio in urine. Monitor the blood pressure, treat hypercholesterolaemia and advise smoking cessation. Recommend physical activity and a diabetic diet. Monitor the glucose and aim for strict glycaemic control.

Marking criteria table

Criteria	Satisfactory	Unsatisfactory
Introduces self, confirms details	1	0
Asks what they know	1	0
Explains disease	2	0–1
Identifies current symptoms	1	0
Covers complications of disease	2	0–1
Assesses background health	1	0
Identifies patient concerns	2	0–1
Provides guidance on education resources	2	0–1

Pass mark: 8

Advanced cardiac life support

Background

Advanced cardiac life support is an algorithm used to optimise the chance of having return of circulation in a patient who has lost cardiac output. It aims to support circulation and open the airway and allow ventilation to occur.

Introduction

You are part of the cardiac arrest Medical Emergency Team (MET)/Code blue team. You are the first to arrive to a 55-year-old male who has had a cardiac arrest. What would you do?

Rationale

Senior students may be asked to outline the principles of advanced life support. Once cardiopulmonary resuscitation (CPR) has been started and the defibrillator attached, cardiac monitoring is available. Further treatment depends on the rhythm. The examiners may show a rhythm strip or describe the rhythm and ask what should be done.

Method

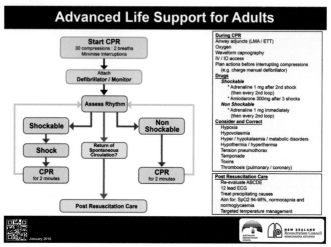

Figure 4.91.1 ANZCOR's advanced life support flowchart (Reproduced with permission from the Australian and New Zealand Committee on Resuscitation. Australian and New Zealand Committee on Resuscitation guidelines. Melbourne: ANZCOR, 2016.)

1. Begin by explaining that advanced life support (ALS) usually involves a resuscitation team and often a certain amount of confusion. One person should direct treatment, usually the senior member of the team but sometimes the patient's treating doctor if he or she is there. If you are first on the scene, ask the patient 'Are you OK?' (See Fig. 4.91.1.) If the patient is unresponsive with no carotid pulse, start CPR (chest compressions) immediately and call for help. As soon as possible, attach the monitor and defibrillator.

2. Ask yourself, is the rhythm 'shockable'? (VF or fast VT) (Fig. 4.91.2). If so, the following protocol is recommended:
   1. Immediate defibrillation with 200 joules.
   2. Recommence CPR at once for 2 minutes.
   3. Check rhythm — normal rhythm restored — check for return of circulation, pulse breathing, responsiveness
      - VF or VT persists — 1 mg adrenaline immediately and after every second shock
      - CPR then shock again

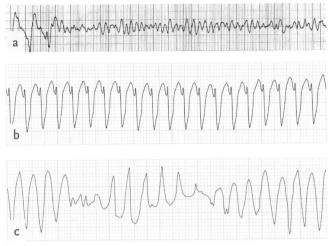

4.91.2 Shockable rhythms: **(a)** Ventricular fibrillation **(b)** Monomorphic ventricular tachycardia **(c)** Polymorphic ventricular tachycardia

- Still VF or VT after third shock — amiodarone 300 mg

Non-shockable rhythms asystole and pulseless electrical activity (PEA) (rhythm but no cardiac output) (Fig. 4.91.3).

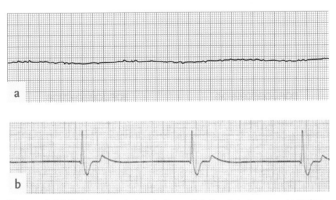

Figure 4.91.3 Non-shockable rhythms: **(a)** Asystole (narrow complex pulseless electrical activity) **(b)** Wide complex PEA (junctional rhythm)

Survival of that hospital admission for a patient who suffered with PEA was 5.9% compared with 1.1% for those with asystole during their admission. In the 12 months following the arrest, nearly 45% of patients will have either died, have severe disability or be in a vegetative state. Non-shockable rhythms carry a worse prognosis. It is worse again for those with asystole (nearly 70%).

Protocol for non-shockable rhythms:

1. CPR 2 minutes.
2. Adrenaline 1 mg and again after every second cycle.
3. Check for return of circulation.

Report your findings

- Tell the examiners about other necessary management.
    1. IV cannula
    2. Oxygen
    3. Fluid replacement, including emergency transfusion if haemorrhage has occurred
    4. Airway management — including intubation
    5. Electrolyte and pH (acidosis) measurements and correction
    6. 12 lead electrocardiogram (ECG).
- Consider a reversible cause — can someone in the patient's treating team give some history?

Use 4 Hs and Ts for a possible reversible cause:

Hypoxia (low levels of oxygen)

Hypovolaemia (shock)

Hyperkalaemia/hypokalaemia/hypoglycaemia/ hypocalcaemia (+ other metabolic disturbances)

Hypothermia

Thrombosis (coronary or pulmonary)

Tension pneumothorax

Tamponade (cardiac)

Toxins

Examiners' likely questions

- You are the ward intern when your patient has a cardiac arrest. The ALS team is managing the patient. What would you think your role should be?
  - You should be able to give the resuscitation team information about the patient's current illness, any recent procedures performed and about resuscitation orders.
  - You should be available to help as directed by the senior member of the team (i.e. do as you are told). This might include inserting a cannula, taking blood samples for urgent testing, giving or recording intravenous (IV) drugs, taking your turn at CPR.

Marking criteria table

Criteria	Satisfactory	Unsatisfactory
Distinguishes shockable from non-shockable rhythms	2	0–1
Understands importance of early cardioversion for shockable rhythm	1	0
Outlines the role of adrenaline and amiodarone	1	0
Explains general management — fluids, oxygen, intubation etc.	3	0–2
Is able to list possible reversible causes	3	0–2
Understands workings of the resuscitation team and knows his or her place in the hierarchy	2	0–1

Pass mark: 8

Atrial fibrillation and anticoagulation

Background

Deciding when to prescribe anticoagulation in a patient with atrial fibrillation is a critical clinical decision with its risks and benefits. You need to know the CHA_2DS_2-VASc score and how to apply it (Table 4.92.1).

Introduction

A 67-year-old man has had a number of episodes of atrial fibrillation (AF). These have resolved spontaneously. He has presented twice to the emergency department with palpitations and

TABLE 4.92.1 CHA_2DS_2-VASc scoring system

Parameter	Points
Congestive heart failure	1
Hypertension	1
Age 75 or over	2
Diabetes mellitus	1
Stroke or transient ischaemic attack (TIA)	2
Vascular disease (peripheral artery disease — PAD)	1
Age 65–74	1
Sex (Female)	1

Score = 0 (no treatment).
CHA_2DS_2-VASc score = 2 or more (anticoagulation with a direct oral anticoagulant (DOAC) is generally indicated).

had AF documented. Please take a history from him and discuss the need for anticoagulation with him.

Rationale

This is a common clinical problem. Students should be able discuss the need for anticoagulation with patients and explain it to them.

Method

1. Introduce yourself and explain that you have been asked to talk about the patient's atrial fibrillation.
   - Are you aware of your heart's beating abnormally when you have this fibrillation? Describe the feeling: heart irregular, or irregular and fast? How badly does it affect you?
   - Has it only been picked up on routine checks, for example electrocardiograms (ECG) or pacemaker checks?
   - How long has it been happening — weeks, months, years?
   - How long do the episodes last — seconds, minutes, hours?
   - Have episodes been recorded on an ECG? What was the longest of them?
   - Have you had treatment to control the fibrillation — drugs, ablation treatment?
2. Now run through the CHA_2DS_2-VASc score.
   - How old are you?
   - Have you had high blood pressure?
   - Have you had diabetes?
   - Have you ever had a stroke?
   - Have you been diagnosed with heart failure?
   - Have you had pains in your calves when you walk or been found to have narrowed arteries in your legs? (peripheral artery disease)
3. Remember here that the question to ask when seeing a patient with atrial fibrillation patients is not 'does this patient really need anticoagulation?' but 'is this a patient who does not need anticoagulation?' In other words, anticoagulation should be the default approach.

4. Remember also that there is no place for aspirin or other anti-platelet drugs for the prevention of embolic events for AF patients.
   - Are you taking any blood thinning tablets at the moment?
   - Have you had problems with your kidney function? (Severe chronic kidney disease (CKD): a dose reduction of a DOAC is usually recommended.)
   - Have you had any heart valve problems? Do you know what the valve problem is?
   - Have you got an artificial heart valve? Is this a metal and plastic valve or one made from animal tissue? (Mechanical heart valves and mitral stenosis must also be managed with warfarin.)
5. Now ask about bleeding risk.
   - Have you had severe high blood pressure that cannot be controlled?
   - Have you ever had a bleed into your brain?
   - Have you had bleeding stomach ulcers? Have they been treated?
   - Have you had bad problems with your liver and bleeding from this, for example into your oesophagus?
   - Do you fall over often and hurt yourself?

Present your findings

Begin by saying that you would recommend anticoagulation to the patient or that this patient is a truly low risk of embolic events and does not need anticoagulation.

Examiners' likely questions

- Are there any investigations you would like to see?
  - You can hardly say 'no', so ask to see an ECG.
- Examiners' comment, 'Here is his ECG we prepared earlier — a few months ago.' See ECG 3, Fig. 4.85.1 (p. 484).
  - This shows atrial fibrillation with a rapid ventricular response rate, about 150 beats per minute, and anterolateral ST segment depression which could be due to ischaemia but is most likely a result of the tachycardia. You should comment that the patient's heart rate was not under control when this ECG was taken.

- Would you recommend warfarin or a DOAC for this patient?
  - Unless there is a contraindication, DOACs are generally preferred. They are at least as effective as and safer than warfarin. They are much more convenient for patients because there is no need to monitor their effect.
- If the patient has a high CHA_2DS_2-VASc score but has had successful ablation treatment for AF, would you still recommend anticoagulation?
  - Yes. As there is still an increased risk of embolisation from thrombus.
- If the AF has only been documented on pacemaker testing and episodes last less than 30 seconds, would you recommend anticoagulation?
  - No. There is controversy about the length of AF associated with increased embolic risk but general agreement that very short episodes require no treatment.
- If the patient has had several falls over the last few months and injured himself slightly, would you still recommend anticoagulation?
  - Yes. Only very frequent and severe falls are considered a contraindication to treatment.

Marking criteria table

Criteria	Satisfactory	Unsatisfactory
Introduces self, explains task, obtains consent	1	0
Obtains a clear history of the patient's symptoms	1	0
Finds out how badly the symptoms affect the patient	1	0
Calculated the CHA_2DS_2VASc score	2	0–1
Makes a reasonable interpretation of the ECG	1	0
Is able to discuss the advantages and disadvantages of anticoagulation	1	0
Makes an assessment of bleeding risk	2	0–1

Pass mark: 6

Background

Heart transplants usually occur in those with end-stage heart failure. The 5-year survival rate is now slightly more than 75% for patients who have received a transplant and the 1-year survival rate is currently about 90%. The average patient survives 15 years, but this rises to 20 years for a 30-year-old and drops to 12 years for a 65-year-old. Patients are likely to have had severe heart failure that has not responded to medical treatment or resynchronisation pacing.

The stem is likely to ask you to focus on a particular aspect of the history rather than a comprehensive history as is expected in a long case.

Introduction

This woman is 45; she has had a heart transplant 3 years ago. Please take a history from her.

Rationale

This seems a daunting case, but keep in mind:

- Medical students do not have to know how to manage heart transplant patients in detail
- You should, however, be aware of some of the general principles of management of any type of transplant and of the main indications and contraindications for having a transplant
- The patient (or actor) is likely to be very well informed about the condition.

Method

1. Introduce yourself.

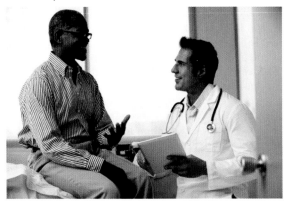

2. Try to establish the original cause of the patient's cardiac failure. 'What was the problem with your heart that led to your needing a transplant?'

In younger patients, cardiomyopathy is more likely to be the problem, but nearly half the patients currently undergoing heart transplantation have ischaemic heart disease. Combined heart and lung transplantation is occasionally carried out for patients with primary pulmonary hypertension or cystic fibrosis. It may also be the treatment of choice for some forms of congenital heart disease, either in childhood or adult life; if pulmonary hypertension is present, these patients have to be considered for combined heart and lung transplantation.

As in all transplantation long cases, the examiners will expect the candidate to be familiar with the contraindications to the procedure:
  - alcoholism
  - severe chronic kidney disease
  - continued smoking
  - interstitial lung disease (consider combined heart and lung transplantation)
  - advanced liver disease
  - old age.

Psychological assessment is always carried out to ensure patients will tolerate this complicated procedure and be adherent to the vital postoperative medications and other treatment.

3. Ask about the patient's symptoms before surgery. Try to allocate a New York Heart Association (NYHA) class to the patient, as listed I–IV below. Obtain an idea of the exercise tolerance and the severity of angina, if present. The patient may know the results of investigations of cardiac function, such as echocardiograms (ECG) and gated blood pool scans, before and after surgery. Many patients know their previous and current ejection fractions (EF) (normal >50%, severe left ventricular dysfunction EF <30–35%).

   I. Cardiac disease, no symptoms with ordinary physical activity
   II. Cardiac disease, slight limitation of physical activity, comfortable at rest
   III. Cardiac disease, marked limitation of physical activity
   IV. Cardiac disease, unable to carry out any physical activity

4. Ask what treatment the patient was receiving before transplantation, particularly the doses of diuretics, angiotensin converting enzyme (ACE) inhibitors and beta-blockers (e.g. carvedilol). There may have been recurrent ventricular arrhythmias before surgery. Treatment may have been with drugs, especially amiodarone or an implanted defibrillator and antitachycardia pacemaker and resynchronisation device. Some patients have undergone previous ablation treatment for arrhythmias. Occasionally, transplantation is used to treat intractable ventricular arrhythmias, particularly for those with a diffuse myocardial disease such as sarcoidosis.

5. Ask whether there were any problems with the surgery — either technical or involving acute rejection. Find out how long the patient was in hospital and what further admissions to hospital have occurred since the operation. Some patients awaiting transplant may have been given a ventricular assist device as a bridge to transplant: ask whether that was necessary.

6. Find out what drugs the patient is taking currently. Transplant patients should not require antifailure treatment,

but will, of course, be taking immunosuppressive drugs. Almost all patients are now maintained on cyclosporin; the dose is determined by its serum level. Cyclosporin and tacrolimus are nephrotoxic and cause hypertension and hyperlipidaemia.

7. Patients are often well informed about symptoms suggesting rejection — often these resemble an attack of pericarditis (pleuritic chest pain). The patient may know of boosts of prednisone that have been given for rejection episodes. Early episodes of rejection are often treated with 1 g of methylprednisolone intravenously (IV) for 3 days. Later rejection tends to be milder and may respond to an increase in oral steroids.

8. Inquire about complications of immunosuppression (Table 4.93.1). Many patients are also taking regular antibiotics to prevent *Pneumocystis jirovecii* (formerly *carinii*) infection. Cotrimoxazole twice daily 3 days a week is a common regimen.

9. The use of steroids for these patients increases the risk of osteoporosis. Ask if she has had bone scans performed and if any treatment has been recommended to prevent osteoporosis.

TABLE 4.93.1   Commonly used immunosuppressants for heart transplant patients

Drug	Side-effects	Monitoring / Avoidance
Steroids	Cushingoid, diabetes, osteoporosis	Minimal dose
Cyclosporin	Renal impairment, hypertension, neurotoxicity	Blood levels, drug interactions
Mycophenolate	Mild marrow suppression, gastrointestinal upset	Reduce dose, check FBC
Methotrexate	Hepato- and marrow toxicity	FBC, liver function tests
Azathioprine	Hepato- and marrow toxicity, pancreatitis	FBC, liver function tests, TPMT

FBC = full blood count; TPMT = thiopurine methyltransferase.

10. Some general questions about the transplant patient's current life are very relevant. Find out how much difference has occurred in the patient's exercise tolerance and whether she has been able to go back to work. If the patient is currently an inpatient, find out why he or she has been admitted to hospital on this occasion. Ask about the patient's family and how they have coped with the illness and the transplant itself. Make some discreet inquiries about the patient's finances and whether there have been any problems returning to the transplant hospital for the various investigations required.

11. Hypertension is another important posttransplant problem. It is associated with the use of cyclosporin. Ask about blood pressure control and treatment.

12. Transplant patients have an increased risk of malignancy. Skin cancers (basal cell and squamous cell carcinomas) are common. Ask if the patient has regular (at least annual) skin checks. There is also a higher incidence of lymphoproliferative disorders.

13. Ask about her mood and whether she has been happy with her treatment.

Present your findings

- Outline the patient's history before the transplant and the events leading up to it. Include her previous NYHA class.
- In chronological order, discuss the posttransplant treatment and change in patient's symptoms, including current NYHA class.
- Mention major complications and how they have been managed.
- Explain how she and her family and work have coped with this chronic illness.

Examiners' likely questions

- What physical examination would you perform on this woman as a routine?
  - Cardiovascular examination for signs of heart failure and median sternotomy scar
  - Skin examination for malignancies
  - Measure the blood pressure

- Lymph node examination
- How well does she understand her condition and treatment?
  - Most patients are very good at this but mention any apparent deficiencies.
- What do you think of her prognosis?
  - If she is symptom-free and has had no serious rejection problems, her prognosis is very good.
- What will be important for her future prognosis?
  - Control of blood pressure
  - Careful maintenance of immunosuppression
  - Protection from osteoporosis (steroids)
  - Regular assessment for malignancy
  - Control of other cardiovascular risk factors
  - Early treatment of infections.

Marking criteria table

Criteria	Satisfactory	Unsatisfactory
Introduces self, explains task, obtains consent	1	0
Obtains history of pre-transplant symptoms	1	0
Asks about the transplant operation and how long the patient was in hospital	1	0
Asks about been any rejection episodes and what happened	1	0
Assesses the success of the procedure from the patient's perspective	1	0
Asks how the patient and her family have coped with the illness and operation	1	0
Is able to discuss patient's understanding of the treatment	2	0–1
Describes the routine examination indicated — skin malignancies, heart failure etc.	1	0
Has some idea of the important complications of the drug treatment, e.g. osteoporosis	1	0

Pass mark: 6 in this difficult case

Low back pain

Background

Low back pain is one of the leading causes of disability world-wide and is the second leading cause of disease burden in Australia. It is a complex problem and a detailed history can help identify a cause and subsequently tailor management to ensure the best patient outcomes.

Rationale

This station aims to ensure that you are able to take a comprehensive history and present it coherently. It is not only important to gather the medical details but also how this affects the patient's function and quality of life.

Introduction

Mrs Chan is a 45-year-old woman who presents with a 4-month history of lower back pain. Please take a history from her about her pain.

Method

1. Introduce yourself.
2. First establish when the pain started and its nature at time of onset. Ask if there was any trauma at this time that instigated the pain.
3. Ask about how the pain has changed over this time period.
4. Ask about the pain as it is currently. This includes:
   ● site of the pain
   ● onset of pain — what brings it on?

- character of the pain:
  - the presence of any neuropathic features (such as numbness, pins and needles, shocks or shooting pain)
  - relieving or exacerbating factors

  Remember that the pain of spinal stenosis is often worse on walking and relieved with sitting and or lying flat.
  - Does the pain radiate?
  - How severe is it?

5. Associated features.
   - Weight loss could indicate underlying malignancy
   - Early morning stiffness could indicate inflammatory conditions (rheumatoid arthritis, ankylosing spondylitis)
   - Sensory changes

6. Ask about its timing. Is it continuous or intermittent? (Neuropathic pain is often spontaneous; worse on use can indicate osteoarthritis.)

7. Ask about the current analgesia regime, including over-the-counter medications. Has there been a problem with dependence on narcotic analgesics?

8. Ask about any interventions in this period and if they had any effect on the patient's pain experience. Specifically ask if any surgery has been performed and what this was for. Ask about which drugs have been tried, for how long and at what dosages. Ask if she has been involved in any physiotherapy, rehabilitation and cognitive behavioural therapies.

9. Ask about the patient's past medical history, such as osteoporosis (increased risk of vertebral fractures) as well as a psychiatric history including depression and anxiety, as this may affect the way the pain is experienced.

10. Take a social history, including how the pain affects the current level of function and the ability to attend to activities of daily living (ADLs). Ask if she partakes in regular exercise. Ask about her current employment and how her pain experience is affecting her ability to work.

11. Ask about her current levels of emotional stress and how that is affecting her friendships and family.

Present your findings

- Summarise the way the patient is currently been affected by the pain, including its effect on normal activities, work and sleep.
- Outline the history of the pain and the effectiveness of previous interventions and therapy.

Examiners' likely questions

- What type of pain is the patient experiencing?
  - Have a differential in regards to spinal stenosis, radicular pain or any neuropathic components to the pain.
- What factors are contributing to this patient's experience of pain?
  - It is important here to discuss not only trigger or mechanical aspects but also the biopsychosocial aspects, which are heavily implicated in chronic pain. Have there been problems with analgesic use?
- What are the red flags for back pain?
  - Cancer
    - unexplained weight loss
    - history of cancer
    - age of onset <20 or >50
  - Infection
    - immunosuppression
    - intravenous (IV) drug use
    - fevers
  - Fractures
    - significant trauma
    - minor trauma in patient with history of osteoporosis
  - Neurological involvement
    - neurological deficits (e.g. urinary retention or incontinence, faecal incontinence, decreased anal tone, saddle paraesthesia)
  - Spondyloarthropathies
    - night pain
    - early morning stiffness
    - worse with rest.

Marking criteria table

Criteria	Satisfactory	Unsatisfactory
Introduces self, explains task, obtains consent	1	0
Asks about onset and character of pain	2	0–1
Asks about associated features	2	0–1
Asks about effect on life, work etc.	1	0
Has a diagnosis been made?	1	0
How effective had treatment been? What has been tried (drug and non-drug)	3	0–2
Makes a reasonable attempt at examiners' questions	3	0–2

Pass mark: 8

Background

Remember that the most common pattern of disease in multiple sclerosis (MS) is called relapsing remitting multiple sclerosis (RRMS). In untreated patients the rate of relapse is 0.65 attacks a year. Episodes of fever or fatigue associated with a temporary worsening of symptoms are not considered to be relapses and are called pseudorelapses. In most cases, complete or almost complete resolution of symptoms occurs in this phase of the disease. After 10 years, up to 50% of patients begin to develop a progressive accumulation of disability — secondary progressive MS (SPMS). Eventually 80% of patients enter this stage.

Introduction

You will probably be told that the patient has multiple sclerosis.

- Please take a history from this woman who has a history of multiple sclerosis.

Rationale

This relapsing condition can affect people throughout their lives. Symptoms are sometimes severe and treatment is complicated. Patients are often well informed (better than most medical students) about the condition. This is a test of your ability to take a comprehensive history and present it coherently. This often severe disease may begin in early adult life, and the effect on the patient may be profound.

Method

The disease usually begins with an episode of acute neurological disturbance, which is called a *clinically isolated* syndrome. However, the clinical diagnosis requires at least two neurological events separated in time and place within the central nervous system (CNS). MS is primarily a clinical diagnosis, but the use of MRI scanning has led to the McDonald criteria for diagnosis. These allow for the diagnosis after a single neurological episode if the MRI shows a separate area typical of MS (see Box 4.95.1).

1. Ask about the presenting symptoms (listed here in approximate order of importance).
   - Episodes of spastic paraparesis, hemiparesis or tetraparesis (may present as gradually progressive disease in late-onset MS)
   - Episodes of limb paraesthesiae (owing to posterior column, medial lemniscus or internal capsule involvement)
   - Episodes of visual disturbance — loss of acuity, pain on eye movement, loss of central visual field (optic neuritis), diplopia on lateral gaze
   - Episodes of ataxia, dysarthria and tremor — Charcot triad (owing to cerebellar or posterior column involvement)
   - Band sensations around trunk or limbs
   - Less common symptoms, such as:
     - vertigo, symptoms of cranial nerve disorders (e.g. tic douloureux)
     - urinary urgency, incontinence of faeces
     - erectile dysfunction
     - depression
     - euphoria
     - dementia
     - seizures
     - bulbar dysfunction (pseudobulbar palsy).

BOX 4.95.1
Sites of demyelinating lesions on MRI scanning

Corpus callosum	Optic nerve
Juxtacortical white matter	Periventricular white matter
Spinal cord	Pons, cerebellar peduncles and cerebellum

1. Ask about precipitating factors, such as:
   - heat (hot baths, etc.)
   - infection
   - fever
   - pregnancy
   - exercise.

     Disease activity tends to be less during pregnancy; relapse is common postpartum.
2. Ask about family history: MS is seven times more common in immediate relatives (sibling risk is 5%).
3. Ask about social disability — sexual function, ability to work, financial problems.
4. Ask about place of birth: MS is more common in subjects who spent their childhood in temperate latitudes than in tropical regions. Smoking is also a risk factor.
5. Find out what treatments have been tried and with what success and side effects. Various unproven treatments are often tried by patients with this incurable disease. Ask whether any of these have been used.
6. Ask about mood and the patient's thoughts about her prognosis and future.

Present your findings

- Try to outline the course of the disease chronologically.
- Discuss major clinical episodes in more detail.
- Summarise the treatment so far and its effects and side effects.
- Discuss the effect of the disease on the patient and her life, family, work and ability to function.
- What is the patient's mood and how does she see her future?

Examiners' likely questions

- Is the disease active at the moment?
  - Comment on any recent symptoms.
- What symptoms currently cause the patient the most trouble?
  - You should have asked about these.
- Is the patient realistic about her prognosis?

Marking criteria table

Criteria	Satisfactory	Unsatisfactory
Introduces self, explains task, obtains consent	1	0
Asks about the symptoms that have led to the diagnosis	1	0
Allows patient to describe these in her own words	1	0
Finds out how the diagnosis was made	1	0
Asks about the time course of the illness	1	0
Asks about treatment given and its side effects	2	0–1
Asks about current symptoms	1	0
Examines the effect of the illness on patient, family, work and ordinary life	2	0–1
Asks about the patient's expectations and thoughts of the future	1	0
Summarises findings coherently	1	0
Answers examiners' questions	1	0

Pass mark: 9

HIV history taking

Background

Human immunodeficiency virus (HIV) infection is now a chronic disease and effective treatment has meant that most patients do not die of the disease. Ischaemic heart disease (IHD) is the most common cause of death. This is due to the effect of chronic inflammation on cardiovascular risk.

You are likely to be directed to take a section of the history in a complex case like this in an OSCE rather than the complete history as would be needed in a long case.

Introduction

This man has HIV infection. Please take a history from him.

Rationale

Taking a history from patients with this chronic disease involves the student in obtaining and presenting information from over a long period in many cases. It is a test of:

- your ability to ask about events in a methodical way and set them out chronologically for the examiners
- your understanding of the important aspects of the disease and it treatment
- your ability to ask questions of the patient tactfully about the way the disease was acquired
- your understanding of the way the disease has affected the patient's life physically, emotionally and personally
- your understanding that many HIV patients have the disease so well controlled that it is not their major health problem — IHD is increasingly a cause of morbidity and mortality for HIV patients.

Method

1. Ask about the presenting symptoms. Ask if the patient minds answering questions about the condition. Begin with a preparatory statement such as 'If you find that any of my questions are about some thing you don't want to talk about please tell me.'

2. Find out about symptoms of a possible seroconversion illness in the past (see Box 4.96.1). Approximately 50% of people have a seroconversion illness. It occurs 3–6 weeks after infection and often resembles glandular fever. Remember that, without treatment, the development of AIDS takes roughly 7–10 years from the time of seroconversion. The occurrence of a seroconversion illness does not seem to be associated with a worse prognosis.

3. Find out what symptoms or complications are currently affecting the patient. These must be assessed in the context of possible longstanding disease affecting many systems of the body.

4. Note from the history any of the conditions likely to occur during the period of mild-to-moderate immunosuppression that precedes the development of AIDS and those related to severe immunosuppression that define the development of AIDS (see Box 4.96.2).

5. If the patient is willing, ask about the mode of acquisition of infection. Comorbidity differs between subgroups, so specific questions about risk factors are essential. For example, coinfections with syphilis or papilloma viruses and Kaposi's sarcoma are often found in the men who have sex with men subgroup, whereas hepatitis B and C

Box 4.96.1
Features of the seroconversion illness

A seroconversion illness occurs in more than 50% of cases. There is usually some combination of the following symptoms:

fever	vomiting
lymphadenopathy	diarrhoea
maculopapular rash	headache
arthralgia	meningism
myalgia	weight loss
pharyngitis	oral candidiasis
nausea	

> **Box 4.96.2**
> **HIV-related conditions with severe immunosuppression**
>
> *Pneumocystis jirovecii* pneumonia (PJP)
> Kaposi sarcoma
> Non-Hodgkin lymphoma
> Disseminated *Mycobacterium avium* complex infection
> Cytomegalovirus infection
> Cerebral toxoplasmosis
> Oesophageal candidiasis
> AIDS dementia complex

Note: This is a representative rather than an exhaustive list.

infection, endocarditis, heroin nephropathy and other disorders related to drug use may complicate the disease in the intravenous drug-using group. Many haemophilia A patients acquired HIV from pooled blood products.

6. Ask about sexual contacts (but again only if the patient is happy to answer these questions). Contact tracing must be mentioned and the possibility addressed of infection of sexual partners without their knowledge.

7. Ask the patient whether family and friends are aware of the diagnosis. Their attitude to this chronic illness may affect the patient's ability to cope.

8. Ask about general constitutional symptoms. Symptoms of fever, lethargy and weight loss may indicate the AIDS-related complex or suggest an underlying opportunistic infection or malignancy.

9. Enquire about specific symptoms:
   - respiratory — cough, dyspnoea, sputum — these may result from *Pneumocystis jirovecii* pneumonia, lymphoid interstitial pneumonitis, tuberculosis, bacterial pneumonia or fungal pneumonia
   - gastrointestinal — diarrhoea or weight loss as a result of cryptosporidiosis, microsporidiosis, mycobacterial infection or cytomegalovirus (CMV) colitis; odynophagia as a result of oesophageal candidiasis, herpes simplex or CMV ulceration; vomiting and abdominal pain owing to biliary tract disease; drug side effects (e.g. pancreatitis) — diarrhoea is usual when patients are treated with protease inhibitors

- neurological — meningism caused by cryptococcal meningitis, focal neurological symptoms or seizures as a result of space-occupying lesions, toxoplasmosis or non-Hodgkin lymphoma; cognitive decline as a result of HIV dementia or multifocal leucoencephalopathy; peripheral nervous system disease owing to peripheral neuropathy, CMV radiculopathy or myopathy
- renal — nephrotic syndrome from HIV-associated nephropathy; renal failure owing to sepsis or drug side effects
- ocular — deteriorating vision, which usually suggests advanced CMV retinitis
- dermatological — rashes may be caused by drug reactions, viral infection (e.g. herpes zoster virus (HZV) or herpes simplex virus (HSV)) or fungal infection; itch may be caused by scabies or drug reaction; and nodules can be caused by Kaposi sarcoma (Fig. 4.96.1) or bacillary angiomatosis. Seborrhoeic dermatitis and psoriasis occur commonly
- cardiac — dyspnoea, chest pain or palpitations owing to myocarditis or pericarditis, angina
- haematological — anaemia (bone marrow suppression or infiltration, treatment with zidovudine); thrombocytopenia and neutropenia are less common.

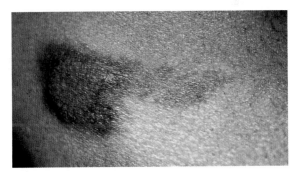

4.96.1 Kaposi sarcoma on the leg. The lesion is reddish-brown because of its vascular nature and accompanying haemosiderin deposition (Piccini JP, Nilsson KR. *The Osler Medical Handbook*, 2nd edn. Baltimore: The Johns Hopkins University, 2019, Plate 19.)

10. Ask about previous treatment. Find out about antiretroviral drug and antibiotic treatment and about any adverse effects of these. Inquire about specific side effects, for example:
    - protease inhibitors — lipodystrophy, diarrhoea
    - non-nucleoside transcriptase inhibitors — rash, hepatitis
    - integrase inhibitors — myopathy, cholesterol elevation.
    - Students will not be expected to know these drugs or their side effects in detail but the patient may. If the disease has recently been diagnosed, ask what treatment options have been discussed with the patient.

11. Ask about previous investigations. The patient may be able to give much helpful information on previous investigations, including viral load results, CD4+ T cell counts, MRI scans, CT scans, lumbar punctures, bone marrow biopsies and endoscopy.

12. Inquire about social, drug and alcohol history. The examiners will expect knowledge of the patient's social, economic and family circumstances.

13. Ask about risk factors and treatment for cardiovascular disease:
    - known IHD — angioplasty, coronary artery bypass graft (CABG)
    - smoking — awareness of risk
    - cholesterol level — statin treatment
    - family history of IHD
    - diabetes
    - hypertension — treatment

Present your findings

- Attempt a chronological outline of the disease.
- Discuss the treatment and its side effects.
- Describe the effect of the disease on all aspects of the patient's life.
- Outline the patient's cardiovascular risk factors and what has been done to control them.

Examiners' likely questions

- How well informed do you think this man is about his illness?

- – This should be obvious to you from your interview. Some patients know much more about their chronic illnesses than most medical students but others pay little attention to it.
- What are the main future risks to this man's health?
  - – Well-treated HIV patients are at risk of dying from cardiovascular disease more than from their HIV infection directly. This is an opportunity to talk about cardiovascular risk factor control.

Marking criteria table

Criteria	Satisfactory	Unsatisfactory
Introduces self, explains task, obtains consent	1	0
Finds out what areas patient is happy to discuss	1	0
Asks details of any seroconversion illness	1	0
If possible, asks about method of contraction	1	0
Asks how diagnosis was made	1	0
Finds out effect of diagnosis on patient and friends and partners	1	0
Asks about the time course of the illness	2	0–1
Asks if there have been serious problems, e.g. admission to ICU	1	0
Asks about current and previous treatment regimens as far as patient can remember	2	0–1
Asks about side effects of treatment	2	0–1
Asks about other associated health problems, e.g. coronary artery disease	1	0
Asks about the patient's current mood and expectations for the future	1	0
Inquires about effect of illness on life, work and friends	1	0
Presents findings and shows understanding of the effect of this illness on the patient	2	0–1

Pass mark: 12

Preoperative assessment history

Background

Modern surgery is generally safe. This is partly because patients' surgical and anaesthetic risk is carefully assessed prior to their operations. Certain aspects of the patient health, medication and the operation itself influence risk. These aspects need to be explored before surgery unless the procedure is an emergency.

The more major the surgery the greater the risk. Examples of major surgical operations include:

- vascular surgery
- thoracotomy and cardiac surgery
- most neurosurgery.
  Of moderate risk:
- abdominal surgery.
  Consider also:
- Is it an emergency? This is always associated with more risk.
- Can it be performed under local anaesthetic? Local anaesthetic is usually associated with lower risk.

Introduction

You have been asked by the surgeon and anaesthetist on your ward to admit this 62-year-old man before his surgery. Please take a history from him.

Rationale

Junior doctors are often asked to admit patients to hospital before planned or urgent surgery. You will be expected to have an approach to this that shows you can safely be allowed to perform this routine but important job. A pass mark would be achieved if most relevant systems and potential problems were asked about. A high mark would come from interpretation and suggested management options.

Method

1. Ask about the operation.
   - What operation are you going to have?
   - What has been the problem that has necessitated the operation?

Ask about comorbidities (most will have been covered during the general history taking).

2. Heart:
   - Have you had any heart problems in the past? Is there a history of ischaemic or valvular heart disease?
   - Have you had angina or a heart attack recently (within the last 6 months)?
   - What treatment have you had for this? (for example, recent coronary artery stenting or a bypass)
   - Are you able to exercise? What do you do for exercise? How much can you do? How many steps can you climb? What stops you from being more active? Arthritis, breathlessness, chest pain?
   - Have you had any tests of your heart, such as exercise test, coronary angiogram, and stress echo? (Describe these to the patient if necessary.)
   - Have you been told your heart is weak or enlarged? Have you had tests to look into this, such as an echocardiogram or chest X-ray? Have you got the results of these with you today?
   - Work out the New York Heart Association (NYHA) class if the patient is breathless;
     - Are you short of breath even doing nothing? (class IV)
     - Are you short of breath when you walk slowly on the flat? (Class III)
     - Are you short of breath if you try to walk fast or uphill? (Class II)

3. Lungs:
   - Have you been a smoker? Still? How many a day? (Current smoking increases the risk of lung

complications in the postoperative period. Stopping even for a few months before surgery improves this risk.)

- Have you been told you have lung problems? Has anyone said you have chronic obstructive pulmonary disease (COPD) or asthma?
- Have you needed cortisone or prednisone for your lungs? When was that? (Patients on long-term steroids will need extra doses in the perioperative period.)
- How good are your lungs at the moment compared with their usual state? (An exacerbation of COPD or asthma will make surgery more risky.)
- Have you been diagnosed with sleep apnoea? Have you got loose teeth? (These can be associated with more difficult intubation.)

4. Endocrine:
   - Are you a diabetic; on insulin? (Insulin requirements will need to be considered pre- and post-surgery.)
   - Have you had any thyroid problems? Has the thyroid been over- or underactive? Have thyroid function tests been performed recently? (Pre-surgery testing is not routine.)
   - Have you been told you have Addison disease? (Steroid replacement will be needed if correct.)

5. Kidneys:
   - Have you had kidney problems? Do you know the cause of the trouble?
   - Do you know your estimated glomerular filtration rate (eGFR)? (Many chronic kidney disease (CKD) patients do. Angiotensin converting enzyme (ACE) inhibitors are often withheld for a few days for these patients.)
   - Severe CKD patients may end up on dialysis temporarily or permanently after major surgery (especially cardiac surgery). They must have this discussed with them before surgery.

6. Blood:
   - Have you been told you have anaemia? Do you know whether you are still anaemic?
   - Have you had clots in your legs (deep vein thrombosis — DVT) or lungs (pulmonary emboli — PE)? (This means an increased risk of perioperative DVT or PE.)

- Have you had low numbers of blood platelets (thrombocytopenia)? Do you have a bleeding tendency (possible increased perioperative bleeding risk)?

7. Liver:
   - Have you had liver problems? Do you know the cause? Have you been told you have had liver failure? (Problems with anaesthetic agents — anaesthetic and other drugs have an increased half-life and may accumulate in these patients.)
   - Are you positive for the hepatitis B or C (or human immunodeficiency — HIV) viruses? (Precautions may be needed by staff in theatre to avoid infection, as always.)

8. Nerves:
   - Have you had problems with muscle-relaxing drugs during previous operations? (myasthenia gravis, malignant hyperthermia)

9. Drugs — ask specifically about allergies or previous adverse drug reactions and about these groups of drugs:
   - anticoagulants
   - antiplatelets
   - beta-blockers
   - steroids
   - insulin
   - oral hypoglycaemics
   - ACE inhibitors
   - anticonvulsants
   - analgesics

   Ask what exactly was the drug reaction. Distinguish anaphylaxis from other reactions.

10. The patient:
    - Has the operation been explained to you? Have been told how long you will be in hospital and about possible complications and risks?

Present your findings

SAMPLE ANSWER 1

'This previously well 62-year-old man has been admitted for a non-urgent cholecystectomy. He has had no problems with previous anaesthetics and there is no history of ischaemic heart disease. He has a good exercise tolerance. He takes no regular medications. He has a good understanding of the proposed surgery and its risks. I feel he is fit for his surgery and has a low perioperative risk.'

SAMPLE ANSWER 2

'This 62-year-old man has been admitted for a colectomy following the recent diagnosis of carcinoma of the colon. He was treated 9 months ago for a myocardial infarction and has been on dual antiplatelet treatment since having an angioplasty and stent at that time. With the permission of his cardiologist, the clopidogrel was stopped 6 days ago but he has continued to take aspirin as instructed. He has had no further cardiac symptoms and was told he did not have significant disease elsewhere in his coronary arteries or left ventricular dysfunction.'

'He has a loose tooth and has discussed this with his anaesthetist.'

'He has been treated for many years with prednisone for inflammatory arthritis and knows he will need steroid supplementation both before and after surgery.'

'I feel he is at some increased cardiovascular risk for his operation but it is now more than 6 months since his infarct and he is free of symptoms.'

(Patients with coronary stents should never come off antiplatelet treatment if at all possible and most surgery can be performed while patients continue to take aspirin — intracranial and spinal surgery are rare exceptions. Heparin is not a safe substitute for aspirin for these patients.)

Be decisive. 'His operation is urgent and should go ahead.'

Examiners' likely questions

There may be much to talk about but questions about anticoagulation and antiplatelet treatment are common.

- You have told us this man takes dabigatran because he is in atrial fibrillation (AF) and has type 2 diabetes. What would be your advice about this treatment before his abdominal surgery?
  - When anticoagulation is being used for patients with AF, cessation 24–48 hours before surgery is routine. These patients do not need to be given heparin or enoxaparin.

- You have found that this man has a mechanical aortic valve replacement and takes warfarin. How would you advise this should be managed?
  - These patients must be protected against valve thrombus.
    For minor surgery the international normalised ratio (INR) can be allowed to fall to 2.0 on the day of surgery by reduction or interruption of the warfarin dose. Otherwise warfarin needs to be stopped 4–5 days before surgery and the patient treated with enoxaparin — last dose 24 hours before surgery. It must be restarted as soon as the surgeon feels this is safe and continued until the INR reaches 2.0.
- You have told us this man has been a heavy smoker until a few weeks ago and has had a diagnosis of COPD. How do think this affects his operative risk?
  - Mull over the risk factors for pulmonary complications of surgery (most often prolonged postoperative intubation) (Box 4.97.1)
- You have told us this man takes insulin. How would you manage this before and after surgery?
  - In general, a fasting patient should have half his usual insulin dose at the usual time, be put on to dextrose infusion and have regular blood sugar measurements. If the blood sugar is difficult to control, an insulin infusion should be started.
  - In general, the risks of surgery or risks of delay of surgery must be weighed up for all patients.

Box 4.97.1
Risk factors for peri-operative pulmonary complications

Patient	Surgery
Age	Intrathoracic or abdominal surgery
COPD	Surgery lasting more than 3 hours
Comorbidities, immobility	Emergency surgery
Smoking	

Marking criteria table

Criteria	Satisfactory	Unsatisfactory
Introduces self, explains task, obtains consent	1	0
Obtains information about the operation and its general risk	1	0
Takes a comprehensive history of patient's medical conditions and comments on their relevance	2	0–1
Discusses patient's medications and their relevance	1	0
Discusses anticoagulation and antiplatelet treatment and whether it can be stopped	1	0
Is able to recommend strategies for management of anticoagulation — this would indicate a very good student	1	0
Takes history about important problems related to anaesthesia and surgery, e.g. lung disease, allergies	2	0–1
Takes history concentrating on other relevant medications, e.g. insulin	1	0

Pass mark: 5

Preoperative assessment examination

Background

Many patients have never been examined until they have a pre-operative assessment. Various abnormalities may be detected here for the first time, such as a cardiac murmur, atrial fibrillation, hypertension, an abdominal mass or poor oral hygiene.

Introduction

Please examine this 74-year-old woman who has been admitted to have a hip replacement tomorrow.

Rationale

The preoperative assessment is an important aspect of surgical care. Often patients have multiple anaesthetic risk factors, which can be identified in this assessment. Once identified, these risk factors can be optimised and can help guide the use of appropriate anaesthetic for their operation.

Method

1. Wash your hands, introduce yourself and ask the patient to undress to her underwear and put on a hospital gown (patients have usually been asked to do this already so that you are not delayed).
2. Look at the general appearance for obesity or signs of Cushing syndrome and immobility; these may slow postoperative recovery. Seriously underweight, malnourished patients may be at risk of slow wound

TABLE 4.98.1 The Modified Mallampati Score

Class	Criteria
Class I	Soft palate, uvula, fauces, pillars visible
Class II	Soft palate, major part of uvula, fauces visible
Class III	Soft palate, base of uvula visible
Class IV	Only hard palate visible

    healing and recovery. Note general frailty, which is associated with an increased risk for any procedure.

3. Look in the mouth for obvious dental problems that will make intubation difficult. You might particularly impress the examiners by estimating the Mallampati score (Table 4.98.1). Ask the patient to open her mouth wide and protrude the tongue as far as possible. Look at the base of the tongue and whether there is a gap between it and the soft palate. A small gap or absence of a gap suggests a more difficult intubation.

4. Take the blood pressure. Uncontrolled severe hypertension will lead to deferral of surgery in many cases.

5. Examine the heart for signs of uncontrolled heart failure or valvular heart disease. Signs of these problems may lead to delay in surgery while cardiac investigations are performed. Severe valvular disease, such as aortic stenosis may be contraindications to surgery.

6. Examine the lungs for signs of chronic obstructive pulmonary disease (COPD) or asthma. Is the patient requiring supplementary oxygen? These conditions severely affect anaesthetic risk.

7. Look for previous surgical scars, particularly abdominal and median sternotomy scars, that mean previous abdominal or cardiac surgery.

Present your findings

Outline any positive findings that may affect operative risk.

Examiners' likely questions

- You have noticed some previous surgical scars. What questions would you like to ask the patient about these?
  - What operations have you had to cause these scars on your chest, abdomen? Have you had a heart operation? What was that for?
  - Did you have any problems recovering from these operations or with the anaesthetic?
- If you found the patient's blood pressure was very high, what would you do?
  - Ask the patient about a previous diagnosis of hypertension.
  - Ask what medications she has been taking for this and whether they have been taken as usual today.
  - 'If she has not taken her usual treatment, I would give these to her now. If she has taken her usual tablets, I would let her rest and retake the blood pressure in 10–15 minutes. If it remains high I would add some immediate additional treatment.'

Marking criteria table		
Criteria	Satisfactory	Unsatisfactory
Introduces self, explains task, obtains consent, washes hands before and after	1	0
Makes a good general assessment of the patient, including frailty, obesity	2	0–1
Performs a cardiovascular and respiratory examination	4	0–3
Has an approach to finding an elevated blood pressure	1	0

Pass mark: 4

Opioid prescription

Background

Opioids are highly effective analgesics often used in acute pain management. However, it associated with significant side effects and complications. Opioid medications act on mu-, kappa- and delta-opioid receptors, producing analgesia, cough suppression, respiratory depression, sedation and constipation.

Issues to be aware of when prescribing opioids include:

- **Side effects:** sedation, respiratory depression, constipation, nausea/vomiting, itch/rash, allergies, impaired psychomotor function and urinary retention
- **Tolerance:** develops within a few days due to receptor desensitisation, meaning increased doses are required to produce the same analgesic effects. Rotation of different agents may be used to overcome this. Tolerance affects the receptors responsible for constipation and pupil constriction less, so these effects are likely to remain present in opioid-tolerant patients.[1]
- **Dependency:** dependence is characterised by withdrawal phenomena of irritability, diarrhoea, weight loss, shakes, aggression and restlessness. These symptoms can be decreased by slowly weaning doses.[1]
- **Reversal:** Naloxone is an opioid antagonist acting on all three receptors (mu > kappa > delta). It blocks endogenous opioid peptides as well as opioid analgesics. Naltrexone is similar but with a longer duration of action.[1]
- **Breakthrough analgesia:** doses of short-acting opioid analgesics for breakthrough pain should be one-sixth of the patient's daily dose of long-acting opioid analgesic.

---

1 Dale MM, Haylett DG. *Rang & Dale's Pharmacology*. Elsevier, 2012.

Introduction

In this station you will be asked to answer a series of questions related to opioid prescriptions. You will be then asked to write an opioid script.

Rationale

Opioids are frequently used medications in both an inpatient and outpatient setting. They can be highly effective analgesic agents but should be used with caution due to their side effect profile and issues with tolerance and dependency.

Method

1. Appropriately convert short-term opioids to a long-term agent. See Table 4.99.1.
   - Seek local guidelines in regard to opioid conversion for equianalgesic doses of different agents
   - Every patient will respond differently to different medications so conversion charts should be used only as a guide
   - When converting from short-acting to long-acting doses of the same agent, the same total dosage can be given across two or three doses of the long-acting agent.

Opioid script writing

- All details must be handwritten by the prescriber, including:
  - patient details: full name, date of birth and address
  - medication: name, strength, route of administration, quantity supplied (in both words and figures)
  - number of repeats to be dispensed (if any) and minimum interval between dispensing
  - directions for use
  - prescriber's signature
  - date of issue.
- Only one medication is to be ordered per script.

Reference: https://www.health.nsw.gov.au/pharmaceutical/Documents/prescriptions-nonhandwritten.pdf.

TABLE 4.99.1 Characteristics of different opioids

Drug	Route of administration	Duration of action (hours)
Morphine	Oral	2–3 (12 or 24 if controlled release)
Codeine	Oral	3–4
Fentanyl	Subcutaneous	1–2
Hydromorphone	Subcutaneous/ Intramuscular	2–4
Hydromorphone	Oral	2–4 (24 if controlled release)
Oxycodone	Oral	3–4 (12 if controlled release)
Pethidine	Intramuscular	2–3
Tapentadol	Oral	4–6 (12 if controlled release)
Tramadol	Intramuscular/ Intravenous	3–6 (12 or 24 if controlled release)
Tramadol	Oral	3–6 (12 or 24 if controlled release)

Examiners' likely questions

1. You are a junior medical officer called to see a patient on the surgical ward who has been charted oxycodone 15 mg/naloxone 7.5 mg (controlled release) twice daily for analgesia following a left total knee replacement. What would be an appropriate breakthrough dose of oxycodone immediate release for this patient?

   • You chart them oxycodone 5 mg (one-sixth of total daily dose of 30 mg) every 4 hours as needed (PRN) to a maximum of 30 mg daily, which provides good control.

2. At the time of discharge, they are using 5 doses daily and you wish to give them 10 doses to take home. Write a discharge script for this patient for 3 days of his long-acting analgesia and 10 doses of his short-acting analgesia. Please ask the examiners for any patient details you need.
   - Patient name: John Smith
   - Patient date of birth: 06/07/1946
   - Patient address: 22 Ocean Street, Bondi, NSW, 2026

Prescribe name: Dr Adam Braye
Prescriber number: x xxxvx
Patient name: John Smith
Date of birth: 06/07/1946
Patient address: 22 Ocean Street
                 Bondi, NSW, 2026
Oxycodone 5 (five) mg PO
   PRN Q4H   Max 30mg (thirty)/
                        24hours

Quantity = 10 (ten) × 5 (five) mg
                        tablets

     NO RE PEATS
Signature:
Date of issue: 01/01/20

Prescriber name: Kirsty Rose
Prescriber number: x xxxxx
Patient name: John Smith
Date of birth: 06/07/1946
Patient address: 22 Ocean Street
                 Bondi, NSW, 2026
Oxycodone 15 (fifteen) mg/
Naloxone 7.5 (seven point five) mg
   (controlled release) PO BD
for 3 (three) days.
Quantity = 6 (six) tablets.

   NO REPEATS

Signature:
Date of issue, 01/01/20

3. Please discuss these medications with Mr Smith, explaining to him the side effects to be aware of and discussing the risks of tolerance and dependence with opioid analgesics. You will need to cover benefits versus risks.

Marking criteria table

Criteria	Satisfactory	Unsatisfactory
Appropriate breakthrough dosing – oxycodone 5 mg	1	0
Script writing		
Separate script for each medication	1	0
PRN script	1	0
Patient's full details handwritten	1	0
Drug name	1	0
Drug dose	1	0
Dose frequency	1	0
Maximum dose per 24 hours	1	0
Quantity	1	0
Repeats	1	0
Prescriber details written, signed and dated	1	0
Regular medication script	1	0
Patient's full details handwritten	1	0
Drug name	1	0
Drug dose	1	0
Dose frequency	1	0
Quantity	1	0
Repeat	1	0
Prescriber details written, signed and dated	1	0
Discusses side effects including constipation, sedation, nausea/vomiting and respiratory depression	1	0
Explains tolerance	1	0
Discusses risk of dependence	1	0

Pass mark: 14

A colleague is reported to be drinking excessively

Background

The impaired colleague represents an ethical issue that you need to be able to manage.

Introduction

You have just started your new rotation and you have become concerned about your senior registrar. Your colleague has recently divorced, smells of alcohol on morning ward rounds and in endoscopy, has missed ward rounds on several occasions, and you found half-empty bottles of whisky in his drawer at work when looking for a reference book. You approach him after a busy endoscopy list and ask to have a discussion with him about a private matter.

Rationale

An ethics and communication station, the issues here are complex and include fitness to practice, patient safety, and the doctor's mental and physical health. Patient safety is above all else the concern, and trumps loyalty and confidentiality in this setting. Be aware that this is not a medical consultation and you should not follow the usual consultation routine.

The colleague will be an actor instructed to play a role, and he may be quite confronting, so be prepared.

Method

1. Ask for the discussions to occur in a quiet, private setting.

2. Describe your observations in a frank, open fashion. Don't patronise. Allow your colleague to talk. Listen actively throughout the discussion. Be non-judgmental and try to show empathy with your words and body language.

3. Ask: have you noticed a problem? Give time for a response and try not to interrupt.

4. Ask: have you sought help?

5. State: you are worried about patient safety. Ask him: what is your view?

6. State: he has a duty of care to seek help. Ask him: what do you plan to do?

7. State: you will support him in seeking care. Ask: do you want support? Mention doctor support organisations that can provide confidential advice.

8. State: you will have to raise these concerns with others. If pressured not to, do not shift your ground but seek to explain while remaining open and honest.

T&O'C hint box

An impaired colleague
- Do not rush. Allow time for the conversation and use prompts to keep it flowing.
- This is not a station testing counselling or health education.
- You may be pressured to keep the conversation confidential. Do not offer any such reassurance (as you can't). Reporting an impaired colleague is mandatory in Australia.

Present your findings

Present the results of your conversation. You may be asked to report the conversation as if you have gone to medical administration.

Examiners' likely questions

You are likely to be asked about your responsibilities if you were to become unwell, and similarly your responsibilities if you have to report concerns.

Marking criteria table

Criteria	Satisfactory	Unsatisfactory
Strong communication of issues	3	0–2
Empathy and understanding	2	0–1
Patient safety discussed	1	0
Supports seeking help	1	0
Understands duty of care	2	0–1
Highlights issue of reporting	1	0

Pass mark: 6

101

Completing a 'do not resuscitate' order

Background

Advanced care planning is an integral part of ensuring patients receive appropriate care that is in line with their wishes and their medical status. It is important to have these conversations before a crisis point so that patients and their family do not make rushed emotional decisions.

Introduction

Mrs Simons is a 75-year-old female who has come into the emergency department with an exacerbation of chronic obstructive pulmonary disease (COPD). She does not require non-invasive ventilation (NIV) this admission. This is her eighth hospital presentation in 6 months, most requiring high-dependency unit (HDU) admission for NIV. She also has a background of chronic kidney disease (stage 4), ischaemic heart disease, congestive heart failure and osteoporosis.

She lives in a nursing home and requires assistance for all personal cares and can mobilise only 5 metres before getting short of breath.

Please speak to her about her limits of care and resuscitation plan.

Rationale

This is a communication station. The issues here are sensitive and there is a strong emotional component. It is important to have these conversations as it allows an avenue for patients to discuss their concerns and fears and understand more about their illness so that they can make the best decisions about their treatment and care.

When these difficult discussion are not done or are done poorly, the quality of life for patients can be at risk.

Method

1. Introduce yourself.
2. It is important to ensure you're at the level of the patient; often it helps to take a seat.
3. Initiate discussion.
   - Assess if she has the capacity to have the conversation and make decisions about her goals of care.
   - Advise the patient about the conversation you are going to have and ask the patient if she would like a support person present.
   - It is important to gauge the patient's end-of-life preferences and if she has thought about this before.
   - Ask the patient about her current quality of life. Explore what she would find acceptable. This is different for all patients, so it is important to ask open-ended questions.
4. Clarify prognosis.
   - Check what the patient knows already. Ask what she would like to know.
   - Avoid using medical jargon; use simple everyday language.
   - Be truthful, direct and caring.
   - Avoid euphemisms, for example use the word 'dying' instead of 'passing away' or 'passing'.
5. Identify end-of-life goals.
   - Allow open discussion about medical care and remaining life goals.
6. Develop a treatment plan.
   - Provide guidance on medical options.
   - Make recommendations regarding appropriate treatment.
   - Clarify resuscitation orders.
   - Offer ongoing assistance if the patient has any further questions.

> **T&O'C hint box**
>
> It is important to recognise and empathise with the patient's emotions.
> Actively listen, explore feelings and express empathy.
> Every patient's resuscitation order will be different.

Present your findings

Present the results of your discussion. You may be expected to complete a resuscitation plan.

Examiners' likely questions

- How confident are you that the patient understands her prognosis?
- Does she know what the plan means?
- Has she been unduly influenced by anyone else — relatives, hospital staff?

Marking criteria table

Criteria	Satisfactory	Unsatisfactory
Makes patient at ease	1	0
Checks knowledge	2	0–1
Assesses quality of life (QOL)	2	0–1
Opens dialogue	2	0–1
Develops treatment plan	2	0–1
Offers follow-up	1	0
Writes resuscitation plan	2	0–1

Pass mark: 7

Confirmation of death

Background

Certification of death is a legal requirement that usually needs to be completed by a medical officer. It is a clinical assessment process undertaken to establish that a person has died.

Introduction

You are the ward junior medical officer at a tertiary hospital. You are called to review a patient to confirm death.

- Mr Timothy Wade is a 67-year-old male who presented with neutropenic sepsis on a background of management for acute myeloid leukaemia. Due to his poor prognosis and multiple recent admissions, on discussion with the patient and his family, a decision was made to cease all active measures of management, taking a palliative approach. The family were present throughout the day and have alerted nursing staff that Mr Wade has stopped breathing.

  Please briefly address Mr Wade's family and certify the death.

  You do not need to counsel the family regarding the diagnosis or treatment approach.

Rationale

Working as a junior doctor, especially on after-hours hospital cover, you will frequently be called to complete death certification. You should be familiar with the process as well as prepared to have a discussion with the patient's family at the time of death certification. See Box 4.102.1.

Method

> ### Box 4.102.1
> ### Tips for talking to the family
>
> - Read the notes first, familiarise yourself with the patient's history.
> - Explain the procedure you are about to perform because the process of death certification may be upsetting for loved ones to witness.
> - Offer for them to remain present or excuse themselves for the procedure.
> - Provide clear and concise information.
> - Use simple language, avoiding euphemisms.
> - If available and appropriate, arrange for someone more senior or more involved in the patient's care to meet with the family.
> - Offer support services as available.

CERTIFICATION OF DEATH

1. Wash hands; don personal protective equipment (PPE) if appropriate.
2. Verify the patient's identity (hospital ID tag).
3. Check for verbal response.
4. Conduct a general inspection — looking for signs of life.
5. Listen for heart and breath sounds.
6. Check with a torch for pupillary response.
7. Assess for response to centralised stimulus, for example supraorbital pressure, or mandibular pressure.
8. Assess for response to painful stimulus.
9. Attend to hand hygiene.
10. Documentation: See Box 4.102.2.

> ### Box 4.102.2
> ### Criteria for death certification
>
> Verification of Death is a clinical assessment to establish that a person has died. This is done by demonstrating all the following:
> - No palpable carotid pulse, and
> - No heart sounds heard for a minimum of 5 minutes, and
> - No breath sounds heard for 5 minutes, and
> - Fixed and dilated pupils, and
> - No response to centralised stimulus, and
> - No motor (withdrawal) response or facial grimace in response to painful stimulus.

(Source: https://www.aci.health.nsw.gov.au/__data/assets/pdf_file/0007/294325/Verification_of_Death_Form_2021.pdf)

The time of death is legally the time you certify the patient dead.

Centralised stimulus may be assessed by trapezius muscle squeeze, supraorbital pressure or sternal rub. No motor (withdrawal) response or facial grimace in response to painful stimulus would be assessed by pinching the inner aspect of the elbow.

Examiners' likely questions

- For how long must you listen for heart sounds?
- For how long must you listen for breath sounds?
- How would you assess a centralised stimulus?
- How would you assess a painful stimulus?

Marking criteria table

Criteria	Satisfactory	Unsatisfactory
Performs hand hygiene at all appropriate moments	1	0
Confirms patient identity	1	0
Checks for verbal response	1	0
General inspection — signs of life	1	0
Checks for carotid pulse	1	0
Listens for heart sounds	1	0
Listens for breath sounds	1	0
Examines pupils	1	0
Checks for response to central stimulus	1	0
Checks for response to painful stimulus	1	0
Discussion with family		
Empathetic and professional approach	1	0
Appropriate language, simple, avoids euphemisms	1	0
Questions sought and answered	1	0
Explains procedure of death certification	1	0

Pass mark: 9

"We are like butterflies who flutter for a day and think it is forever."

Carl Sagan

Index

Note: Page numbers followed by *f* indicate figures, *t* indicate tables, and *b* indicate boxes.